Case Studies in Orthodontics

Editor: Wyatt Cook

AMERICAN
MEDICAL PUBLISHERS
www.americanmedicalpublishers.com

AMERICAN
MEDICAL PUBLISHERS
www.americanmedicalpublishers.com

Cataloging-in-Publication Data

Case studies in orthodontics / edited by Wyatt Cook.
p. cm.
Includes bibliographical references and index.
ISBN 979-8-88740-612-1
1. Orthodontics. 2. Orthodontics--Disgnosis. I. Cook, Wyatt.
RK522 .078 2023
617 .643--dc23

American Medical Publishers,
41 Flatbush Avenue,
1st Floor, New York,
NY 11217, USA

ISBN 979-8-88740-612-1 (Hardback)

Contents

Preface

Orthodontics is a specialized branch of dentistry that focuses on dental and facial irregularities as well as their diagnosis, prevention and treatment. The goal of orthodontic treatment is to correct misaligned teeth and jaws, in order to improve oral function and aesthetics. Some of the prominent issues which are treated within this area of dentistry are crowded teeth, crooked teeth, overbites, underbites and gaps between teeth. Orthodontic treatment involves the use of various appliances to gently move teeth into their proper positions over time, using implements such as braces and aligners. By correcting dental and facial irregularities, orthodontic treatment improves chewing efficiency, speech, and self-confidence. It also facilitates better oral hygiene, reducing the risk of tooth decay, gum disease, and other dental problems. This book unfolds the innovative aspects of orthodontics which will be crucial for the progress of this field in the future. It will provide comprehensive knowledge to the readers.

The information shared in this book is based on empirical researches made by veterans in this field of study. The elaborative information provided in this book will help the readers further their scope of knowledge leading to advancements in this field.

Finally, I would like to thank my fellow researchers who gave constructive feedback and my family members who supported me at every step of my research.

Editor

1

A Multidisciplinary Approach to Malocclusion Caused by Facial Multiple Fracture

Daishi Arai,[1] Akihiro Yasue,[2] Shinya Horiuchi,[3] and Eiji Tanaka[2]

[1]*Department of Orthodontics and Dentofacial Orthopedics, Tokushima University Graduate School of Oral Sciences, Tokushima, Japan*
[2]*Department of Orthodontics and Dentofacial Orthopedics, Tokushima University Graduate School of Biomedical Sciences, Tokushima, Japan*
[3]*Department of Orthodontics and Dentofacial Orthopedics, Tokushima University Hospital, Tokushima, Japan*

Correspondence should be addressed to Eiji Tanaka; etanaka@tokushima-u.ac.jp

Academic Editor: Darko Macan

In the case of multiple facial fractures, a simple open reduction occasionally causes various disorders during healing process after the surgery. Moreover, esthetic disturbance of a facial deformity might be induced. Therefore, the acquisition of facial symmetry and the recovery of occlusal and masticatory functions become increasingly important. This case report presents a successful treatment of facial multiple fracture induced by a car accident. A 20-year-old male was diagnosed with suffered multiple midface and mandibular fractures induced by a car accident. Midface fractures included the LeFort I and II type fractures, as well as sagittal fracture at midline and fractures from right maxillary sinus anterior wall to orbital wall. In the mandible, midline and left body fractures were detected. The patient underwent open reduction and rigid fixation of the fractured left zygoma, comminuted LeFort I and II fractures, and midline and left body of the mandible with intermaxillary fixation by multibracket appliance; maxillary osteotomy with iliac bone grafting; orthognathic two-jaw surgery with coronoid process grafts onto the depressed zygoma; and onlay graft of hydroxyapatite block on mandible. As the result, the multidisciplinary treatments successfully recover functions and esthetics to the satisfactory level of the patient with multiple facial fractures. As treatments for multiple facial fractures are required complexity due to the extent of trauma, multidisciplinary approach under the close cooperation between hospital departments is thought to be important.

1. Introduction

Patients involved in motor vehicle accidents often suffer from multiple midface and mandibular fractures including the damage of both hard and soft tissues [1]. In the case of multiple facial fractures involving maxilla, mandible, and zygomatic bone, a simple open reduction occasionally causes various disorders during healing process after the surgery such as trismus, masticatory disturbance, swelling, and post-operative morbidity, leading to a decrease of a patient's quality of life [2]. Moreover, esthetic disturbance of a facial deformity might be induced. These sequelae are often caused by the malunion of fracture sites, and long-term treatment is needed in some cases. Therefore, the acquisition of facial symmetry and the recovery of occlusal and masticatory functions become increasingly important. Even if the operation for the purpose of functional and esthetic recovery was executed, refracture of malunion, scar tissue dissection, and subsequent bone mass insufficiency and dead space may cause another malunion. Hence, multilateral diagnoses and advanced treatments are required for these improvements.

This article demonstrates a clinical experience of multidisciplinary approach to oral and esthetic rehabilitation from maxillofacial fracture induced by a car accident.

2. Case Presentation

A 20-year-old male was first sent to an emergency hospital after a car accident. His maxillofacial injuries had included dehiscence wounds on the left temporal region, right frontal

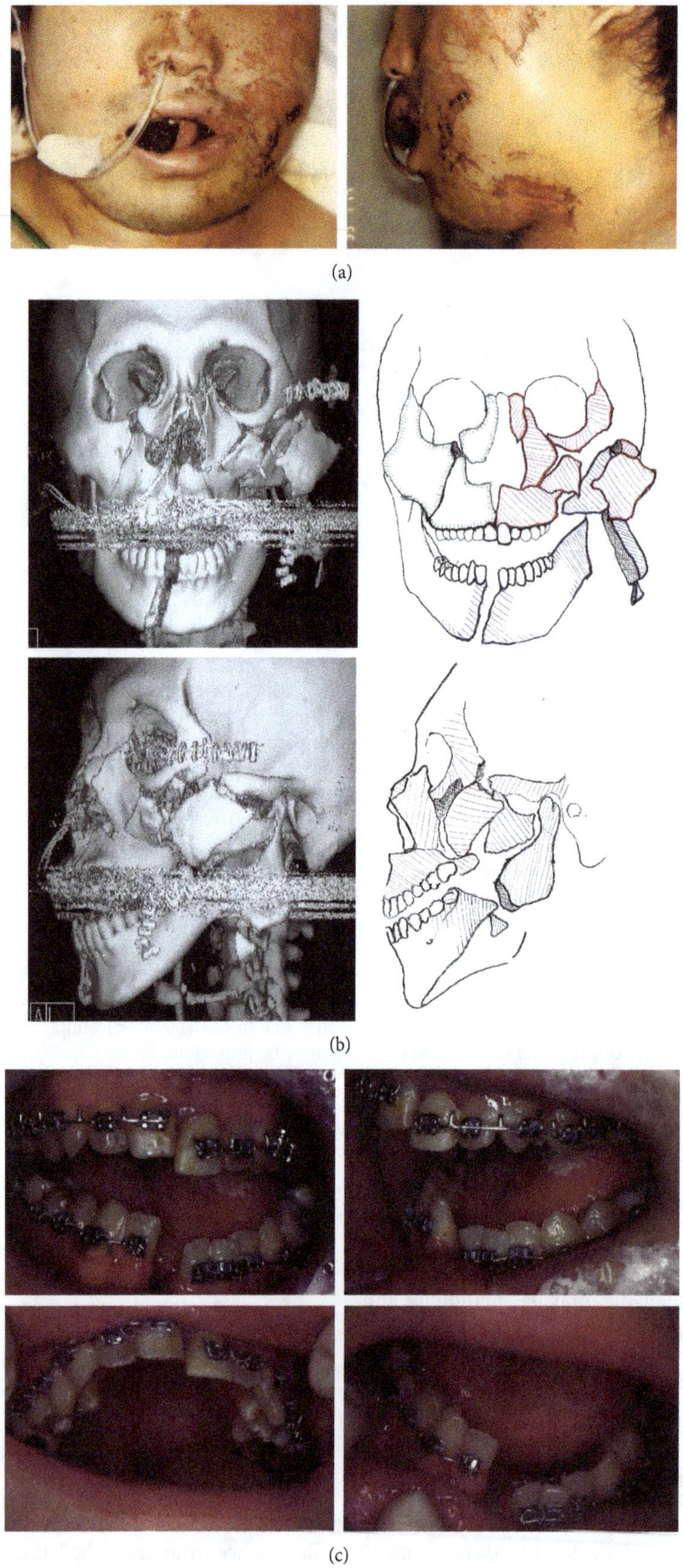

Figure 1: Facial photographs (a) and cephalic CT images with schematic illustrations immediate after injury (b) and intraoral photographs taken after placement of surgical braces for the intermaxillary fixation (c).

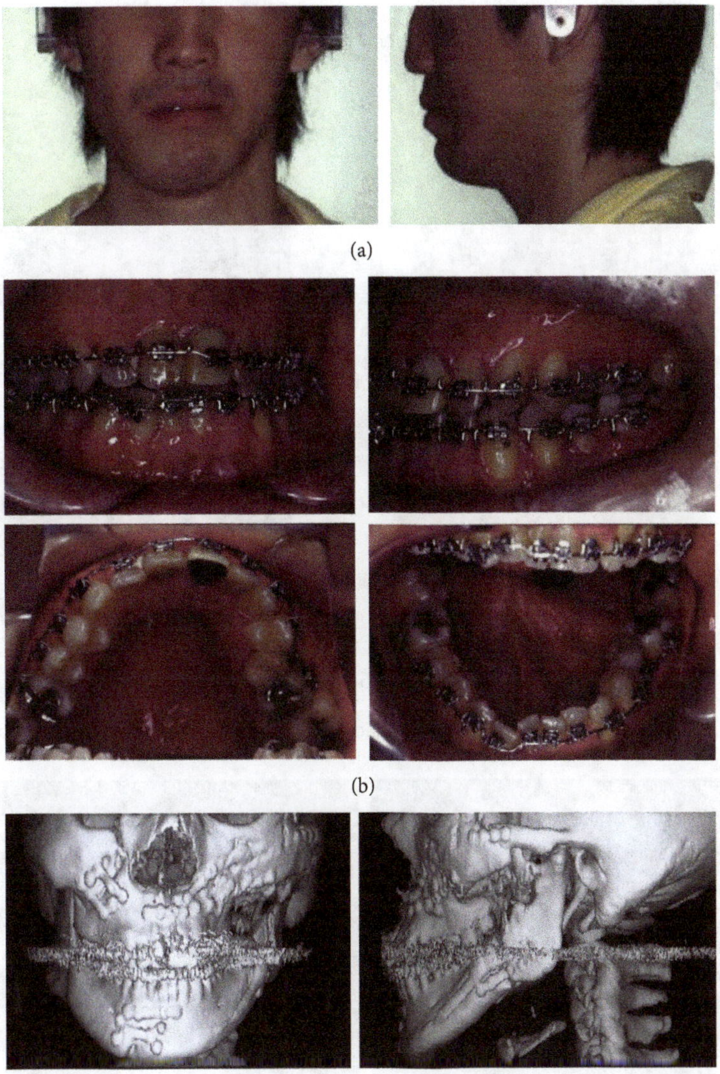

(a)

(b)

(c)

FIGURE 2: Facial (a) and intraoral photographs after 9 months (b) and cephalic CT images after open reduction (c).

region, left lower eyelid, and buccal region (Figure 1(a)). Furthermore, as arterial bleeding from the nose and mouth was observed, wound suturing and astriction were then performed. Symptoms of cranial nerves were not confirmed regardless of the clouding of his consciousness. He had his normal eyesight, and abnormal findings were not observed even in cephalic computed tomography (CT) images. Fracture of fifth rib was found by chest radiography. On the other hand, tracheotomy had been performed to avoid suffocation due to airway constriction caused by severe swelling and subcutaneous bleeding from the left cranium to submandibular region. Four days after injury, his physical status was recovered, then he was transferred to the Tokushima University Hospital for close inspection and medical treatment of gnathic bone fractures.

From the cephalic CT images, midface fractures included fractures of the Le Fort I and II planes, as well as sagittal fracture at midline and fractures from right maxillary sinus anterior wall to orbital wall (Figure 1(b)). In the mandible, the body was completely separated off at midline, distal region of the left third molar, coronoid process, and condylar process. The fractured end of condylar process was displaced to the outer side. As in the intraoral findings, the laceration on the fracture line at mandibular incisor area and the submucous bloody spots on left sublingual region were observed, the continuous dental arch was lost with mobility, and the cross bite on the left molar region and anterior open bite were observed (Figure 1(c)). A clinical diagnosis was made of malocclusion due to facial multiple fractures, and the following treatment plans were determined: (1) closed reduction by intermaxillary elastics, (2) open reduction, and (3) intermaxillary fixation using a multibracket appliance. The patient gave written informed consent before beginning treatment.

To tract both dentitions and maxilla, the intermaxillary elastics and the maxillary protraction headgear were started. The fractures were operated on open reduction one week after closed reduction. The mandible with a fewer fracture was first reduced and fixed temporarily to establish a yardstick for the occlusal plane that the original position is

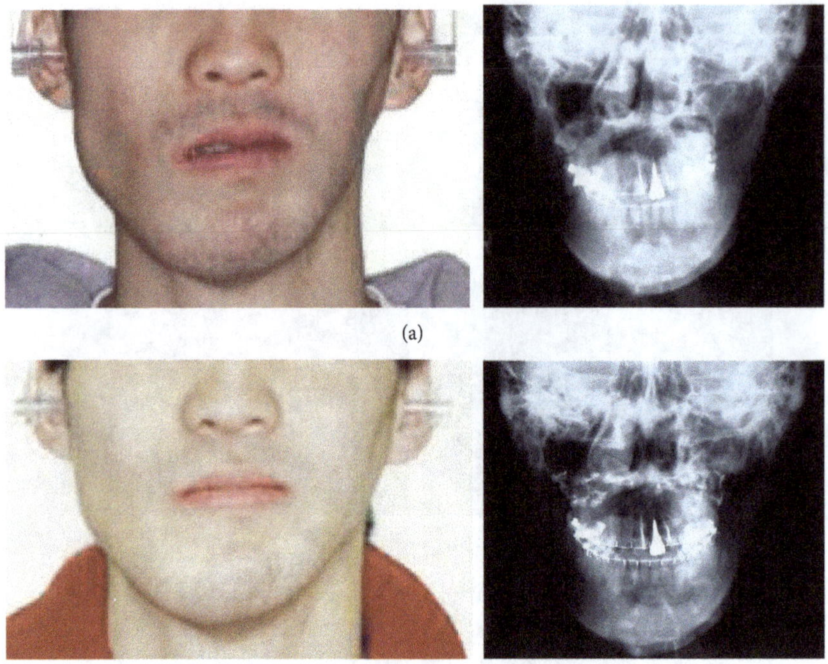

(a)

(b)

Figure 3: Facial photographs and frontal cephalograms before (a) and after two-jaw surgery (b).

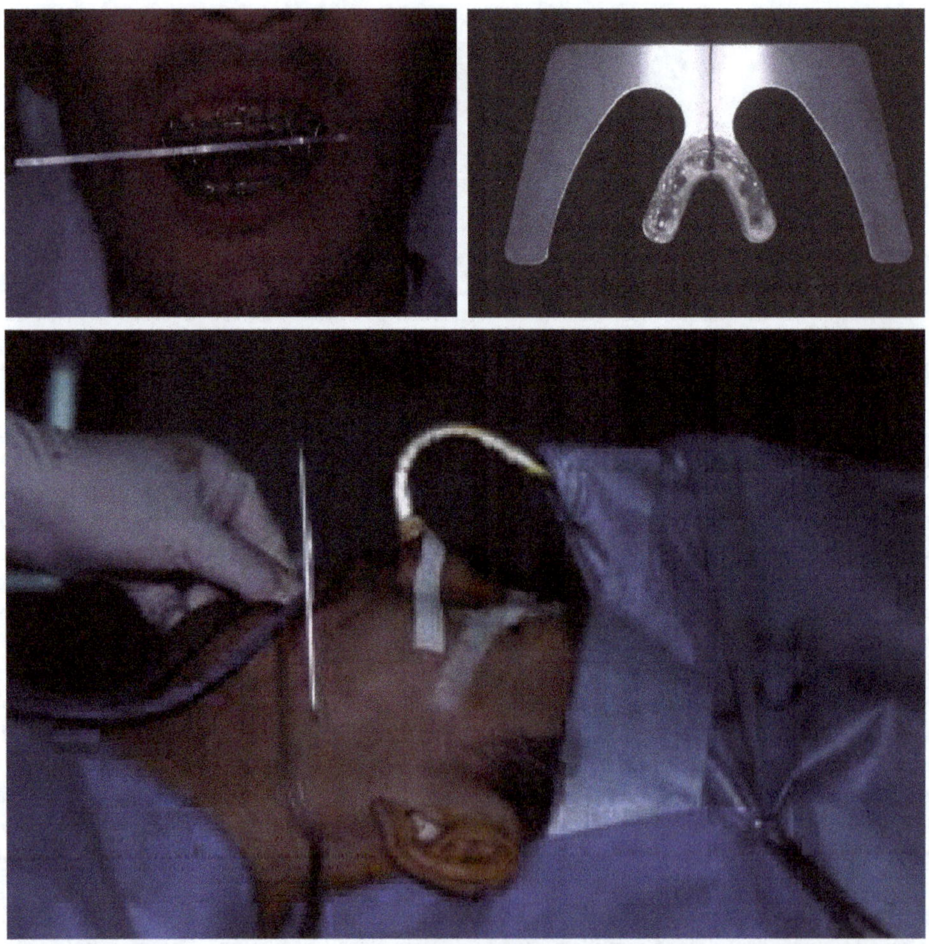

Figure 4: Maxillary positioning using an occlusal plane table as a parallel indicator to Frankfort horizontal plane.

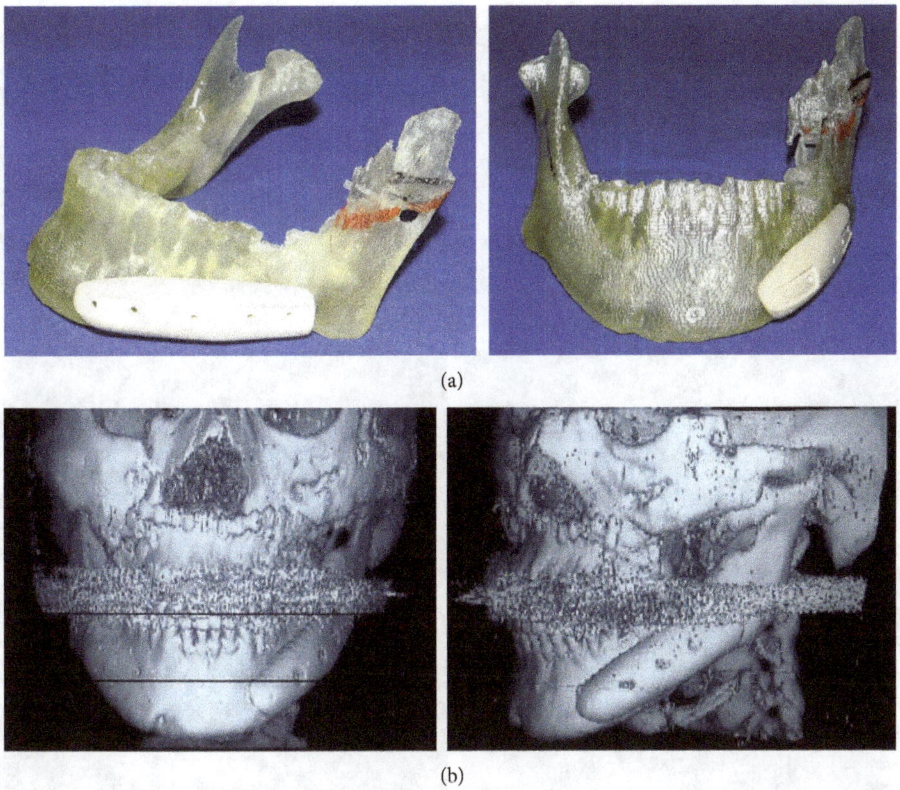

Figure 5: HAP-TCP blocks for onlay grafting on three-dimensional model (a) and cephalic CT images after onlay grafting of HAP-TCP block (b).

unclear, then shifted to the reduction and fixation of the maxillary and zygomatic bones. After that, the mandible was reduced again following to a plaster model reconstructed as a prospective occlusion. The operation was completed with intermaxillary fixation. After 31 days of internal fixation, postsurgical orthodontic treatment was executed for 9 months. Maximum mouth opening without pain was 30 mm within 3 months after surgery; meanwhile, the scar revision surgery on the left buccal region and the correction of the left lower eye lid ectropion were performed by plastic surgeons. The submucous resection of nasal septum by otolaryngologists was also undergone. Although almost stable and functional occlusion was obtained, asymmetric frontal view caused by occlusal cant in the frontal plane was remained (Figures 2(a) and 2(b)). At the same time, upper left maxillary osteotomy with iliac bone grafting was executed as the left molar crossbite was impossible to improve with tooth movement alone (Figure 2(c)). At this time, the patient reported to be fairly satisfied with pronouncing words and eating foods; however, he strongly requested the improvement of his facial asymmetry. Then, two-jaw surgery was decided to undergo with onlay grafting of right coronoid process onto the left side of depressed buccal area. The application of hydroxyapatite blocks for skeletal reconstruction was explained to the patient in the case that the asymmetry still remained after surgery. Before surgery, the blood flow changes due to injury were suspected and examined by angiography. Then, it was ascertained that the blood flow where the left external carotid artery branches off into the lingual, facial, and maxillary artery was not identified. Next, preoperative three-dimensional model was prepared to understand the accurate prediction. As a result, Le Fort I osteotomy was adopted for the modification of the maxillary cant. As to mandible, bilateral intraoral vertical ramus osteotomy (IVRO) was chosen as sagittal split ramus osteotomy (SSRO) was estimated to be difficult because of malunion from the former open reduction. Another reason was to decrease the bleeding risk from scar tissue. After 1 year and 5 months of preorthodontic treatment, two-jaw surgery was executed (Figure 3(a)). As a surgical procedure, an occlusal plane table was used as a parallel indicator to Frankfort horizontal plane for fixing maxilla (Figure 4). Then, IVRO was performed bilaterally. Confirming 40 mm of maximum jaw opening during operation, the bone fragment removed from right coronoid process was shaped into 3×2 cm block for onlay grafting in the depression of left buccal region. After two-jaw surgery, although the shifted chin point and occlusal cant were improved, the patient still complained the meagerness of his left mandibular angle region (Figure 3(b)), then decided to undergo another onlay graft of hydroxyapatite-tricalcium phosphate composite (HAP-TCP) blocks (Figures 5(a) and 5(b)) and free vascularized fat graft following patient's wishes. At the end of postoperative treatment, facial asymmetry was improved to his satisfactory level, and an acceptable occlusion with adequate interincisal relationship was obtained (Figures 6(a) and 6(b)). From CT images, bone healing was completed (Figure 6(c)).

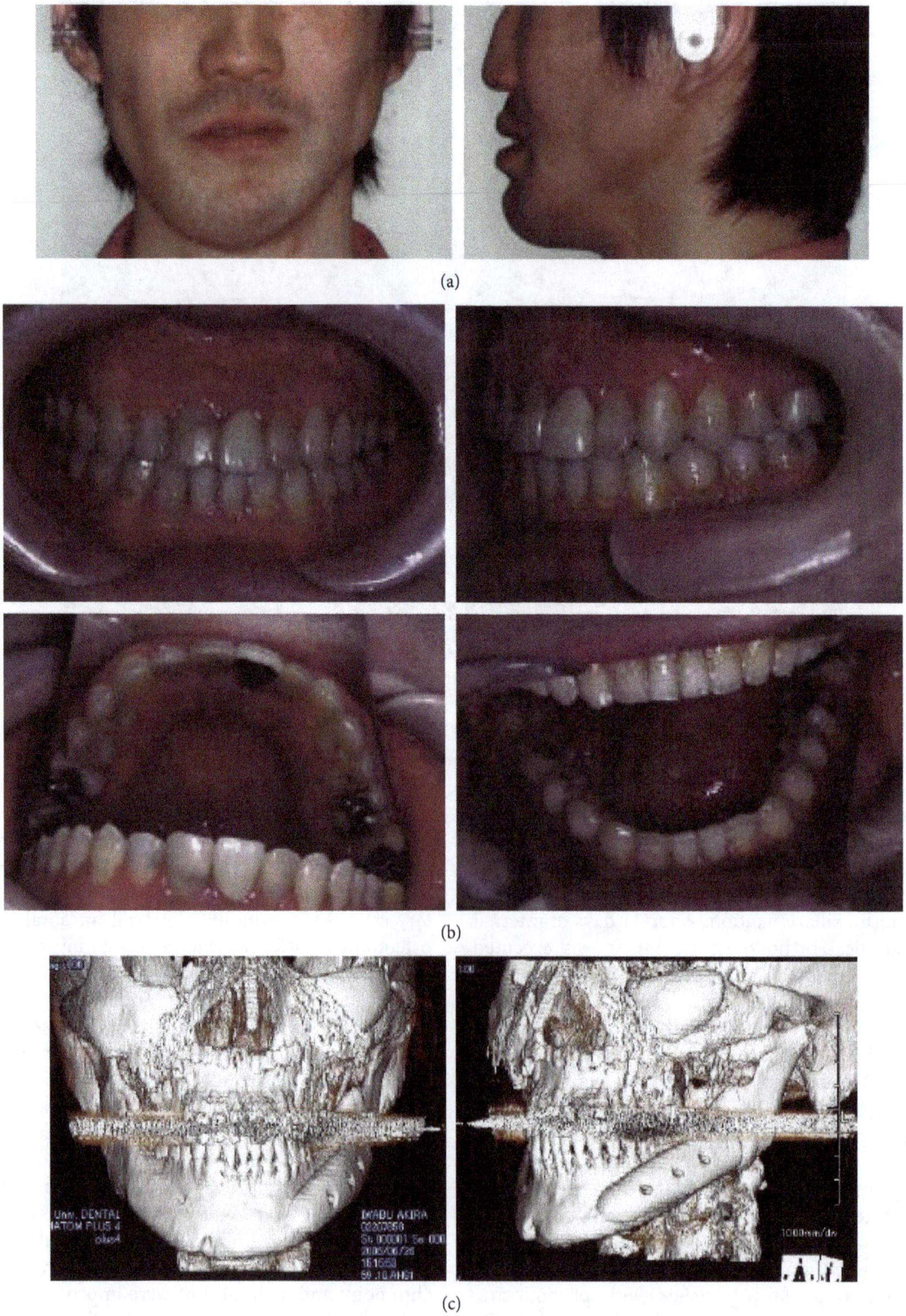

FIGURE 6: Facial (a) and intraoral photographs (b) and CT images after postoperative orthodontic treatment (c).

3. Discussion

Jaw deformity could be induced by not only acquired skeletal deformation but also malunion after traumatic bone fractures. For these patients, comprehensive treatment involving multiple disciplines is needed to successfully restore esthetics and functions and allow the patient to regain their self-esteem; on the other hand, several points such as soft tissue injury and displacement of bone fragment should be considered in orthognathic surgery. For example, bleeding risk increases. There are not a few cases of anatomical change in blood streams in scar tissue caused by injury. In this case, blood streams in the site of injury were examined before surgery by angiography to choose the safer and more reliable operative method. On the other hand, blood storage by autotransfusion was prepared in advance.

Since surgical movements of the jaws are complicated three-dimensional shifts of geometrically complex structures, the establishment of a yardstick for osteotomy is serious. An intermediate splint using the mandible to place the maxilla is generally adopted to reach the predictable destination in bimaxillary orthognathic surgery [3]. The splint was generally fabricated on the articulator to relate the repositioned maxillary cast to the preoperative mandibular cast before surgery. In the surgery, after maxilla is fixed to the mandible with the intermediate splint interposed, vertical dimension was determined by external reference measure to avoid the accidental error. A vertical measurement is recorded from the medial palpebral fissure to the maxillary orthodontic arch wire between incisors as it is a very stable reference point which is easily accessed pre- and intraoperatively [4]. Moreover, it eliminates the need for placement of a wire or a screw at nasion and the possible soft tissue scarring. This external vertical measurement is about as accurate as the placed rigid fixation [5, 6], and is useful in all Le Fort I maxillary osteotomies. In this case, medial palpebral fissure is used as a standard to avoid scarring soft tissue.

Obtaining prearranged occlusal plane angle is also one of the most important points for acquisition of a good treatment outcome. A splint combined with occlusal plane table was used to determine occlusal plane in this case. Thus far, the following indices have been used for occlusal plane alteration, such as the angular relationship between the occlusal and Frankfort horizontal plane [7–9], the facial appearance in harmony with the chin, upper lip position, and lower facial height by the rotation of the maxilla-mandible complex around ANS, point A, and the incisal edge of maxillary central incisor [10, 11], and parallel to naso-auditory meatus line. In this case, the confirmation of occlusal plane was easily achieved anteroposteriorly with the occlusal plane table equipped to the splint established parallel to Frankfort horizontal plane. As was estimated before surgery, postsurgical occlusal plane angle was decreased 4.2°. The improvement of asymmetry was also verified by occlusal plane table. For the procedure of osteotomy, SSRO seemed to be difficult because of the malunion of mandible, and to minimize bleeding from scar tissue and operative duration, IVRO was executed.

Facial asymmetry still kept the patient feel dissatisfaction even if occlusal function was recovered. After the two-jaw surgery, although bone grafting from right coronoid process to left depressed cheek area was performed, patient insisted the enlargement of left mandibular body. As the modification of the mandibular asymmetry required huge bone mass, an artificial bone grafting with free vascularized fat grafting from femur was chosen for the augmentation. Many studies have confirmed the osteoconductivity of composite biomaterials. Gosain et al. [12] compared volume maintenance of onlay grafts and bone replacement of implants in sheep among hydroxyapatite ceramic, HA/TCP, and hydroxyapatite cement past. The HA/TCP, then, demonstrated good scores in both maintenance and replacement [12]. We also used hydroxyapatite/beta-tricalcium phosphate (HA/β-TCP; NGK SPARK PLUG CO., LTD., Japan), which is a ceramic composed of a combination of hydroxyapatite [$Ca_{10}(PO_4)_6(OH)_2$] and beta-tricalcium phosphate [$Ca_3(PO_4)_2$], heated at 900 to 1300 degree Celsius and has a porous structure including large pores. Symmetrical mandible is still retained 1 year and 4 months after grafting, and the HA/TCP efficacy was confirmed. It was reported that the transplants of autologous culture-expanded bone marrow stromal cells (BMSCs) combined with HA/TCP scaffolds formed cortico-cancellous bone in dog craniofacial skeleton and showed long-term stability; meanwhile, HA/TCP particles alone underwent a high degree of resorption [13]. Long-term careful observation is then required for the patient. Recently, the use of polylactic acid/polyglycolic acid (PLA/PGA) biodegradable membranes in the form of volumetric chambers to carry an underlying HA/TCP onlay graft was also reported [14]. PLA/PGA is already known as biocompatible, geometrically stable, and favourably degradable product. Almasri et al. showed its great osteoconductivity of the distribution of bone arranged in multiple semicircular deposits and significant bony surface area by onlay graft in rabbit, indicating that this method would be an excellent option to overcome disadvantages of autogenous bone grafts, such as morbidity at donor site, limited quantity, and rapid resorption when compared with nonautogenous grafts.

The final results with regard to facial contour, maxillomandibular relationship, and symmetrical feature were satisfactory for the patient, which indicates the importance of multidisciplinary treatment for the correction of malocclusion due to maxillofacial bone deformities from fractures.

4. Conclusion

The patient with deformities of the maxillofacial bones that were caused by facial multiple fractures are reported. Multidisciplinary treatment was successfully used to achieve cosmetic reconstruction and recovery of maxillomandibular function and occlusion for the patient. In this case, the esthetics and functions were difficult to recover only with the first open reduction, and then, the secondary correspondence was needed. As treatments for multiple facial fractures are required complexity due to the extent of trauma, multidisciplinary approach under the close cooperation between hospital departments is thought to be important.

Consent

Written informed consent was obtained from the patient for publication of this case report and any accompanying images.

References

[1] K. T. Chuang, F. Hsieh, and H. T. Liao, "The correlation of age and patterns of maxillofacial bone fractures and severity of associated injuries caused by motorcycle accidents," *Annals of Plastic Surgery*, vol. 83, no. 6, pp. e28–e34, 2019.

[2] A. Dongol, M. R. Jaisani, L. Pradhan, S. Dulal, and A. Sagtani, "A randomized clinical trial of the effects of submucosal dexamethasone after surgery for mandibular fractures," *Journal of Oral and Maxillofacial Surgery*, vol. 73, no. 6, pp. 1124–1132, 2015.

[3] E. Ellis, "Bimaxillary surgery using an intermediate splint to position the maxilla," *Journal of Oral and Maxillofacial Surgery*, vol. 57, no. 1, pp. 53–56, 1999.

[4] T. H. Lapp, "Bimaxillary surgery without the use of an intermediate splint to position the maxilla," *Journal of Oral and Maxillofacial Surgery*, vol. 57, no. 1, pp. 57–60, 1999.

[5] M. R. Cope, "Measuring changes in maxillary height during osteotomy surgery," *The British Journal of Oral & Maxillofacial Surgery*, vol. 32, no. 4, pp. 257–259, 1994.

[6] J. W. Ferguson and N. H. Luyk, "Control of vertical dimension during maxillary orthognathic surgery," *Journal of Cranio-Maxillo-Facial Surgery*, vol. 20, no. 8, pp. 333–336, 1992.

[7] L. M. Wolford, P. D. Chemello, and F. W. Hilliard, "Occlusal plane alteration in orthognathic surgery," *Journal of Oral and Maxillofacial Surgery*, vol. 51, no. 7, pp. 730–741, 1993.

[8] L. M. Wolford, P. D. Chemello, and F. Hilliard, "Occlusal plane alteration in orthognathic surgery–part I: effects on function and esthetics," *American Journal of Orthodontics and Dentofacial Orthopedics*, vol. 106, no. 3, pp. 304–316, 1994.

[9] P. D. Chemello, L. M. Wolford, and P. H. Buschang, "Occlusal plane alteration in orthognathic surgery–part II: long-term stability of results," *American Journal of Orthodontics and Dentofacial Orthopedics*, vol. 106, no. 4, pp. 434–440, 1994.

[10] A. G. McCollum, J. P. Reyneke, and L. M. Wolford, "An alternative for the correction of the class II low mandibular plane angle," *Oral Surgery, Oral Medicine, and Oral Pathology*, vol. 67, no. 3, pp. 231–241, 1989.

[11] D. M. Sarver, S. M. Weissman, and M. W. Johnston, "Diagnosis and treatment planning of hypodivergent skeletal pattern with clockwise occlusal plane rotation," *The International Journal of Adult Orthodontics and Orthognathic Surgery*, vol. 8, no. 2, pp. 113–121, 1993.

[12] A. K. Gosain, P. A. Riordan, L. Song et al., "A 1-year study of hydroxyapatite-derived biomaterials in an adult sheep model: III. Comparison with Autogenous Bone graft for facial augmentation," *Plastic and Reconstructive Surgery*, vol. 116, no. 4, pp. 1044–1052, 2005.

[13] S. A. Kuznetsov, K. E. Huang, G. W. Marshall, P. G. Robey, and M. H. Mankani, "Long-term stable canine mandibular augmentation using autologous bone marrow stromal cells andhydroxyapatite/tricalcium phosphate," *Biomaterials*, vol. 29, no. 31, pp. 4211–4216, 2008.

[14] M. Almasri and M. Altalibi, "Efficacy of reconstruction of alveolar bone using an alloplastic hydroxyapatite tricalcium phosphate graft under biodegradable chambers," *The British Journal of Oral & Maxillofacial Surgery*, vol. 49, no. 6, pp. 469–473, 2011.

2

A Novel Temporary Anchorage Device Aided Sectional Mechanics for Simultaneous Orthodontic Retraction and Intrusion

Adith Venugopal,[1] Paolo Manzano,[2] and Sri Rengalakshmi[3]

[1] *Section of Orthodontics, University of Puthisastra, Phnom Penh, Cambodia*
[2] *10:10 Dental Clinic, Mandaluyong, Manila, Philippines*
[3] *Department of Orthodontics, Saveetha Dental College, Tamil Nadu, India*

Correspondence should be addressed to Adith Venugopal; avenugopal@puthisastra.edu.kh

Academic Editor: Giuseppe Alessandro Scardina

Closing spaces on light wires with inadequate knowledge and inappropriate mechanics can cause a "roller coaster" effect leading to an improper occlusion. Current knowledge of biomechanics, along with the incorporation of TADs, has made this process less challenging and more predictable. Resistance to sliding is considered the most prominent inhibitor of space closure in archwire-guided space closure or sliding mechanics, in turn delaying treatment duration considerably. In our case, resistance to sliding, primarily binding of the wire in the bracket slot, was nullified with the use of loop and sectional mechanics. This case report is aimed at showcasing the successful treatment of a young lady with a novel clinical setup to retract the canines into the premolar extraction space and simultaneously retract and intrude the anterior segment using sectional archwires and TADs in just under nine months. The current setup with sectional wires and TADs produced an uprighting, and an intrusive effect on the upper incisors during space closure. Additionally, the anchorage design avoided any significant change in the vertical dimension during sagittal correction of the Class II malocclusion. The occlusal plane remained almost stable with good amount of uprighting of the lower incisors following lower space closure too. The use of good biomechanical principles helped us achieve all the treatment goals and objectives in a very short period of time.

1. Introduction

Closing edentulous sites in orthodontics is a challenging task. Using light wires with inadequate knowledge and inappropriate mechanics in this task can cause a "roller coaster" effect leading to an improper occlusion [1]. Current knowledge of biomechanics, along with the incorporation of temporary anchorage devices (TADs), has made this process less challenging and more predictable [1–4].

"Friction" has received much attention in orthodontics, especially when it comes to space closure. Resistance to sliding is considered the most prominent inhibitor of space closure in archwire-guided space closure or sliding mechanics. Resistance to sliding is caused due to three components. These are (1) classical friction, (2) binding, and (3) notching. Binding and notching have been proved to play an essential role in the resistance to sliding [5]. It is clear from the current literature that resistance to sliding is an unavoidable concern in archwire-guided tooth movement or sliding mechanics, especially in closing extraction spaces and in turn prolongs the treatment duration considerably [6].

Segmented arch mechanics was proposed to have better-controlled tooth movement than archwire-guided tooth movement and is multifactorial, as reflected in the literature. Segmented arch mechanics suggests dividing the dental arch into three major segments (especially in extraction cases) [3]. These three segments are one anterior (incisors and canines) and two posteriors (teeth posterior to the extraction site). The canines are retracted first into the extraction spaces, followed by retraction of the incisors. This technique is aimed at minimizing posterior teeth movement forward, also known as maximum anchorage [7, 8]. Unfortunately, this technique also prolongs treatment duration due to its two-step nature.

This case report is aimed at showcasing the successful management of the spaces required to improve the esthetics and function of an adult female through the simultaneous retraction and intrusion of the whole anterior segment. This technique was achieved through the retraction of the canines with the posterior teeth and TADs as anchorage, while the four incisors were retracted and intruded using the TADs combined with sectional archwires in just under nine months.

2. Diagnosis and Treatment Planning

A 25-year-old female patient presented to our office with prior braces. On clinical examination, she presented with a convex profile, vertical growth pattern, slight gummy smile, extracted teeth 1.4 and 2.4, noncoincident midlines, increased overjet of 8 mm, and a deep bite. Canines were retracted half-way through on a 0.016″ nickel-titanium (NiTi) wire on 0.022″ slot MBT prescription brackets (Figure 1).

The patient had brought along her pretreatment records along for evaluation. Initial pretreatment extraoral records revealed a convex profile with incompetent lips. Pretreatment intraoral records revealed an overjet of 5 mm, visible buccal corridors, and narrow maxillary arch with Class II canines on the left and the right. Root stumps in relation to 4.6 and spaces between her lower anterior teeth were present (Figure 2).

Radiographic evaluation of the initial pretreatment records revealed a slightly retrognathic mandible (SNB, 78.88°), steep mandibular plane angle (FMA, 28.94°) with proclined upper and lower incisors (U1-SN, 109.45°; IMPA, 101.07°). Tooth numbers 2.4 and 3.6 had undergone prior endodontic treatment (Figure 2 and Table 1).

2.1. Treatment Objectives. The patient had been undergoing orthodontic treatment for two years already before visiting our practice. The patient expressed psychological frustration with the existing treatment due to its duration and the mounting pressure for her need to leave the country in the next nine months. She stressed it enough that she was not willing to continue her orthodontic treatment elsewhere and would have the appliance removed, whether completed or not.

With the patient's wishes in mind, we decided to fabricate realistic goals and objectives, which were to correct the severe deep bite, close the residual spaces on the upper and lower arches to achieve ideal overjet and overbite, achieve Class I canine relationships, and achieve a pleasant profile. One of the objectives was also to maintain space for an extra premolar prosthesis in the 4th quadrant as there was insufficient time to close the molar space.

2.2. Treatment Alternatives. Three alternatives were constructed in order to achieve the treatment objectives successfully.

(a) The first option would be to bond the second molars and relevel and align the arches followed by using an intrusion arch to correct the deep bite. Then, the canine retraction could be continued on a heavy stainless steel archwire followed by anterior retraction using loop or sliding mechanics by using the posterior segment as anchorage

(b) The second option was to bond the second molars and use an intrusion arch to correct the deep bite followed by protraction of the canines. Then, two TADs could be placed between the upper second premolars and first molars (1.5–1.6, 2.5–2.6) followed by en masse retraction by sliding mechanics

(c) The third option was to design a mechanotherapy which would allow simultaneous canine retraction using a section of wire with a closing loop along with simultaneous anterior intrusion and retraction using sectional wires and three TADs. Two of which would be placed between the upper first and second molars (1.6–1.7, 2.6–2.7) and the third between the two upper central incisors (1.1–2.1)

After careful consideration of all the three treatment options, the third option was finalized due to the given time constraints and was thoroughly explained to the patient.

2.3. Treatment Progress

2.3.1. Canine Retraction, Anterior Retraction, and Simultaneous Intrusion. The design consisted of three segments of wires. One segment of 0.019″ × 0.025″ SS wire extended from tooth 1.2 to 2.2. Hooks were extended on the wire distal to the lateral incisor brackets to reach close to the center of resistance of the anterior segment.

Posterior segments consisted of a segment of 0.019″ × 0.025″ SS extending from the first molar to the canines on either side. A closing loop was fabricated on the segment just distal of the canines (Figure 3).

Three TADs (1.6 × 8 mm) were inserted, two of them were placed between the upper first and second molars (1.6-1.7, 2.6–2.7) and the third between the two upper central incisors (1.1–2.1) (Figure 3).

2.3.2. Activation. Elastic traction using a power chain from the posterior TADs was directed to the hooks fabricated on the anterior segment of wire just distal to the lateral incisor brackets in order to retract the anterior segment. The force was measured to be 150 grams per side using a Dontrix force gauge. Elastic traction using an elastic thread was applied from the anterior miniscrew to the sectional archwire between the two incisors in order to prevent the uncontrolled tipping, which would be a direct result of the posterior traction. At the same time, this would help intrude the anterior segment eventually correcting the deep bite. The force for intrusion was measured to be 60 grams.

The posterior segment was activated by cinching the wire posteriorly distal to the first molar and anteriorly mesial to the canines, thereby activating the closing loop, eventually

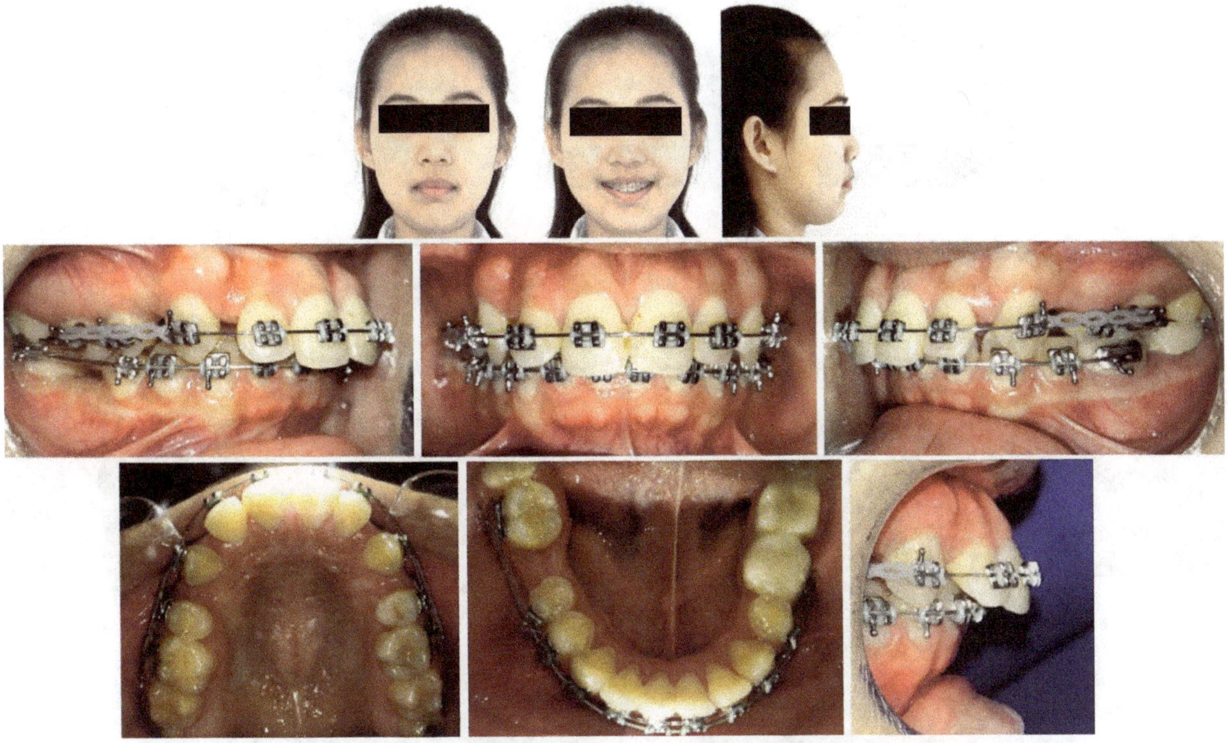

FIGURE 1: Pretreatment records with prior braces. 0.22″ MBT prescription brackets seen with canines half retracted on a 0.016″ NiTi archwire.

retracting the canines. A passive ligature was tied from the posterior TADs to the second premolar brackets for indirect anchorage in order to prevent molar mesialization during canine retraction.

In six months, the anterior segment and the canines were retracted, and the deep bite was also corrected. The lower arch was stabilized passively with a 0.019″ × 0.025″ SS wire from the third month itself as the arch had leveled and the minor spaces had closed early in the treatment (Figure 4).

2.3.3. Leveling and Alignment. Following space closure, the arch was releveled using a 0.017″ × 0.025″ NiTi archwire for two months. The wire was tightly engaged in the bracket slots, and a power chain was placed from the upper first molar to the first molar on the other side to prevent space opening. This helped in paralleling the roots without opening up spaces (Figure 5).

2.3.4. Finishing and Retention. Finishing was done on a 0.019″ × 0.025″ SS with light settling elastics following which the brackets were debonded. The anterior TAD was not removed and still kept in place to aid in the retention (Figure 6).

Essix retainers were planned on the upper and lower arches with the addition of a lingual button embedded in the upper Essix between the two central incisors. The patient was informed to wear the retainers for 24 hours for the next 2 years. In addition, she was instructed to attach a light intermaxillary elastic (3/16″, 2 Oz) from the anterior TAD to the button on the Essix at night for the next two years to retain the intrusion of the anterior segment.

3. Results

A balanced profile with an esthetic and pleasing smile was achieved along with harmony between the upper and lower lips, lip competence, and bilateral Class I canine relationships (Figure 6). The dental midlines were corrected, and no muscle or joint problems had developed during the treatment.

A panoramic radiograph taken after debonding showed acceptable root angulations with no evidence of root resorption, and stable bone levels.

Posttreatment cephalometric analysis showed that the sagittal jaw relationship improved while facial height remained almost constant (Table 1). There was a marked decrease in the upper and lower incisor inclination (IMPA, 97.48°; U1-SN, 100.76°) (Figure 7). The overjet was corrected, addressing the patient's initial complaint of protrusive teeth and protruding lips.

4. Discussion

Poor choice of dental procedures, incorrect treatment indication, adoption of hazardous treatment strategies, inadequate treatment performance, wrong estimation of treatment time, not changing treatment plan when necessary, and not establishing good communication with the patient are failures that may significantly affect outcomes, quality, and stability of correction. Moreover, these factors delay the treatment by a significant amount of time [9].

Retracting teeth on a light, flexible, round NiTi wire with large forces causes a phenomenon called "roller coaster" effect [1]. The "roller coaster" effect is observed when a wire

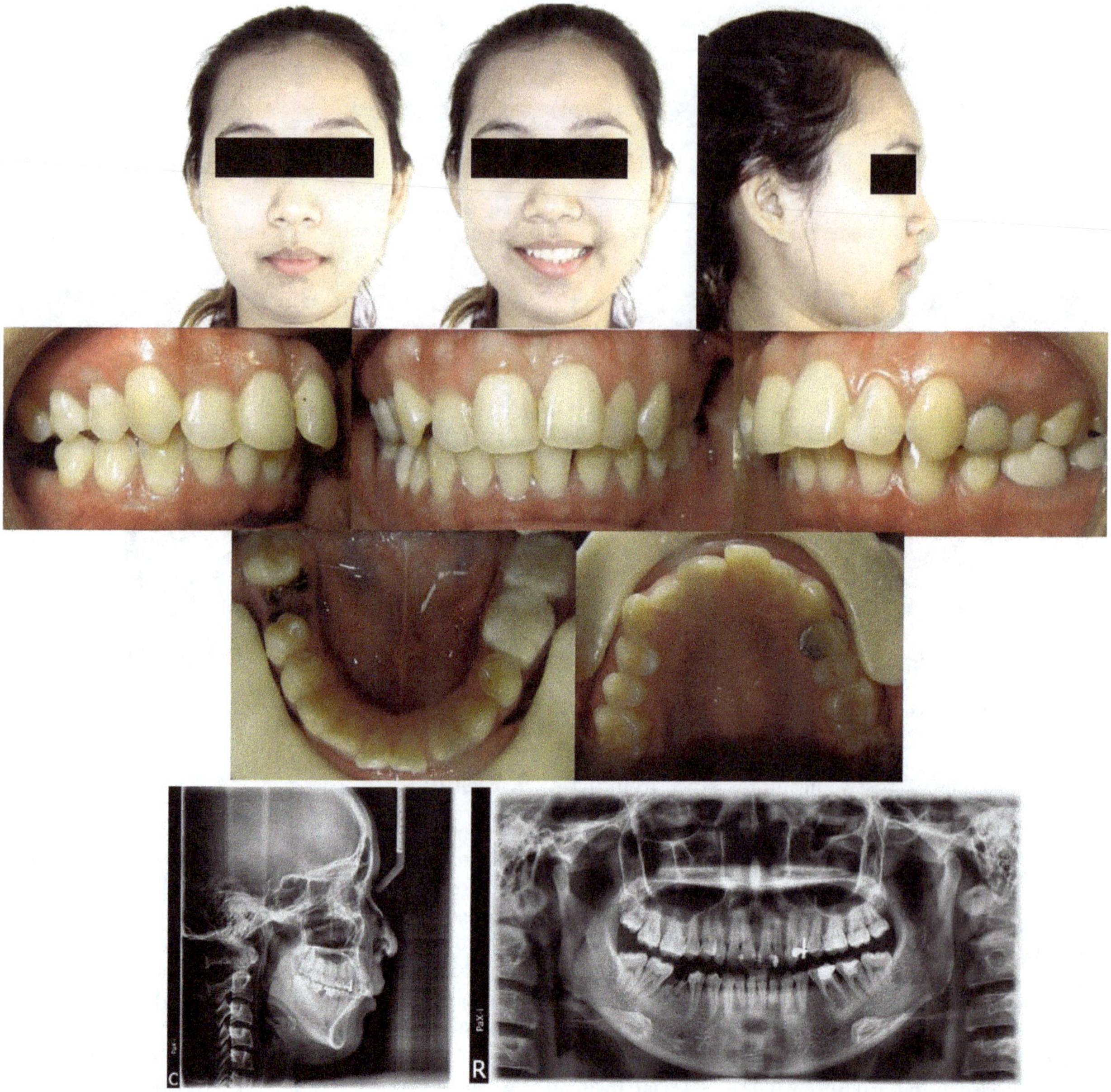

FIGURE 2: Initial treatment records prior to bonding with her previous orthodontist from two years ago.

TABLE 1: Cephalometric analysis.

Variable	Pretreatment	Posttreatment
FMA (dg)	28.94	29.43
FMIA (dg)	49.99	53.09
SNA (dg)	83.22	81.25
SNB (dg)	78.88	77.17
ANB (dg)	4.34	4.08
IMPA (dg)	101.07	97.48
Occlusal plane (dg)	5.54	7.30
U1-SN (dg)	109.45	100.76
Upper facial height	43.3%	42.6%
Lower facial height	57.7%	57.4%

of low strength such as NiTi archwire is used for canine retraction. NiTi does not have the stiffness to remain rigid when a retracting force such as an elastic chain is stretched from the molar to the canine. The molar and premolar crowns tend to tip mesially and extrude distally. The flexible NiTi then bends gingivally and, as a result, tends to tip the canine crown distally. The orientation of the canine bracket when the crown tips distally tend to extrude the incisors and deepen the bite. The use of proper biomechanics to overcome the iatrogenic side effects and satisfactorily complete the case is paramount in such situations [10].

In our case, prior use of high forces to retract the upper canines bilaterally on a 0.016″ NiTi wire resulted in such "roller coaster" effects. In the recent decade, many studies have shown a surge in the usage of TADs as direct anchorage for correction of transmigrated lower canines [11], upper

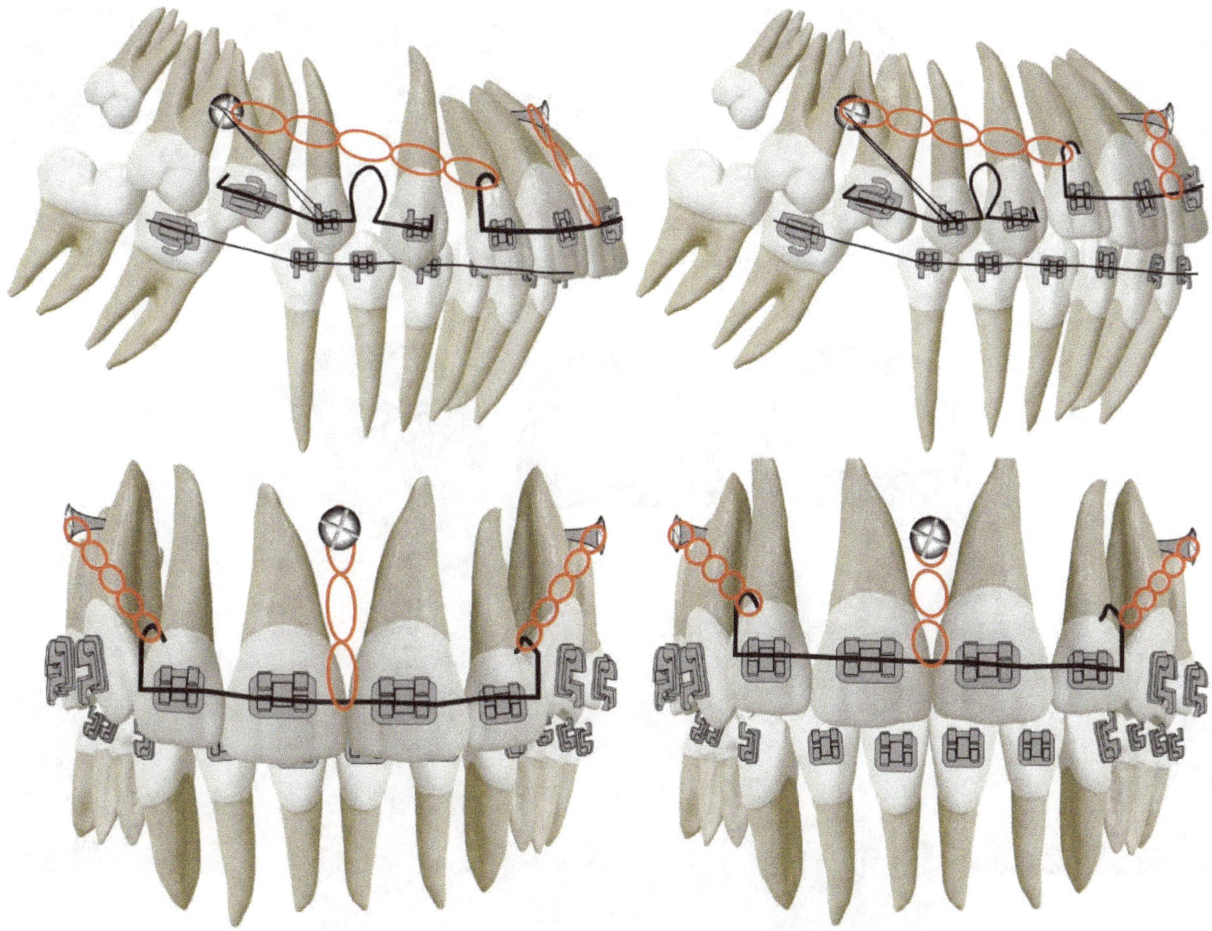

Figure 3: Biomechanical setup for canine retraction and simultaneous anterior retraction and intrusion. TADs placed between upper second premolar and first molars and also between upper central incisors. Sectioned 0.019″ × 0.025″ SS archwires anteriorly and posteriorly.

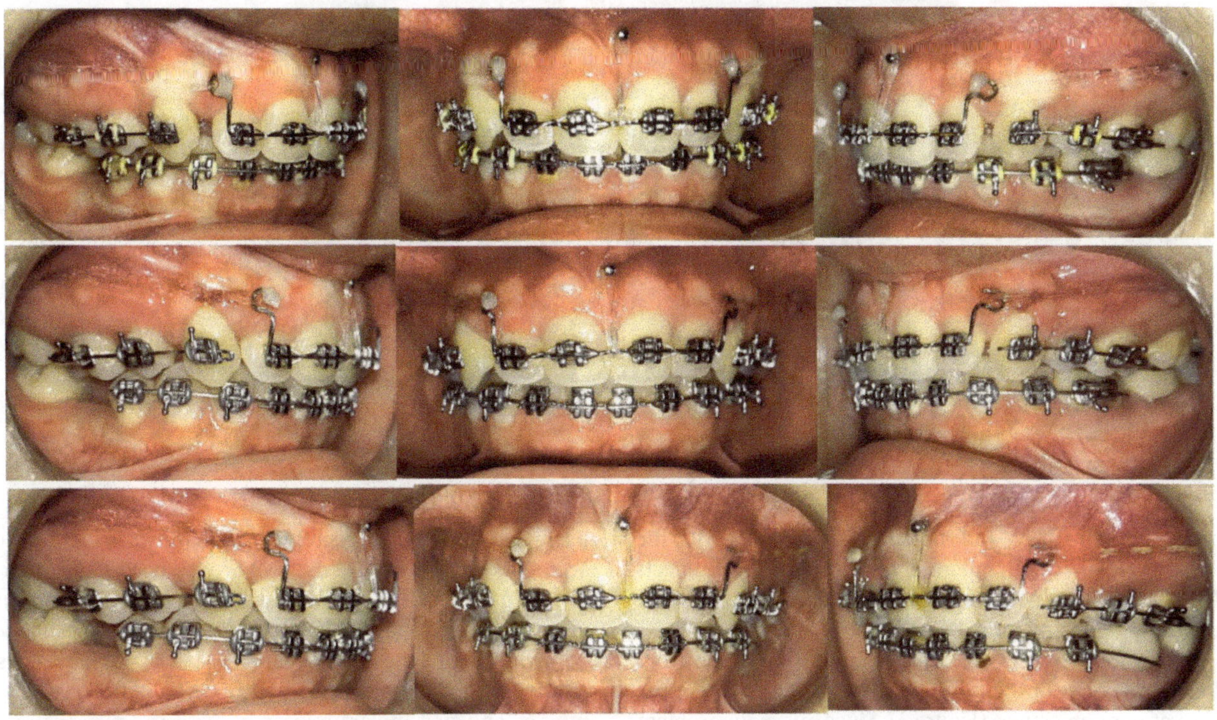

Figure 4: Retraction and simultaneous intrusion of anterior segment.

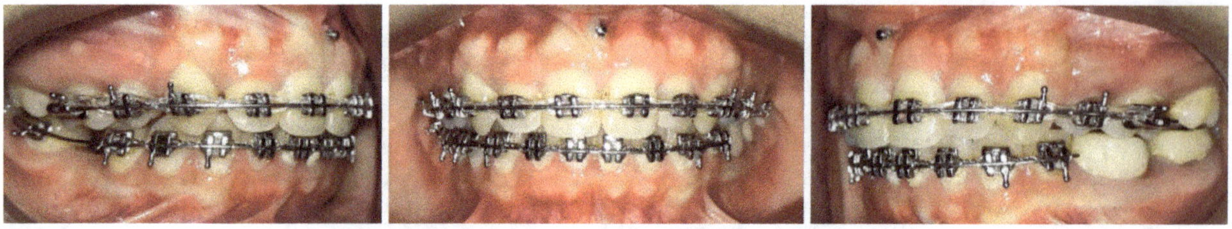

Figure 5: Finishing on a $0.019'' \times 0.025''$ SS archwire.

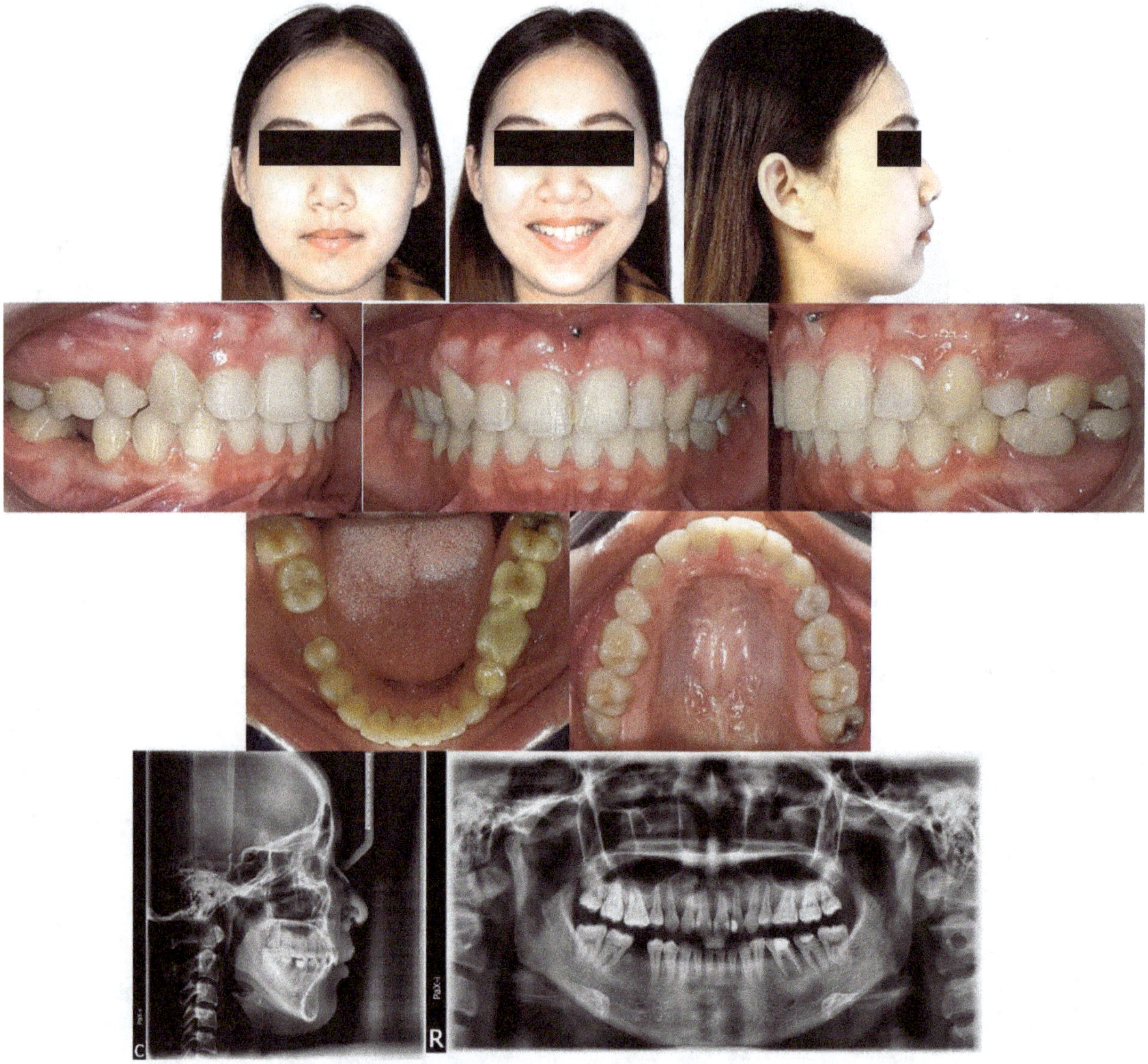

Figure 6: Posttreatment records.

canine impactions [12], and molar uprighting [13] with the aid of sectional mechanics to nullify the unwanted side effects which accompany the use of archwire-guided mechanics or the usage of opposing dental components as anchorage.

The current clinical biomechanical setup would be more of a customization of the required mechanics to achieve the ideal treatment objectives (Figure 3). Since our main problem was time underscored by the demands and duration of preparing the anchorage, segregating the maxillary arch into 3 segments (1.6–1.3; 1.2–2.2; 2.3-2.6) was needed in order to prudently negate the demands of time, anchorage, and force vectors required to achieve the ideal treatment objectives. By performing this, the canines could be positioned in a Class I relationship by the independent utilization of the second premolars, and first molars reinforced with indirect anchorage from the posterior TADs as anchorage. The incisors could

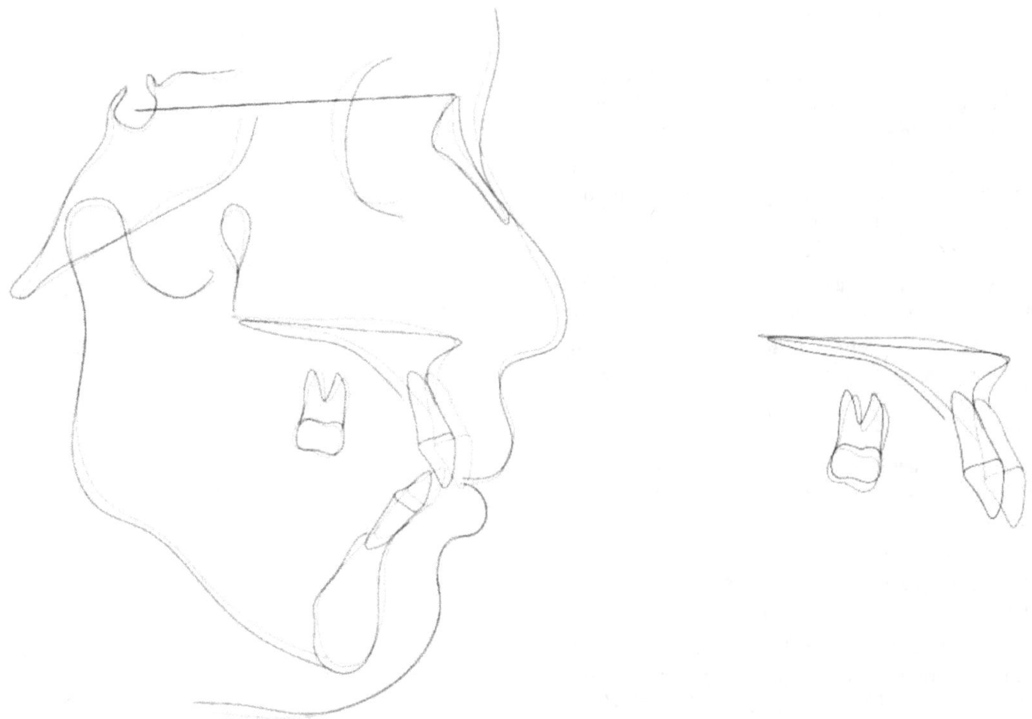

Figure 7: Superimpositions of pre- and posttreatment cephalograms showing almost constant mandibular planes, marked decrease in the upper and lower incisor inclination and upper incisor intrusion.

be retracted and intruded with the use of TADs, which could provide an ideal anchorage to support absolute anchorage demands and provide the ideal force vector required to correct the overjet and gingival show.

In the presented case, resistance to sliding, primarily binding of the wire in the bracket slot, was nullified with the use of loop and sectional mechanics. Power chains from the TADs posteriorly delivered forces of 150 grams to the anterior hooks per side, and the elastic thread from the third TAD (between the upper central incisors) delivered 60 grams of intrusive force to the anterior segment.

The advantage of this setup was that force delivered onto the anterior segment was completely utilized in the retraction and simultaneous intrusion unlike in archwire-guided mechanics wherein most of the force is unaccounted for and is probably lost in binding and notching [8].

Canine retraction was performed using a segment of $0.019'' \times 0.025''$ SS with closing loops distal to the canines with appropriate antirotational bends to prevent the distobuccal rotation of the canines.

Evidence has suggested that anterior intrusion is very hard to retain [14]. Therefore, it was decided to maintain the third TAD (between the upper central incisors) in place during the retention period, and the patient was instructed to wear $3/16''$ 2 Oz elastics from the TAD to the lingual button incorporated in the Essix between the central incisors at night time during the retention phase.

In our case, this setup with sectional wires and TADs produced an uprighting, and intrusive effect on the upper incisors during space closure (9° reduction in the U1-SN). Additionally, the anchorage design avoided any significant change in the vertical dimension during sagittal correction of the Class II malocclusion (Figure 7 and Table 1). The occlusal plane remained almost stable (2° increase). There was a good amount of uprighting on the lower incisors (4° decrease in the IMPA) following lower space closure. The apt use of sound biomechanical principles helped us achieve all the treatment goals and objectives in under nine months.

5. Conclusion

We should always have in mind our limitations and the importance of proper orthodontic training while treating patients. This clinical biomechanical setup of sectional archwires with TADs helped us achieve all the treatment goals (canine retraction, retraction, and intrusion of the anterior segment) in a short period of time.

References

[1] R. P. McLaughlin and J. C. Bennett, "Evolution of treatment mechanics and contemporary appliance design in orthodontics: a 40-year perspective," *American Journal of Orthodontics and Dentofacial Orthopedics*, vol. 147, no. 6, pp. 654–662, 2015.

[2] C. J. Burstone, "The segmented arch approach to space closure," *American Journal of Orthodontics and Dentofacial Orthopedics*, vol. 82, no. 5, pp. 361–378, 1982.

[3] C. J. Burstone and H. A. Koenig, "Optimizing anterior and canine retraction," *American Journal of Orthodontics and Dentofacial Orthopedics*, vol. 70, no. 1, pp. 1–19, 1976.

[4] A. J. Kuhlberg and D. N. Priebe, "Space closure and anchorage

control," *Seminars in Orthodontics*, vol. 7, no. 1, pp. 42–49, 2001.

[5] R. P. Kusy and J. Q. Whitley, "Friction between different wire-bracket configurations and materials," *Seminars in Orthodontics*, vol. 3, no. 3, pp. 166–177, 1997.

[6] G. A. Thorstenson and R. P. Kusy, "Effects of ligation type and method on the resistance to sliding of novel orthodontic brackets with second-order angulation in the dry and wet states," *Angle Orthodontist*, vol. 73, no. 4, pp. 418–430, 2003.

[7] C. J. Burstone, "The mechanics of the segmented arch techniques," *Angle Orthodontist*, vol. 36, no. 2, pp. 99–120, 1966.

[8] S. Braun and M. R. Marcotte, "Rationale of the segmented approach to orthodontic treatment," *American Journal of Orthodontics and Dentofacial Orthopedics*, vol. 108, no. 1, pp. 1–8, 1995.

[9] A. M. Nazeer, "Iatrogenic possibilities of orthodontic treatment and modalities of prevention," *Journal of Orthodontic Science*, vol. 2, no. 3, pp. 73–86, 2013.

[10] R. S. Kulshrestha, R. Tandon, and P. Chandra, "Canine retraction: a systematic review of different methods used," *Journal of Orthodontic Science*, vol. 4, no. 1, pp. 1–8, 2015.

[11] S. Cavuoti, G. Matarese, G. Isola, J. Abdolreza, F. Femiano, and L. Perillo, "Combined orthodontic-surgical management of a transmigrated mandibular canine," *Angle Orthodontist*, vol. 86, no. 4, pp. 681–691, 2016.

[12] F. Heravi, H. Shafaee, A. Forouzanfar, S. H. Zarch, and M. Merati, "The effect of canine disimpaction performed with temporary anchorage devices (TADs) before comprehensive orthodontic treatment to avoid root resorption of adjacent teeth," *Dental Press Journal of Orthodontics*, vol. 21, no. 2, pp. 65–72, 2016.

[13] N. Derton, A. Perini, S. Mutinelli, and A. Gracco, "Mandibular molar uprighting using mini-implants different approaches for different clinical cases- two case reports," *Orthodontics*, vol. 13, no. 1, pp. 138–145, 2012.

[14] C. Gioka and T. Eliades, "Orthodontic dental intrusion: indications, histological changes, biomechanical principles, possible side effects," *Hellenic Orthodontic Review*, vol. 6, pp. 129–146, 2003.

3

Long-Term Outcome of Autotransplantation of a Complete Root Formed a Mandibular Third Molar

Hiroyuki Kimura[1] **Yusuke Hamada**[2] **Taro Eida,**[3] **Tsuyoshi Kumano,**[1] **Kazutoshi Okamura,**[3] **and Makoto Yokota**[4]

[1]*Private Practice, Kumamoto, Kyushu, Japan*
[2]*Department of Periodontology, Indiana University School of Dentistry, Indianapolis, IN, USA*
[3]*Faculty of Dental Science, Kyushu University, Japan*
[4]*YDA Yokota Juku, Japan*

Correspondence should be addressed to Hiroyuki Kimura; dokimura@mocha.ocn.ne.jp

Academic Editor: Sreekanth Kumar Mallineni

Autogenous tooth transplantation is a procedure to reposition an autogenous tooth to another extraction area or surgically created recipient site. The autotransplantation procedures have been documented well in the literature, and the survival rate of the transplanted teeth was reported to be more than 90% after ten years. Therefore, autotransplantation might have been overlooked as a treatment option. The purpose of this case report is to evaluate the long-term (29-year) success and periodontal stability of the tooth autotransplantation from the mandibular third molar to the second molar. A 24-year old female presented to a clinic with a large caries lesion with periapical radiolucnecy on to tooth #18. The tooth was extracted with the site and treated with autogenous tooth transplantation from #17 with a complete root form. Endodontic treatment was completed 3 months post autotransplantation; the final prosthesis was placed 6 months postoperatively. The patient has shown excellent oral hygiene care and high compliance with the regular maintenance recall program. The transplanted tooth has been still functioning without any symptoms. Radiographic and clinical examinations revealed stable periodontal and endodontic conditions over the 29 years after the procedure. This case report showed the long-term success of autotransplantation of the mandibular third molar with a closed root apex to the second molar site. Autotransplantation can be an option when an adequate donor site is available to reconstruct the occlusion after the tooth extraction.

1. Introduction

One of the dental treatment goals is reconstructing the partial and complete edentulism with satisfactory functional and esthetical outcomes. Although dental implants and fixed prostheses have been utilized to replace the missing teeth, tooth autotransplantation can be a viable option to reestablish stable occlusion when an appropriate donor site is available [1, 2]. Autogenous tooth transplantation is a procedure to reposition an autogenous tooth to another extraction area or surgically created recipient site [3, 4]. The transplantation of the teeth has multiple benefits compared to other treatment modalities such as dental implants or fixed prosthesis. The advantages include that the procedure is indicated to children and young adults who have not completed the maxillofacial growth [5]. Furthermore, the transplanted tooth can stimulate alveolar bone growth with the eruption process due to the presence of periodontal ligament. Besides, the transplanted teeth can be moved to the ideal position with orthodontic treatment if necessary [5, 6]. However, multiple factors affecting results need to be taken into account with the procedure, such as surgeons' skill and knowledge, patient selections, local inflammatory status, endodontic treatments, and availability of periodontal ligament in both donor and recipient sites [7–10]. The autotransplantation procedures have been documented well, and systematic reviews and meta-analysis showed that the survival rate of the transplanted teeth was more than 90%

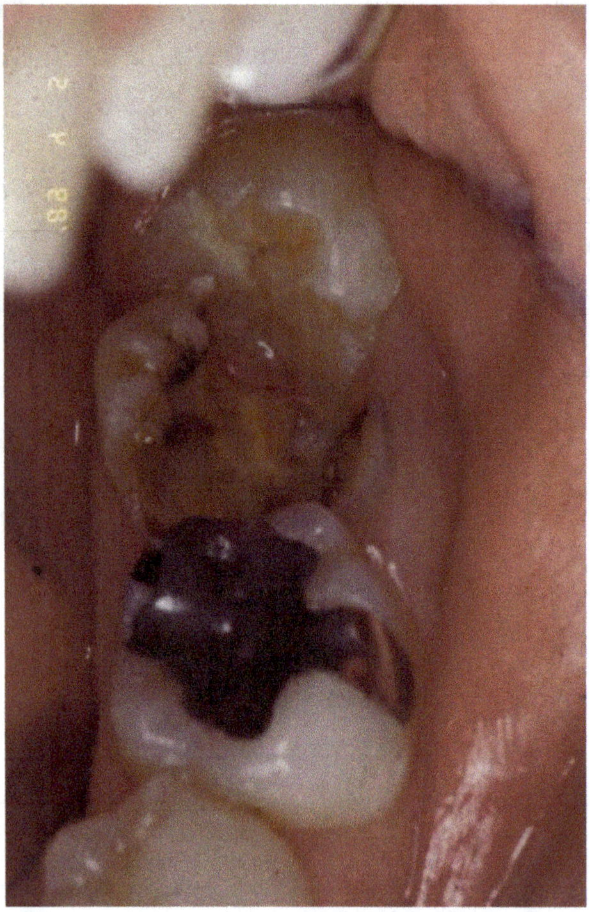

FIGURE 1: The initial clinical presentation of #18 with gross caries extending to the subgingival margin.

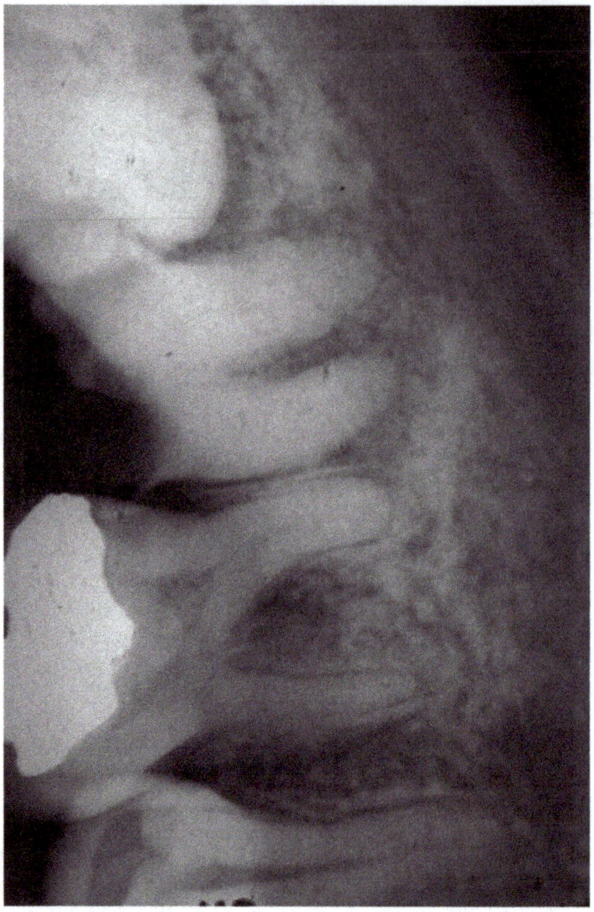

FIGURE 2: Periapical radiograph at the initial appointment. Large periapical radiolucency was present on the second molar. The gross caries reached to the almost alveolar bone level on the radiograph. This was deemed as a nonrestorable tooth.

after ten years [8, 11]. Moreover, a systematic review by Machado et al. included studies that had more than six years of follow-up period to analyze the long-term prognosis [7]. The meta-analysis revealed an 81% survival rate, and this rate showed an excellent long-term therapeutic prognosis of autotransplantation.

However, the evidence of the very long-term outcome of autotransplantation is still limited. Therefore, this case report is aimed at demonstrating the 29-year follow-up of the successful autotransplantation of the mandibular third molar to the second molar.

2. Clinical Presentation

A 24-year-old Asian female presented to private practice on March 29, 1989. She was with the chief complaint of caries treatment in the lower left second molar. She was classified as ASA I, and no history of smoking was noted. Tooth #18 was considered as a nonrestorable tooth based on the clinical and periapical radiograph (Figures 1 and 2). Panoramic radiograph showed large periapical radiolucency on #18 and relatively a conical shape of the #17 root form (Figure 3). Since she was not interested in having a dental implant at the time, this patient chose autologous tooth transplantation from #17 to #18.

The patient was fully informed of all possible adverse events, and she consented to the procedure before the procedure. The procedure was completed under local anesthesia in April 1989. Initially, #18 was extracted in a minimal traumatic manner and meticulous debridement was completed in the socket. Following the extraction of #17 with the caution of saving periodontal regiment, the removed #17 was temporarily stored in a glass petri dish with 0.9% of saline solution (Figure 4). The recipient site was prepared with a low-speed handpiece (20,000 rpm) with carbide round bur under copious irrigation. This process was repeated until the root shape of #17 fit well in the recipient site. Since the transplanted tooth did not show any mobility after the insertion, the temporary fixation was completed with the 4-0 silk sutures in an interrupted manner. The total duration from extraction to stabilization of #17 in the recipient site was less than 10 minutes. An occlusal adjustment was completed to remove any contacts to the opposing arch on the transplanted tooth (Figure 5). This patient was prescribed bacampicillin 250 mg and diclofenac 25 mg three times a day for three days and was instructed to refrain from using the left side for mastication. Suture removal was completed one week postoperatively. Approximately 3 months after the

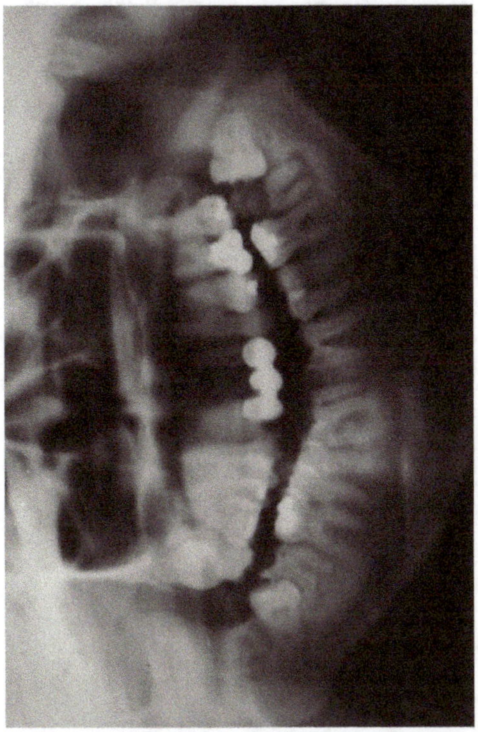

FIGURE 3: Panoramic radiograph showed that horizontal impaction of #17 was noted. The apical part of #17 was fully formed.

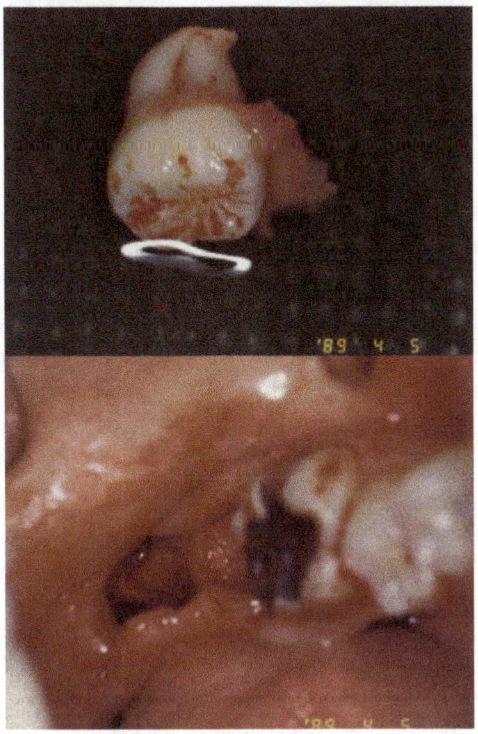

FIGURE 4: Immediate after of minimal traumatic extractions of #17 and 18. #17 was kept in the saline until this was used.

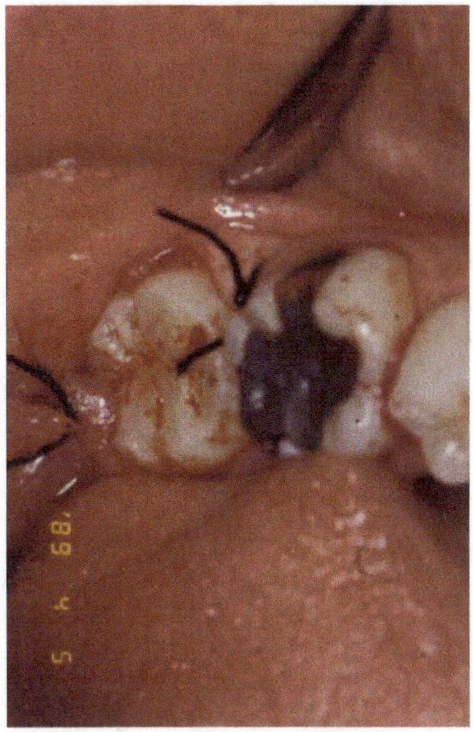

FIGURE 5: Tooth #17 was transplanted into the #18 site. Interrupted sutures were rendered to proximate the gingival tissues.

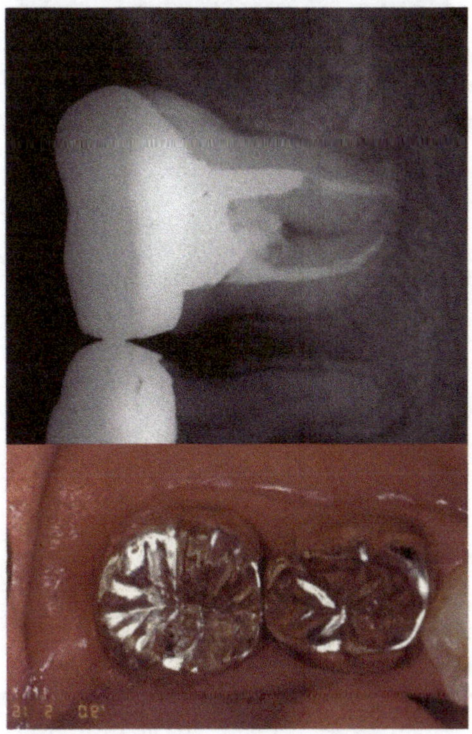

FIGURE 6: One year follow-up from the surgical procedure. Slight apical radiolucency was noted in the transplanted tooth. Soft tissue healing was uneventful. Slight inadequate root canal filing material was noted on the distal root of the transplanted tooth.

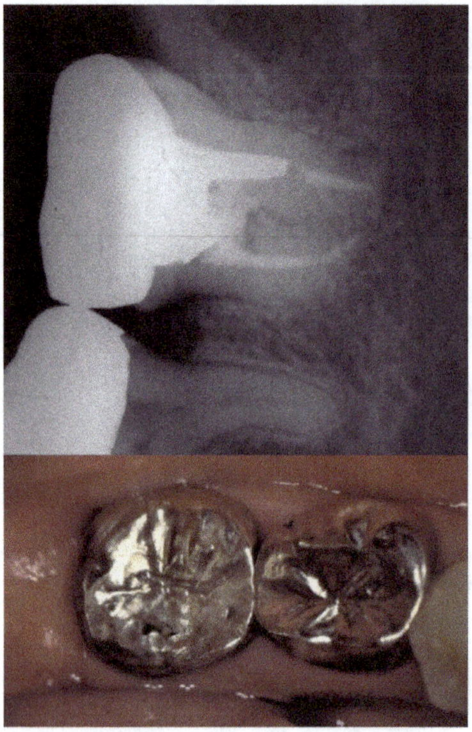

FIGURE 7: Ten-year follow-up after the transplantation. The size of the apical radiolucency reduced from one year after the procedure.

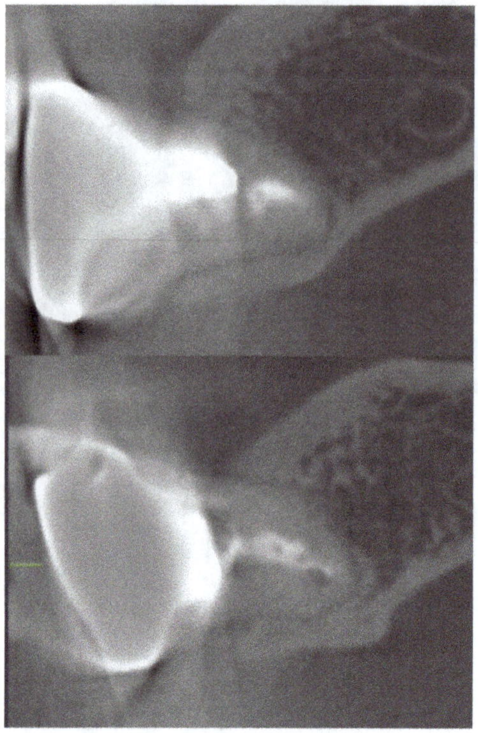

FIGURE 9: CBCT revealed the presence of buccal and lingual bone on both mesial (a) and distal (b) roots of the transplanted tooth.

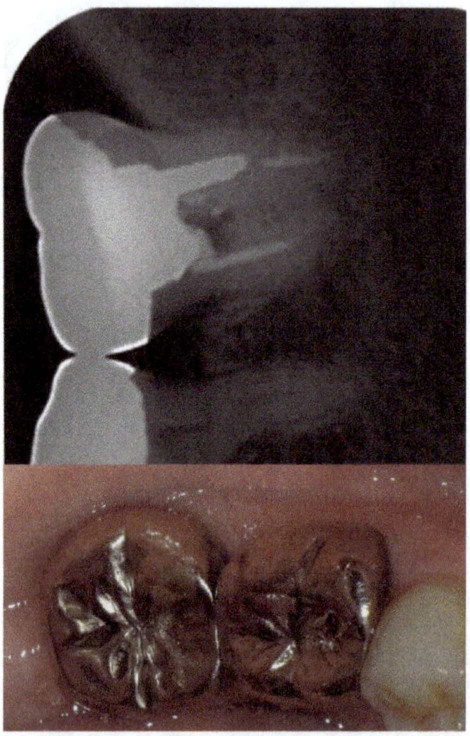

FIGURE 8: Twenty-eight years after the transplantation. Probing depth was less than 3 mm and gingival health was confirmed. There is no alveolar bone loss that was noted around the transplanted tooth. A radiolucency was noted in the pulp chamber which reached to the furcation area. However, no clinical pathological changes were noted.

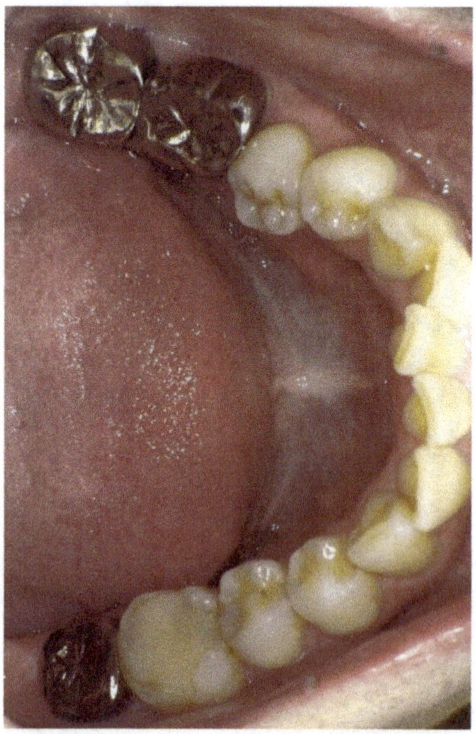

FIGURE 10: Twenty-nine years after the procedure, this patient maintains good oral hygiene and gingival health.

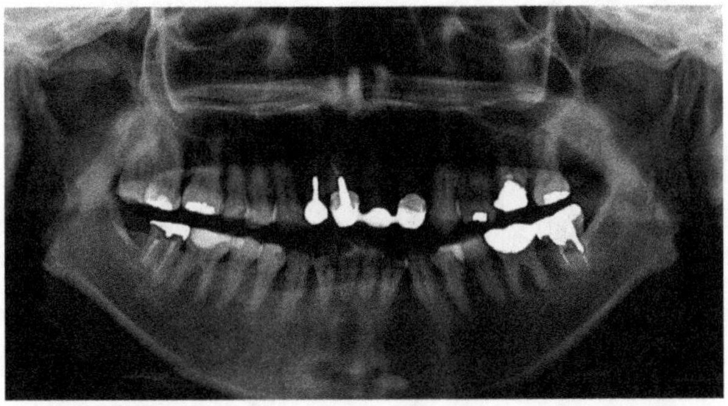

FIGURE 11: Panoramic radiograph demonstrated the no sign of alveolar bone loss on the transplanted tooth. This patient has maintained all the teeth for almost 30 years from initial appointment.

surgical procedure, the swelling was noted on the buccal surface of the tooth. The transplanted tooth was diagnosed with pulp necrosis. On the same day, endodontic treatment was rendered. Since periodontal tissue was fully stabilized within 6 months after the surgical procedure, the final prosthesis was delivered on the transplanted tooth in October 1989.

One year following the autotransplantation, slight periapical radiolucency was still noted. However, since the tooth was not symptomatic and probing depth was within 3–4 mm without any alveolar bone loss, the maintenance and oral hygiene program began one year postoperatively. Slightly inadequate root canal filling material was noted on the distal root of the transplanted tooth (Figure 6). A periapical radiograph and clinical examinations showed reduced periapical radiolucency and periodontal stability ten years after the procedure (Figure 7). At the 28-year follow-up in 2017, probing depth around the tooth showed within 3 mm without bleeding on probing and the interdental bone level was within 2 mm from cement enamel junction (Figure 8). Cone beam computed tomography (CBCT) showed the absence of root resorption and the presence of buccal and lingual bone on the transplanted tooth (Figure 9).

After 29 years of the procedure, in February 2018, the transplanted tooth was still functioning without any discomfort or symptoms (Figures 10 and 11). This patient has complied every 4–6 months of the maintenance program, and occlusal check and adjustment have been rendered if necessary, at each visit. The patient was delighted with the outcome of the treatments over these years.

3. Discussion

This case report demonstrated the long-term success and periodontal stability of the transplanted tooth. Even with this patient's age and suitability of a dental implant on #18 after the extraction, the autotransplantation was attempted because this procedure included a single surgical intervention; the tooth presented a conical root shape, even if the root form was almost completed. The total cost of autotransplantation can be lower compared to that of implants because the procedure is performed in one stage, and a prosthesis may not be needed in some cases [12]. The predictability of the procedure needs to be considered for the choice of treatments. Fugazzotto reported that the cumulative success rate of implants in the mandibular second molar was 85% and the rate was slightly lower than other molars [13]. On the other hand, the total success rates of autotransplantation were 94% with the open apex teeth and 84% with closed apex groups [14]. The other retrospective study showed 92% of the survival rate of the immature root form-autotransplanted teeth for midterm length [15]. In this study, the authors utilized the enamel matrix derivatives (EMD) to apply the root surface to enhance the healing process if necessary. The additional biologic modifiers might play a crucial role in regenerative therapy. Based on these previously reported high predictabilities, the toot autotransplantation should be considered as one of the treatment options when an adequate donor site is available. However, the autotransplantation procedure is not complication free. Unsuccessful autotransplantation is more likely associated with excessive surgical trauma and contaminated donor tooth and when the periodontal probing depth is more than 4 mm and patients are older than 40 years [16]. A retrospective study reported that the main reasons for autotransplantation failure were periodontal attachment loss (54.9%), root resorption (26.5%), dental caries (4.0%), and root fracture (2.9%) [17]. In this case, the patient was 24 years old at the time of the procedure and did not present evidence of periodontitis. Patient selection factors, including stable systemic conditions, excellent oral hygiene, and high compliance with the regular dental visits with occlusal adjustments, play essential roles in achieving the ideal outcomes.

Authors' Contributions

Drs. Kimura, Eida, and Kumano have contributed to this patient care. Dr. Hamada completed the literature review, developed the conception, and did paper writings. Drs. Okamura and Yokota contributed to the radiographic analysis and conceptions. All authors contributed to the paper revision and final approval.

References

[1] J. H. Bae, Y. H. Choi, B. H. Cho, Y. K. Kim, and S. G. Kim, "Autotransplantation of teeth with complete root formation: a case series," *Journal of Endodontia*, vol. 36, no. 8, pp. 1422–1426, 2010.

[2] Q. Yan, B. Li, and X. Long, "Immediate autotransplantation of mandibular third molar in China," *Oral Surgery, Oral Medicine, Oral Pathology, Oral Radiology, and Endodontics*, vol. 110, no. 4, pp. 436–440, 2010.

[3] J. R. Natiella, J. E. Armitage, and G. W. Greene, "The replantation and transplantation of teeth: A review," *Oral Surgery, Oral Medicine, and Oral Pathology*, vol. 29, no. 3, pp. 397–419, 1970.

[4] M. Tsukiboshi, "Autotransplantation of teeth: requirements for predictable success," *Dental Traumatology*, vol. 18, no. 4, pp. 157–180, 2002.

[5] S. Kvint, R. Lindsten, A. Magnusson, P. Nilsson, and K. Bjerklin, "Autotransplantation of teeth in 215 patients. A follow-up study.," *Angle Orthodontist*, vol. 80, no. 3, pp. 446–451, 2010.

[6] J. O. Andreasen, H. U. Paulsen, Z. Yu, R. Ahlquist, T. Bayer, and O. Schwartz, "A long-term study of 370 autotransplanted premolars. Part I. surgical procedures and standardized techniques for monitoring healing," *European Journal of Orthodontics*, vol. 12, no. 1, pp. 3–13, 1990.

[7] L. A. Machado, R. R. do Nascimento, D. M. T. P. Ferreira, C. T. Mattos, and O. V. Vilella, "Long-term prognosis of tooth autotransplantation: a systematic review and meta-analysis," *International Journal of Oral and Maxillofacial Surgery*, vol. 45, no. 5, pp. 610–617, 2016.

[8] K. Almpani, S. N. Papageorgiou, and M. A. Papadopoulos, "Autotransplantation of teeth in humans: a systematic review and meta-analysis," *Clinical Oral Investigations*, vol. 19, no. 6, pp. 1157–1179, 2015.

[9] E. Kim, J. Y. Jung, I. H. Cha, K. Y. Kum, and S. J. Lee, "Evaluation of the prognosis and causes of failure in 182 cases of autogenous tooth transplantation," *Oral Surgery, Oral Medicine, Oral Pathology, Oral Radiology, and Endodontics*, vol. 100, no. 1, pp. 112–119, 2005.

[10] P. Ravi kumar, M. Jyothi, K. Sirisha, K. Racca, and C. Uma, "Autotransplantation of mandibular third molar: a case report," *Case reports in dentistry*, vol. 2012, Article ID 629180, 5 pages, 2012.

[11] E. C. M. Rohof, W. Kerdijk, J. Jansma, C. Livas, and Y. Ren, "Autotransplantation of teeth with incomplete root formation: a systematic review and meta-analysis," *Clinical Oral Investigations*, vol. 22, no. 4, pp. 1613–1624, 2018.

[12] J. B. Baviz, "Autotransplantation of teeth: a procedure that gets no respect," *Oral Surgery, Oral Medicine, Oral Pathology, Oral Radiology, and Endodontics*, vol. 110, no. 4, p. 441, 2010.

[13] P. A. Fugazzotto, "A comparison of the success of root resected molars and molar position implants in function in a private practice: results of up to 15-plus years," *Journal of Periodontology*, vol. 72, no. 8, pp. 1113–1123, 2001.

[14] T. Lundberg and S. Isaksson, "A clinical follow-up study of 278 autotransplanted teeth," *The British Journal of Oral & Maxillofacial Surgery*, vol. 34, no. 2, pp. 181–185, 1996.

[15] C. Raabe, M. M. Bornstein, J. Ducommun, P. Sendi, T. von Arx, and S. F. M. Janner, "A retrospective analysis of autotransplanted teeth including an evaluation of a novel surgical technique," *Clinical Oral Investigations*, vol. 25, no. 6, pp. 3513–3525, 2021.

[16] T. Sugai, M. Yoshizawa, T. Kobayashi et al., "Clinical study on prognostic factors for autotransplantation of teeth with complete root formation," *International Journal of Oral and Maxillofacial Surgery*, vol. 39, no. 12, pp. 1193–1203, 2010.

[17] K. Yoshino, N. Kariya, D. Namura et al., "A retrospective survey of autotransplantation of teeth in dental clinics," *Journal of Oral Rehabilitation*, vol. 39, no. 1, pp. 37–43, 2012.

4

The "Prosthetic Orthodontic Approach": An Application of the Biologically Oriented Preparation Technique Protocol

Luca Casula

Vita Salute University, Milan, Italy

Correspondence should be addressed to Luca Casula; lucacasula.nu@gmail.com

Academic Editor: Giuseppe Alessandro Scardina

In this study, three cases involving patients who required multidisciplinary treatment for the aesthetic and functional rehabilitation of the maxillary or mandibular arch are described. In particular, an indication for preprosthetic orthodontic treatment, such as orthodontic extrusion, tooth realignment, correction of malocclusion, and diastemata closure, was present in all cases. Preprosthetic orthodontic treatment to resolve these issues before the restorative procedures was proposed; however, all patients refused preprosthetic orthodontic treatment. Thus, to restore aesthetics and function, solely a feather-edge prosthetic protocol has been used. The biologically oriented preparation technique was used to prepare the teeth that were moved in the established direction by preparing the abutment more on one side than the opposite. This so called "prosthetic orthodontic approach" allowed resolving clinical issues that would typically require preprosthetic orthodontic treatment, such as complete clinical crown loss, occlusal vertical dimension loss, tooth misalignment, malocclusion, tooth agenesis, and severe multiple diastemata. The degree of reciprocal movement of the prepared teeth achievable through this approach was minor and not comparable to a traditional wide-range orthodontic movement. Besides, the technique resulted in a modification of the gingival tissues and improvement of their thickness although it is unclear what effect this technique has on the gingival biotype. None of the patients had prosthetic or periodontal complications for at least 12 months following the procedure. Gingival health was excellent, and the prosthetic procedure did not affect the pulp survival of the vital teeth. The biologically oriented preparation technique used with a prosthetic orthodontic approach can effectively manage complicated cases without the need for preprosthetic orthodontics.

1. Introduction

The biologically oriented preparation technique (BOPT) is a prosthetic protocol which consists of a feather-edge subgingival preparation whereby the gingival profile adapts itself to the new prosthetic coronal emergence profile [1]. This is made possible by the elimination of an emergence profile of the tooth or any preexisting finish line. A new prosthetic emergence profile is created by placing the prosthesis in such a way that leaves the gingival margin at the desired position [2, 3].

The BOPT protocol has been shown to increase gingival thickness and achieve stable and healthy soft and hard tissues in natural teeth [3, 4]. The same protocol has been described for dental implants showing good clinical outcomes [5, 6].

An example of soft tissue adaptation to the new prosthetic emergence profile after the BOPT protocol is shown in Figures 1 and 2. In Figure 1, the central incisor (Figure 1(a)) was prepared with a feather-edge preparation using a flame-shaped bur on the bottom of the previously probed sulcus and eliminating the preexisting finishing line. A new emergence profile was created with the interim restoration that was positioned 1.5 mm coronally to the gingival margin (Figure 1(b)). After one month of soft tissue maturation, the gingiva adapted itself to the new emergence profile (Figure 1(c)). In Figure 2, the canine (Figure 2(a)) was prepared with the same technique and the interim crown restoration was left 0.5 mm subgingivally for one month (Figure 1(b)). After this period, the interim crown restoration was shortened (Figure 1(c)), and one month later, the gingiva adapted itself to the new emergence profile (Figure 1(d)). In this series of clinical cases, the teeth were moved by means of the feather-edge preparation, avoiding a preprosthetic orthodontic treatment, and the BOPT protocol was then used

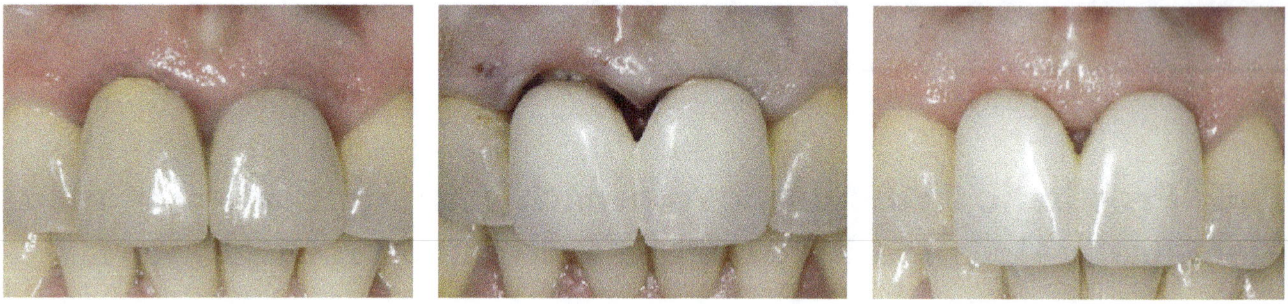

(a) (b) (c)

Figure 1: Adaptation of the soft tissue after the feather-edge preparation: (a) disparallelism of the gingival margin before BOPT; (b) right incisor shortened after BOPT; (c) coronal growth of the gingiva after one month.

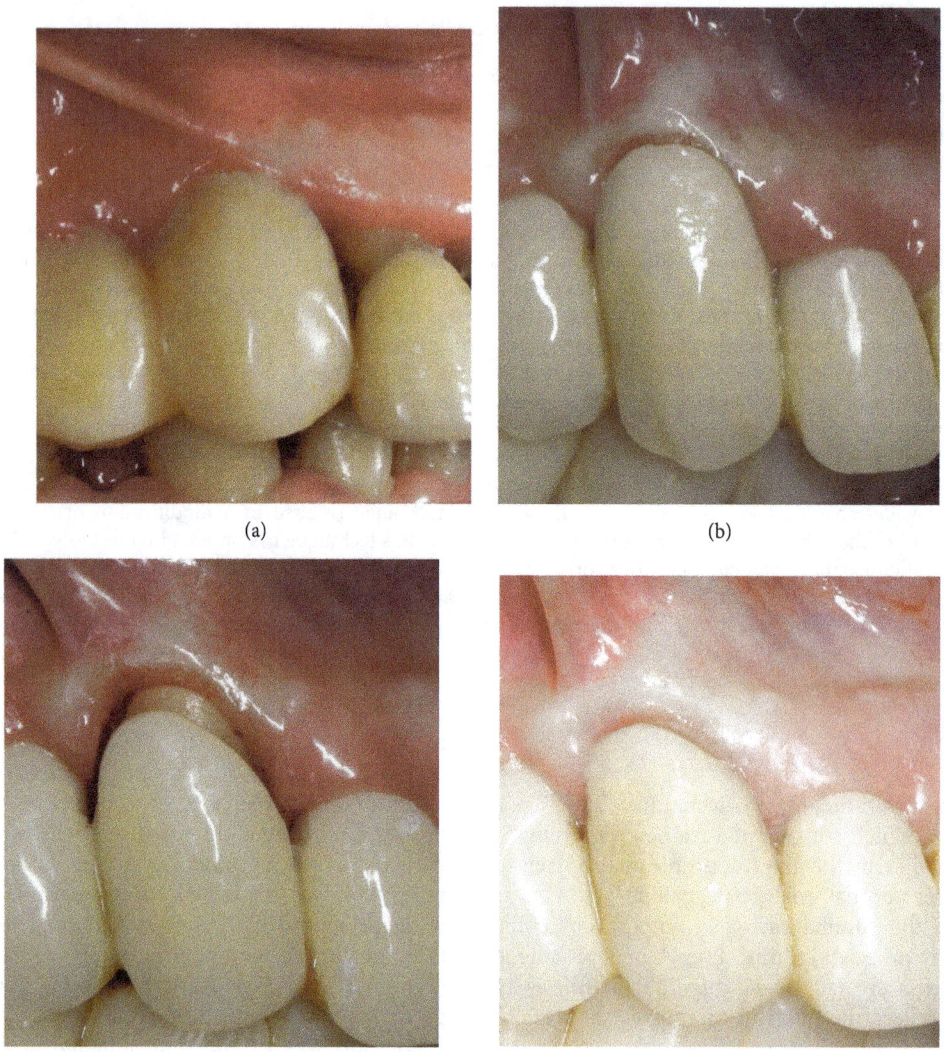

(a) (b) (c) (d)

Figure 2: Adaptation of the soft tissue after the feather-edge preparation: (a) old complete crown restorations; (b) new interim restoration with the BOPT protocol; (c) right canine shortened after BOPT; (d) coronal growth of the gingiva after one month.

to guide the soft tissue maturation to the new tooth position. This tooth movement solely by means of the dental preparation was termed the "prosthetic orthodontic approach (POA)." The approach allowed only small tooth movements and is not suitable to perform complex orthodontic movements with a large range of action. In the clinical cases described, we presented all thick gingival biotypes with the exception of the lower incisors in case number two where

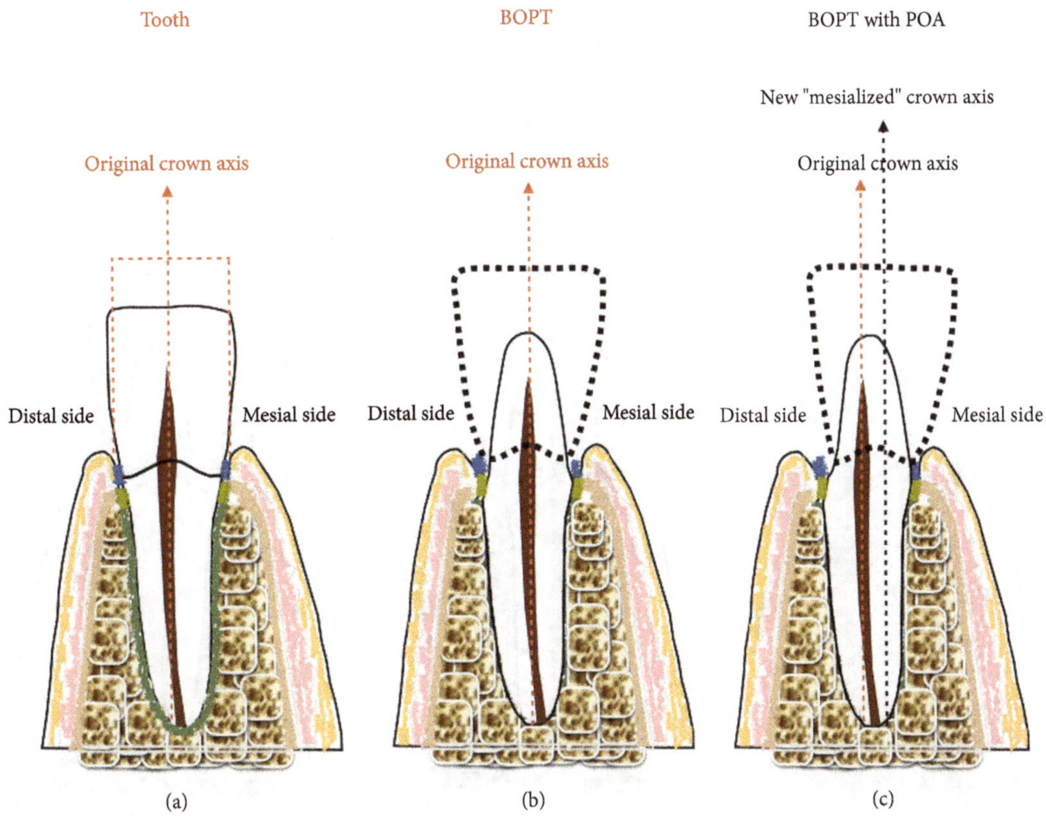

FIGURE 3: Mesialisation of the abutment tooth using the biologically oriented preparation technique (BOPT): (a) tooth; (b) the tooth is prepared without a finish line (BOPT), equally on the distal and mesial sides, such that the tooth axis remains unchanged; (c) the tooth is prepared without a finish line (BOPT), more on the distal than on the mesial side: this allows the mesialisation of the crown axis.

we also made a diagnosis of severe gingival recession. The procedural technique followed would seem to result in a thickening of the gingiva [1–6]. The phenotype after therapy appeared pink and healthy, although it is unclear what effect this technique has on the gingival biotype itself [1–6]. Further studies, both clinical and histologic, are needed to elucidate what the biological mechanisms are for gingival tissue to be modified.

2. Methods

The prosthetic procedure, laboratory stages, and used materials were the same for all three clinical cases described below.

The preparation technique we used in all cases followed the BOPT protocol described by Loi in 2013. This technique involves the use of a diamond flame-shaped bur (6863D.314.016, Komet, Italy) for the abutment tooth preparation mounted in a high-speed handpiece. Before starting the dental preparation, the gingival sulcus was sounded with a calibrated probe (Hawe Click-Probe®, KerrHawe SA, Switzerland) to establish the preparation depth. The tooth was prepared until the bottom of the probed sulcus. A vertical area without a finish line was created, and the interim restoration was relined using a self-curing methacrylate resin (Sintodent, Italy). The new emergence profile was positioned in the gingival sulcus without violating the biologic width. The movement of the crown axis of the abutment teeth was achieved by means of the BOPT with the POA in all cases where tooth movement was required. The tooth movement was obtained by preparing the abutment teeth with the feather-edge preparation (BOPT) more on the one side than the opposite. For example, if mesial movement of the abutment tooth was required, the tooth was prepared more on the distal side so that the abutment tooth could be moved mesially (Figure 3). In this way, the crown could be moved in the desired direction while simultaneously maintaining the tooth proportion, simulating an orthodontic treatment. In the preparation without a finish line (vertical preparation), the crown is positioned in a vertical area of the abutment tooth so that when the vertical area is moved in a given direction, the crown can be moved together with the abutment tooth and the same tooth proportion can be maintained. Contrarily, in the horizontal finish line preparation, the crown margin is continuous with the external root profile, so that even if the distal side is prepared more than the mesial side, the crown axis cannot be moved without altering the tooth proportion (Figure 4). During the interim stage, the crown margins of the interim crown restorations were shortened if signs of inflammations (redness, bleeding) were detected, and the final impressions were taken only when the soft tissue appeared healthy and free from inflammation at every point.

2.1. Case 1. A 71-year-old man, American Society of Anesthesiologists (ASA) type I, presented to a hospital dental department hoping to correct aesthetic and functional

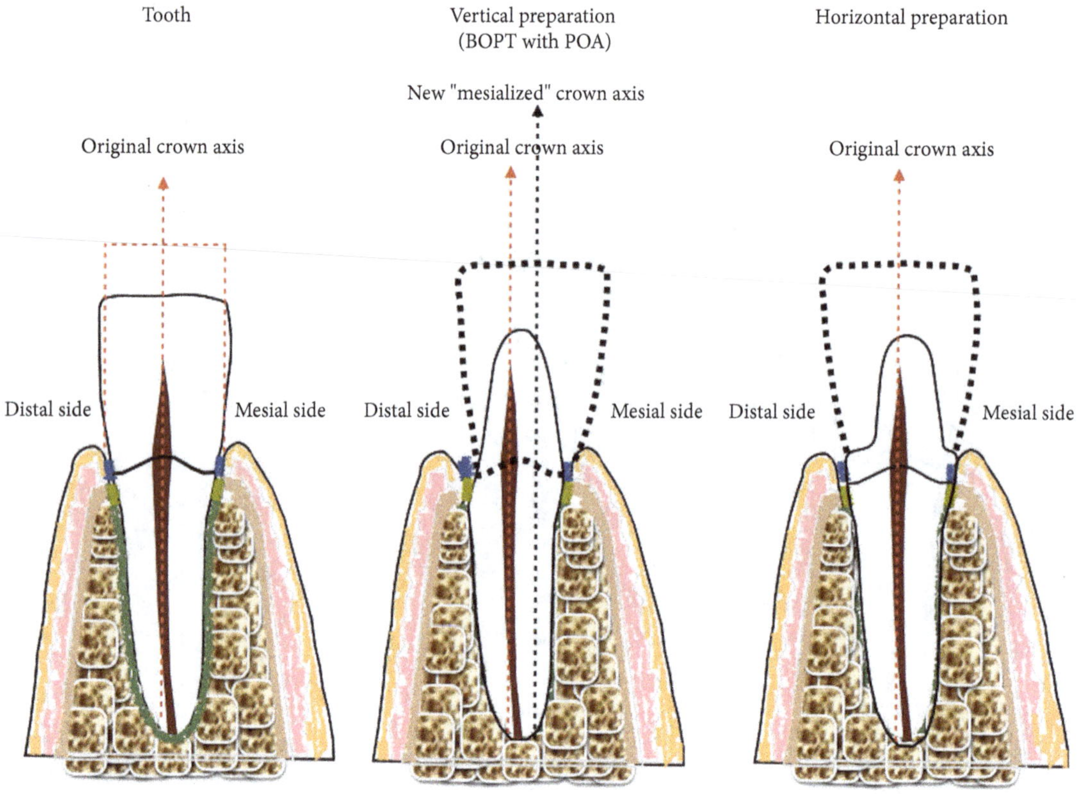

FIGURE 4: Mesialisation of the abutment tooth using the biologically oriented preparation technique (BOPT): (a) tooth; (b) the tooth is prepared without a finish line (BOPT), more on the distal than on the mesial side: this allows the mesialisation of the crown axis; (c) the tooth is prepared with a horizontal finish line, such that the crown restoration is in continuity with the external profile of the root. Therefore, the crown axis cannot be moved without altering the tooth proportions, even if the distal side is prepared more than the mesial side.

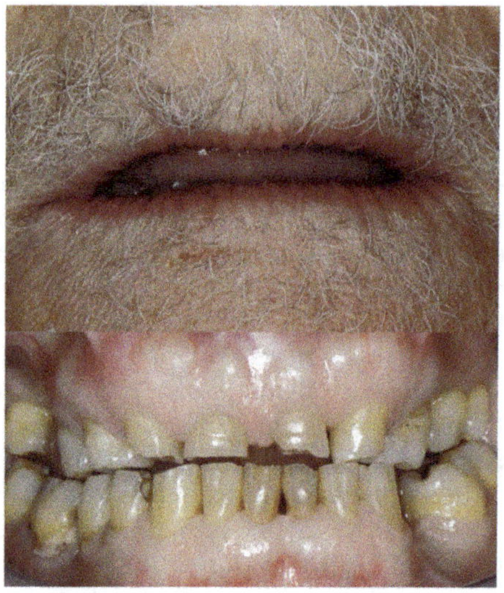

FIGURE 5: Extraoral and intraoral view of the severely worn dentition.

problems of the maxillary arch (Figure 5) where the teeth were severely worn and with the lateral incisor agenesis (Figure 6). The full-arch interim crown restoration was fabricated with the correct tooth proportion and position, in such a way that the lateral incisors replaced the misaligned canine.

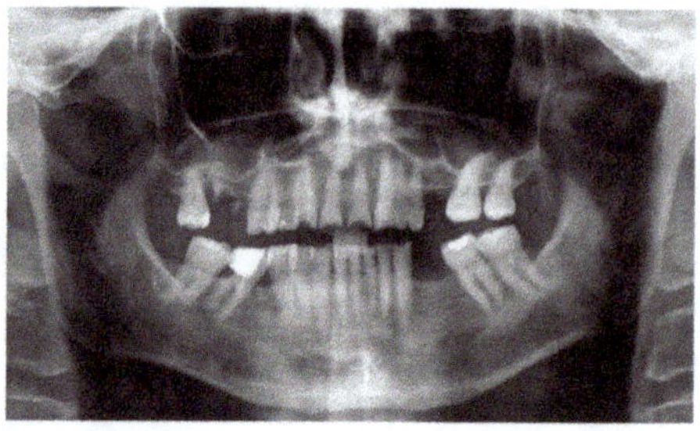

FIGURE 6: The panoramic radiograph showing the lateral incisor agenesis.

The correct tooth proportions were achieved by preparing the distal side of the canines more than the mesial side with the BOPT and POA, so that the abutment teeth were adapted to the interim restoration and not the opposite (Figure 7). The full-arch interim restoration was positioned in the maxillary arch with the crown margin 0.5 mm subgingivally, and after one month of soft tissue maturation, the soft tissue appeared healthy without signs of inflammation (Figure 8). A panoramic radiograph was made with the interim restoration showing that the dental pulp was not involved after the prosthetic procedure (Figure 9). The definitive impression was taken using a double retraction cord (Ultrapack™, Ultradent Products, USA) soaked in a haemostatic solution

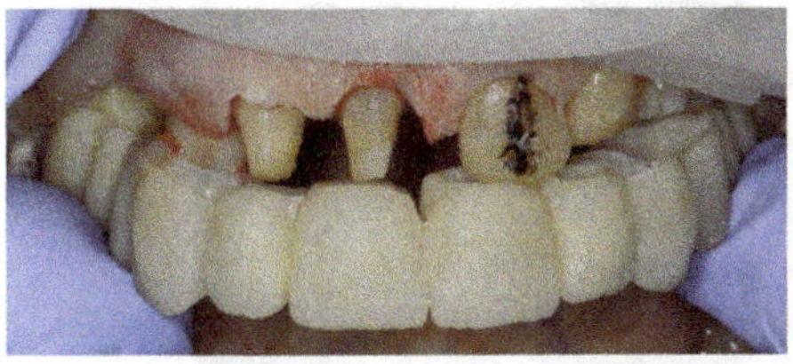

Figure 7: The abutment teeth were adapted to the interim restoration used as a guide for the dental preparation.

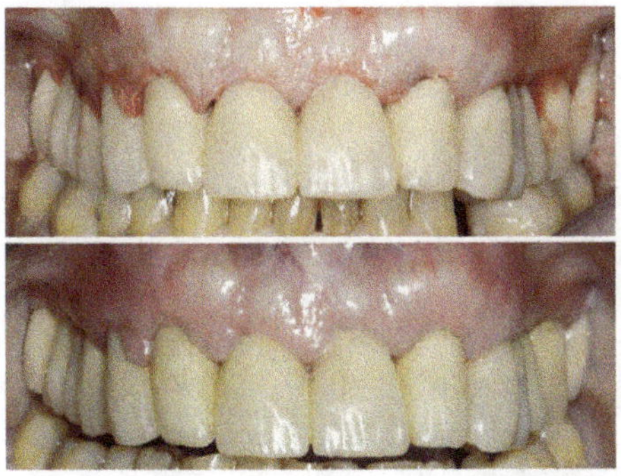

Figure 8: The interim restoration immediately after the prosthetic procedure and after one month of soft tissue maturation.

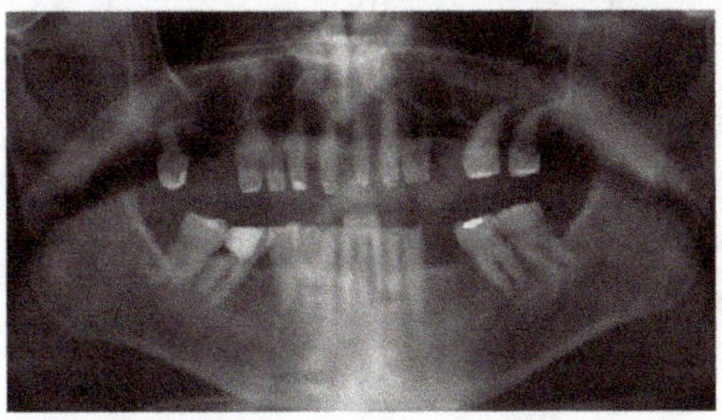

Figure 9: The panoramic radiograph with the interim restoration showing that the dental pulp was not involved after the prosthetic procedure.

(Gengistal, Ogna, Italy) and a one-step light body and putty polysiloxane impression (Putty and Light Elite HD, Zhermack, Italy). The impression was sent to the dental technician with a request that the final restorations be shaped in a manner that allowed the emergence profile to sustain the mature soft tissues. In the dental laboratory, the final restoration was fabricated with a zirconia framework veneered with feldspathic porcelain (VITAVM 9, VITA Zahnfabrik, Germany). The final restorations were clinically checked and sent for the final glaze and at the final appointment were cemented (placed 0.5 mm into the gingival sulcus) with a self-adhesive resin cement (RelyX Unicem; 3 M ESPE, USA). At the one-year follow-up visit, no biological or technical complications were noted, and the gingiva appeared thick, pink, healthy, and completely adapted to the definitive restoration (Figure 10).

2.2. Case 2. A 70-year-old healthy woman presented at a private practice dental office, unsatisfied with her smile; this was due to excessive maxillary gingival display (a gummy smile), concomitant with short clinical crowns (Figure 11). Intraoral

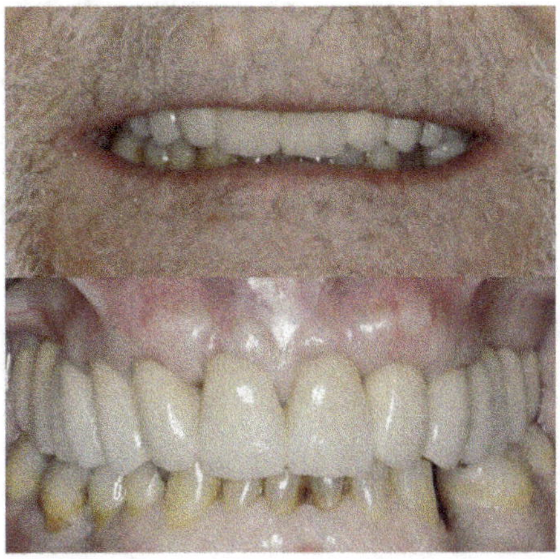

Figure 10: Extraoral and intraoral views of the final restoration after the 1-year follow-up.

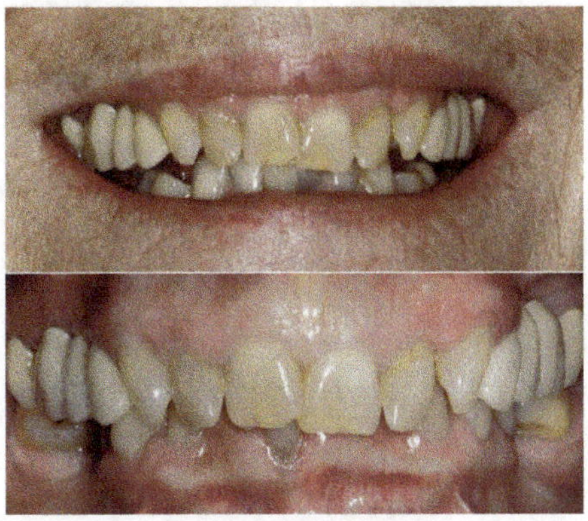

Figure 11: Extraoral and intraoral views showing deep bite and gummy smile.

examination revealed partial edentulism, rotated anterior maxillary teeth with incisal erosion, and enamel wear (Figure 11). The mandibular molars were mesially inclined, resulting in the collapse of the occlusal vertical dimension (OVD) [7, 8]. The remaining mandibular teeth were severely worn. The right central incisor was rotated in the buccal position, with gingival recession and loss of gingival height (Figure 11).

During the next appointment, the anterior maxillary teeth were prepared with the BOPT, and the interim restoration was cemented. Next, two 3.8 mm diameter implants (WINSIX® BIOSAF IN Srl, Milan, Italy) were placed in the area of the mandibular first molar and left submerged during the osseointegration period. At the end of the session, two alginate impressions and a new centric relation record were obtained and mounted in an articulator to fabricate a mandibular full-arch restoration corresponding to the increased OVD.

The mandibular full-arch restoration was fabricated using a 3 mm OVD increment, and the curve of Spee was harmonized with the opposing arch. The mandibular teeth were prepared with the BOPT, and the complete restoration was placed in the mandibular arch from the right to the left second molar. The mandibular left second molar was

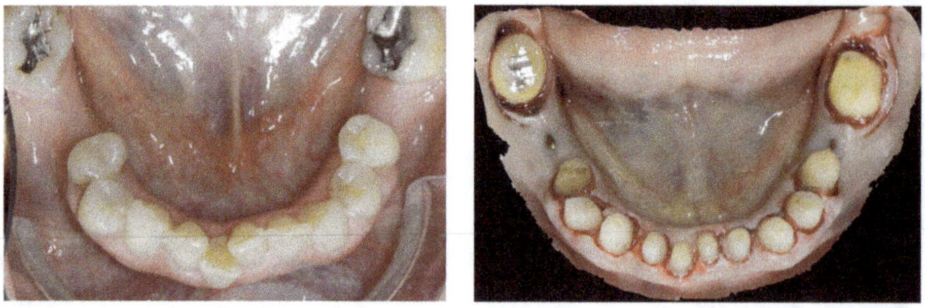

(a) (b)

FIGURE 12: The mandibular arch showing the right central incisor and the second molars before the prosthetic preparation (a) and realignment after the POA (b).

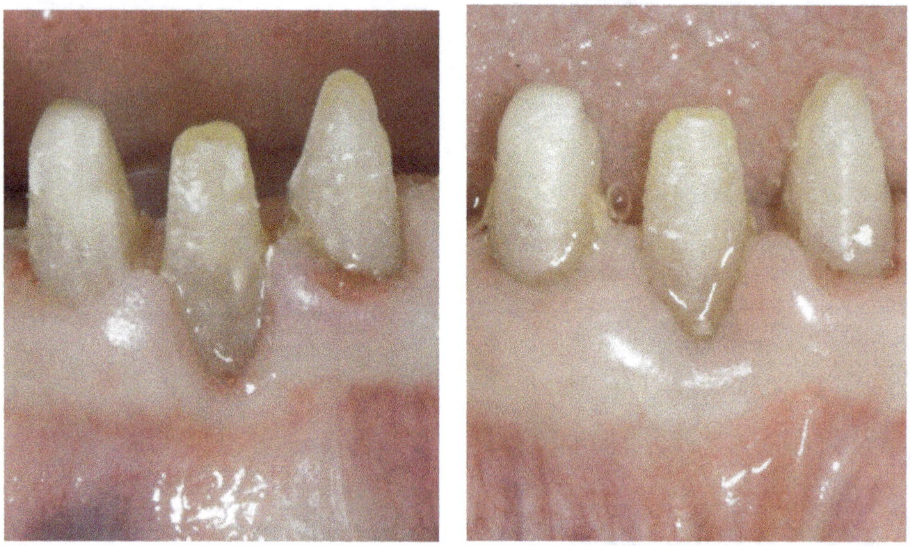

(a) (b)

FIGURE 13: The mandibular right central incisor without the interim restoration: (a) gingival recession; (b) healing of the gingival recession and thickening of the gingiva after the BOPT protocol with POA.

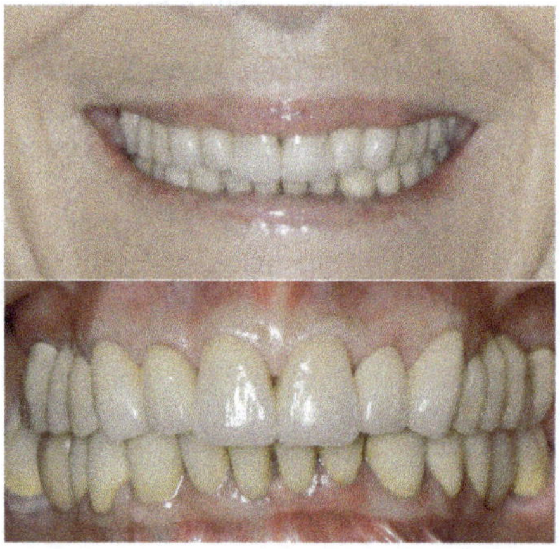

FIGURE 14: Final rehabilitation at the two-year follow-up with the new smile after the correction of the deep bite and gummy smile.

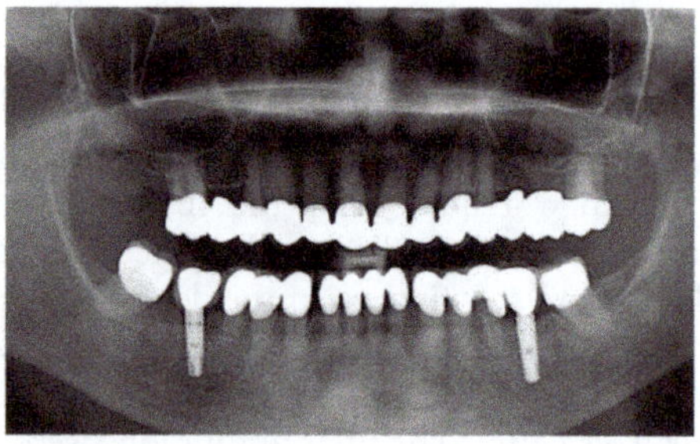

FIGURE 15: Panoramic radiograph taken two years after the procedure showing that the dental pulp was not involved after the prosthetic procedure.

mesially inclined, so it was prepared more on the mesial side than on the distal one using the BOPT with the POA to move the dental axis distally, thereby creating an adequate space for the first molar parallel to the path of prosthesis insertion (Figure 12). The POA was also used for the mandibular right central incisor by preparing it more on the vestibular side to realign it with the adjacent teeth (Figure 13). The interim mandibular full-arch restoration was cemented and corresponded to the new OVD. One month after soft tissue maturation, the definitive impression of the maxillary abutment teeth was taken, and zirconia ceramic full-crown restorations

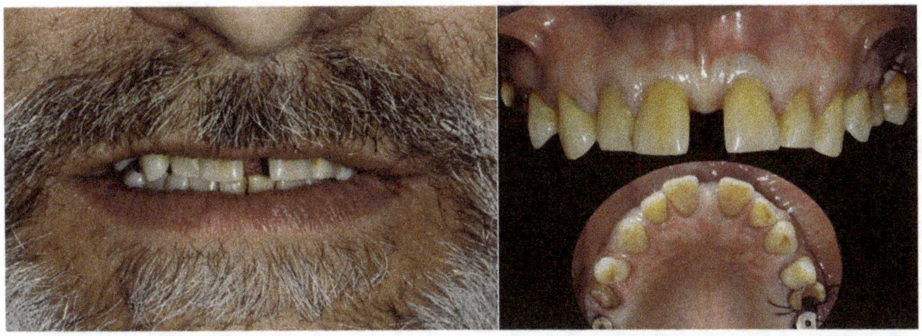

FIGURE 16: Preoperative extraoral and intraoral views showing 6 mm midline diastema.

were fabricated in the dental laboratory. The gingival sulcus was probed again and found to be 2 mm on the vestibular side. The dental technician was instructed to position the crown margin 1.5 mm subgingivally only on the vestibular side, using all of the available gingival sulcus, thus improving the gummy smile (Figure 14). In the interdental spaces and on the palatal side, the crown margin was placed 0.5 mm into the gingival sulcus. The patient expressed satisfaction with the results. Healthy gingiva, with an ideal scalloped architecture, was observed at the 2-year follow-up. No gingival recession or inflammation was noted. The restoration accomplished three goals: (1) correction of the deep bite, (2) realignment of the teeth, and (3) elimination of the gummy smile. The procedure did not affect the pulp vitality, and no endodontic complications were observed at the 2-year follow-up (Figure 15).

2.3. Case 3. A 63-year-old man, ASA type I, presented at a hospital dental department. The subject wanted to improve their dental aesthetics and function. Intraoral examination revealed a 6 mm maxillary midline diastema and multiple diastemata, rampant caries, radicular fractures, and periodontal involvement of the first molars, which were immediately extracted and replaced with 3.8 diameter implants (WINSIX® BIOSAF IN Srl, Milan, Italy) that were loaded 3 months after placement (Figure 16).

The correct tooth proportions were achieved by preparing the distal side more than the mesial side with the BOPT and POA. Thus, during abutment preparation, the vertical area was moved toward the centre of the tooth, and the mesialisation of the teeth concurrently facilitated diastema closure and maintained the correct tooth proportions (Figure 17). As previously described, the interim restoration was used as a guide during tooth preparation, and the distal side of the teeth was prepared until a point previously marked with a pencil to put the interim crowns on the abutment teeth (Figure 17). The BOPT was completed, and the crown margins were positioned 0.5 mm within the gingival sulcus (Figure 17).

Eight weeks after soft tissue maturation, the gingival tissues appeared healthy (Figure 18), and the definitive restorations were completed. The patient showed healthy gingiva, no probing depths more than 3 mm, no bleeding upon probing, and no signs of inflammation at the 2-year follow-up. Further, the prosthetic restorations were functionally integrated with the soft tissues, and the gingiva and interdental papillae were pink and stippled (Figure 19). Diastemata closure was achieved, and the prosthetic crowns were well

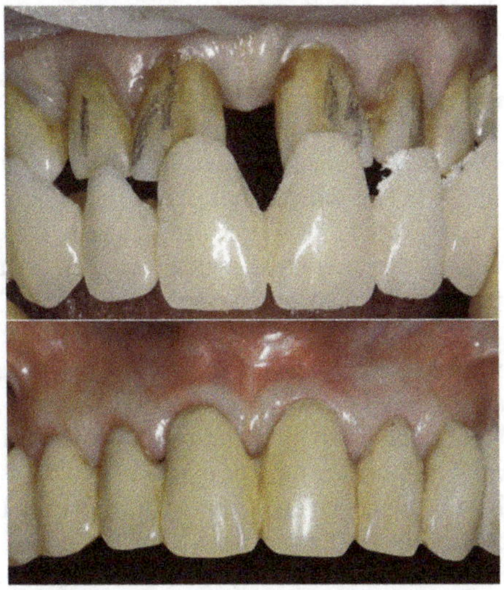

FIGURE 17: The full-arch interim crown restoration used as a guide for the dental preparation and the correct tooth proportion achieved after BOPT with POA.

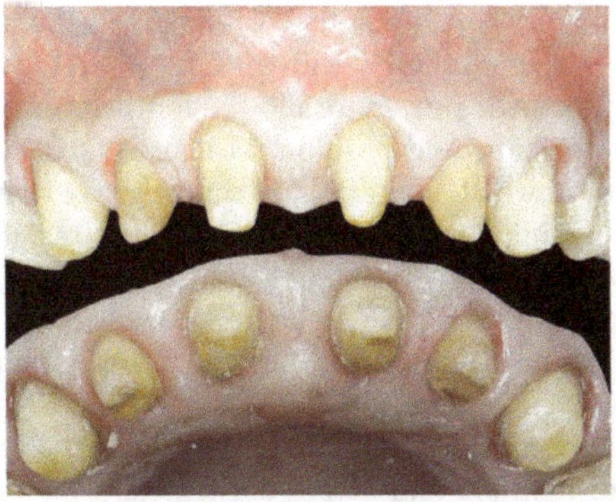

FIGURE 18: Abutment teeth 8 weeks after soft tissue maturation.

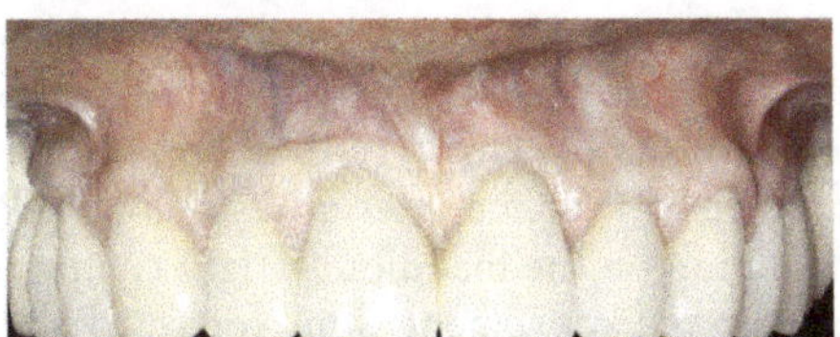

FIGURE 19: Definitive restoration 2 years after the procedure.

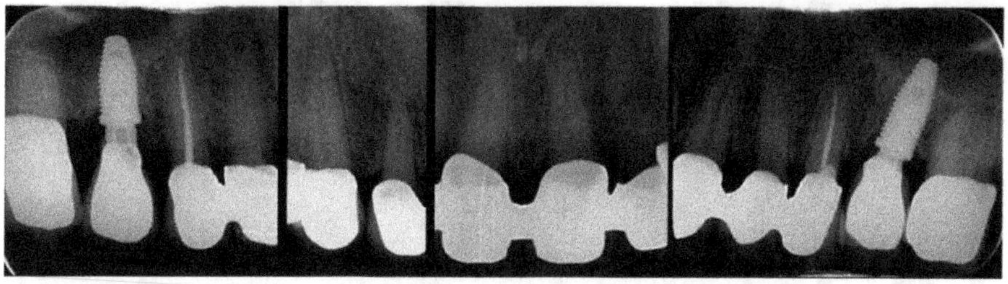

FIGURE 20: Periapical radiograph taken 24 months after the procedure.

proportioned. The procedure did not affect the pulp vitality, and no endodontic complications were observed at the 2-year follow-up (Figure 20).

3. Discussion

The BOPT provides a feather-edge subgingival preparation on natural teeth, for which good clinical periodontal outcomes and thickening of keratinized tissues are reported [1–6]. Feather-edge preparation offers a good marginal fit with similar outcomes to other designs, and it was recently reported that restoration margins located within the gingival sulcus do not cause gingivitis if the patient practices appropriate oral hygiene [9–11].

This abutment tooth preparation consists of a vertical area in which the crown margin is positioned. This vertical area can be moved in a given direction by preparing the abutment tooth more on the one side than the other, and the crown restoration is moved together, allowing the clinician to move the tooth axis in a mesio-distal or buccal-lingual direction (Figure 3). These concepts were applied in the present clinical cases, in which orthodontics would have been a primary treatment option [12–15]. However, orthodontic treatment was refused by the patients; thus, an alternative treatment plan was proposed, which comprised a prosthetic procedure using the BOPT with a POA.

This prosthetic procedure allowed for the transformation of the tooth shape and position, as is presented in the first case report in which the maxillary canines were transformed into the missing lateral incisors and the first maxillary premolars were moved mesially and transformed into canines. In the other cases, the BOPT with a POA was able to facilitate significant improvements in function and aesthetics in patients with a collapsed OVD with a limited prosthetic space, tooth misalignment, gingival recession, a gummy smile, and multiple and severe diastemata. This procedure was adopted in these cases because tooth wear and aesthetic problems were also present. The vertical area without a finish line, in contrast to the horizontal finish line, allowed clinicians to move the interim restoration in an apical or coronal direction, which greatly facilitates tissue adaptation to the emergence profile of the crown restoration [1–6]. In the second case, movement of the interim restoration allowed the gingival recession on the mandibular right central incisor to be closed (coronal movement) and corrected the gummy smile in the anterior maxillary sector (apical movement) [16]. Nevertheless, this approach is limited to cases where rehabilitation with complete clinical crown restorations is required for teeth with unsuitable clinical crown restoration or in severely worn teeth or those with aesthetic problems. A drawback to this technique is that it involves the use of crown margin restoration placed in a subgingival position that has serious implications for the health of the supporting periodontal tissues [17–19]. Inflammation of the gingival tissues was avoided by placing the crown margin only in the gingival sulcus and not in the junctional epithelium or supracrestal connective tissue [11]. This was achieved before tooth preparation by probing the gingival sulcus with the calibrated dental probe and thus deciding the preparation depth. During the dental preparation, the depth was observed by preparing the abutment tooth with a calibrated bur (graduated into millimetres). During the interim stage, tissue inflammation was avoided by shortening the crown margins of the interim crown restorations if signs of inflammation (redness, bleeding) were detected, and the final impressions were taken only when the soft tissue appeared healthy and free from inflammation. In the vertical preparation, there is no dental finish line to refer to, and it is difficult for the dental technician to place the crown margin adequately. To avoid problems related to this, the crown margin of the definitive restoration was controlled during the clinical framework examination, and if necessary, was shortened. After the framework-soft tissue relationship was captured with an impression, the dental technician who was aware of the depth rechecked all of the crown margins before veneering.

Orthodontic treatment with a multidisciplinary approach would have been recommended as the primary treatment option for all of the clinical situations described in this study; however, in cases in which a patient is unable or unwilling to undergo preprosthetic orthodontic treatment, it is possible to instead use the BOPT with a POA to simulate multidisciplinary treatment [20–24]. This approach allowed only small reciprocal tooth movements and not really extensive range orthodontic outcomes. Previous studies describe how this technique is beneficial to obtain gingival modifications especially in the presence of gingival recessions [3, 17]. Indeed, the technique is prone to affect both the gingival thickness and the height of the keratinized gingiva [1–6, 17]. Our clinical outcomes resulted in gingival thickening with acquisition of an excellent pink and healthy gingiva, and the same protocol showed good clinical outcomes for dental implants [5, 6, 25]. Further studies, both clinical and histological, are needed to clarify what mechanisms underlie the biological conditioning of gingival tissues and their biotype.

4. Conclusion

In the present case report, the BOPT used with a POA effectively managed complicated cases without the need for preprosthetic orthodontic treatment. The absence of a finish line in natural abutment teeth offers many possibilities to clinicians for solving situations in which a multidisciplinary approach is usually required. After at least one year, none of the patients experienced prosthetic or periodontal complications; the gingival tissues were healthy, and the odontotomies did not affect the pulp survival of the vital teeth. Nevertheless, long-term clinical studies are needed to validate the results of these cases.

Acknowledgments

The author wishes to express his gratitude to Prof. Ignazio Loi for teaching the BOPT.

References

[1] I. Loi and A. Di Felice, "Biologically oriented preparation technique (BOPT): a new approach for prosthetic restoration of periodontically healthy teeth," *The European Journal of Esthetic Dentistry*, vol. 8, no. 1, pp. 10–23, 2013.

[2] R. Agustín-Panadero, M. F. Solá-Ruíz, C. Chust, A. Ferreiroa et al., "Fixed dental prostheses with vertical tooth preparations without finish lines: a report of two patients," *The Journal of Prosthetic Dentistry*, vol. 115, no. 5, pp. 520–526, 2016.

[3] B. Serra-Pastor, I. Loi, A. Fons-Font, M. F. Solá-Ruíz, R. Agustín-Panadero et al., "Periodontal and prosthetic outcomes on teeth prepared with biologically oriented preparation technique: a 4-year follow-up prospective clinical study," *Journal of Prosthodontic Research*, vol. 63, no. 4, pp. 415–420, 2019.

[4] R. Agustín-Panadero, B. Serra-Pastor, A. Fons-Font, M. F. Solá-Ruíz et al., "Prospective clinical study of zirconia full-coverage restorations on teeth prepared with biologically oriented preparation technique on gingival health: results after two-year follow-up," *Operative Dentistry*, vol. 43, no. 5, pp. 482–487, 2018.

[5] R. Agustín-Panadero, N. Bustamante-Hernández, M. F. Solá-Ruíz, Á. Zubizarreta-Macho, A. Fons-Font, L. Fernández-Estevan et al., "Influence of biologically oriented preparation technique on peri-implant tissues; prospective randomized clinical trial with three-year follow-up. Part I: hard tissues," *Journal of Clinical Medicine*, vol. 8, no. 12, p. 2183, 2019.

[6] R. Agustín-Panadero, N. Bustamante-Hernández, C. Labaig-Rueda, A. Fons-Font, L. Fernández-Estevan, and M. F. Solá-Ruíz, "Influence of biologically oriented preparation technique on peri-implant tissues; prospective randomized clinical trial with three-year follow-up. Part II: soft tissues," *Journal of Clinical Medicine*, vol. 8, no. 12, p. 2223, 2019.

[7] F. Vailati and S. Carciofo, "Treatment planning of adhesive additive rehabilitations: the progressive wax-up of the three-step technique," *International Journal of Esthetic Dentistry*, vol. 11, no. 3, pp. 356–377, 2016.

[8] J. Abduo, "Safety of increasing vertical dimension of occlusion: a systematic review," *Quintessence International*, vol. 43, no. 5, pp. 369–380, 2012.

[9] S. Patroni, G. Chiodera, C. Caliceti, and P. Ferrari, "CAD/-CAM technology and zirconium oxide with feather-edge marginal preparation," *The European Journal of Esthetic Dentistry*, vol. 5, no. 1, pp. 78–100, 2010.

[10] J. H. Schmitz, D. Cortellini, S. Granata, and M. Valenti, "Monolithic lithium disilicate complete single crowns with feather-edge preparation design in the posterior region: a multicentric retrospective study up to 12 years," *Quintessence International*, vol. 48, pp. 601–608, 2017.

[11] C. Ercoli and J. G. Caton, "Dental prostheses and tooth-related factors," *Journal of Periodontology*, vol. 89, pp. S223–S236, 2018.

[12] P. Goenka, N. Marwah, and S. Dutta, "A multidisciplinary approach to the management of a subgingivally fractured tooth: a clinical report," *Journal of Prosthodontics*, vol. 20, no. 3, pp. 218–223, 2011.

[13] E. Moslehifard, S. Nikzad, F. Geraminpanah, and F. Mahboub, "Full-mouth rehabilitation of a patient with severely worn dentition and uneven occlusal plane: a clinical report," *Journal of Prosthodontics*, vol. 21, no. 1, pp. 56–64, 2012.

[14] A. S. Bidra and F. Uribe, "Preprosthetic orthodontic intervention for management of a partially edentulous patient with generalized wear and malocclusion," *Journal of Esthetic and Restorative Dentistry*, vol. 24, no. 2, pp. 88–100, 2012.

[15] N. Şen and S. Işler, "Multidisciplinary management of a severe maxillary midline diastema: a clinical report," *Journal of Prosthodontics*, vol. 28, no. 3, pp. 239–243, 2019.

[16] L. Casula, A. Gillone, and D. Musu, "Correction of gingival architecture using the biologically oriented preparation technique in two patients with human immunodeficiency virus," *Case Reports in Dentistry*, vol. 2020, Article ID 8830949, 7 pages, 2020.

[17] C. J. Goodacre, W. V. Campagni, and S. A. Aquilino, "Tooth preparations for complete crowns: an art form based on scientific principles," *The Journal of Prosthetic Dentistry*, vol. 85, no. 4, pp. 363–376, 2001.

[18] G. M. Newcomb, "The relationship between the location of subgingival crown margins and gingival inflammation," *Journal of Periodontology*, vol. 45, no. 3, pp. 151–154, 1974.

[19] B. Reitemeier, K. Hänsel, M. H. Walter, C. Kastner, and H. Toutenburg, "Effect of posterior crown margin placement on gingival health," *The Journal of Prosthetic Dentistry*, vol. 87, no. 2, pp. 167–172, 2002.

[20] M. Wishney, "Potential risks of orthodontic therapy: a critical review and conceptual framework," *Australian Dental Journal*, vol. 62, pp. 86–96, 2017.

[21] J. Kim, S. Chu, G. Gürel, and G. Cisneros, "Restorative space management: treatment planning and clinical considerations for insufficient space," *Practical Procedures & Aesthetic Dentistry*, vol. 17, pp. 19–25, 2005.

[22] A.-M. Bollen, J. Cunha-Cruz, D. W. Bakko, G. J. Huang, and P. P. Hujoel, "The effects of orthodontic therapy on periodontal health: a systematic review of controlled evidence," *Journal of the American Dental Association (1939)*, vol. 139, no. 4, pp. 413–422, 2008.

[23] M. Baricevic, M. Mravak-Stipetic, M. Majstorovic, M. Baranovic, D. Baricevic, and B. Loncar, "Oral mucosal lesions during orthodontic treatment," *International Journal of Paediatric Dentistry*, vol. 21, no. 2, pp. 96–102, 2011.

[24] S. L. Walker, L. D. Tieu, and C. Flores-Mir, "Radiographic comparison of the extent of orthodontically induced external apical root resorption in vital and root-filled teeth: a systematic review," *European Journal of Orthodontics*, vol. 35, no. 6, pp. 796–802, 2013.

[25] L. Casula, A. Gillone, and D. Musu, "Peri-implant tissue adaptation after implant rehabilitation with shoulderless abutments with 24 months of follow-up," *Case Reports in Dentistry*, vol. 2021, Article ID 6689446, 8 pages, 2021.

5

Combined Orthodontic and Surgical Management for Treatment of Severe Class III Malocclusion with Anterior and Posterior Crossbites

Yahya A. Alogaibi,[1,2] Fahad F. Alsulaimani,[3] Basem Jamal,[4] and Rania Mitwally[5]

[1]*Orthodontist, Bisha Dental Center, Ministry of Health, P.O. Box 418, Bisha 61922, Saudi Arabia*
[2]*Orthodontics Resident, Department of Orthodontic, King Fahad Hospital, Specialized Dental Center, Madina, Saudi Arabia*
[3]*Consultant and Professor, Department of Orthodontics, Faculty of Dentistry, King Abdulaziz University, P.O. Box 80209, Jeddah 21589, Saudi Arabia*
[4]*Consultant and Associate Professor, Oral & Maxillofacial Surgery Department, King Abdulaziz University, Jeddah, Saudi Arabia*
[5]*North Dental Specialty Center, Orthodontic Department, Orthodontist, Ministry of Health, Jeddah, Saudi Arabia*

Correspondence should be addressed to Yahya A. Alogaibi; y1010@hotmail.com

Academic Editor: Andrea Scribante

Severe class III malocclusion can be a great challenge, especially in adult patients. This case report describes an adult patient with severe skeletal class III malocclusion and with an obvious maxillary deficiency and mandibular excess causing both anterior and posterior crossbites in addition to a shift in the upper and lower midlines to the left concerning the facial midline. This was complicated by compensatory mechanisms such as the proclination of upper incisors and retroclination of lower incisors. Decompensation of the upper and lower arches was performed combined with upper arch expansion to relieve crowding in the upper arch and correct the posterior crossbite. This was followed by double jaw surgeries, including Le Fort I osteotomy in the maxilla and bilateral sagittal split osteotomy (BSSO) in the mandible. Orthodontic finishing procedures were then used to correct any other dental discrepancies. Remarkable esthetic and functional results were achieved with high patient satisfaction.

1. Introduction

Skeletal class III malocclusion is considered to be one of the most difficult cases to treat especially if a severe form is found in adult patients. The deformity was found to be caused by class III malocclusion, which is not always restricted to the dental arches and may involve the total craniofacial complex, and the etiology of this malocclusion is mainly influenced by genetic factors [1]. Most of the patients with class III malocclusions show a combination of both skeletal and dento-alveolar components. These components may act synergistically or in isolation to increase or decrease the severity of the condition [2].

There are three available treatment options for management of skeletal class III malocclusions. These are modification of growth, orthodontic camouflage treatment, or combination of orthodontic treatment and orthognathic surgery. Modification of growth by utilizing orthopedic appliances is only effective for treatment of skeletal class III discrepancies in growing patients [3]. Camouflage orthodontic therapy can be considered to correct mild skeletal class III patients with acceptable profiles. However, management of this problem in adult patients will usually require considering the option of orthognathic surgery, especially if the problem was severe [4, 5].

In severe adult cases with class III malocclusion, a combination of both orthodontic treatment and orthognathic surgery is usually needed to achieve a proper outcome. However, the skeletal type of class III malocclusion usually affects the type of surgery. It was found that 43% of class III cases had only mandibular prognathism with a normal-sized maxilla, while 19.6% had a normal-sized mandible with deficiency and retrognathism of the maxilla, and the smallest

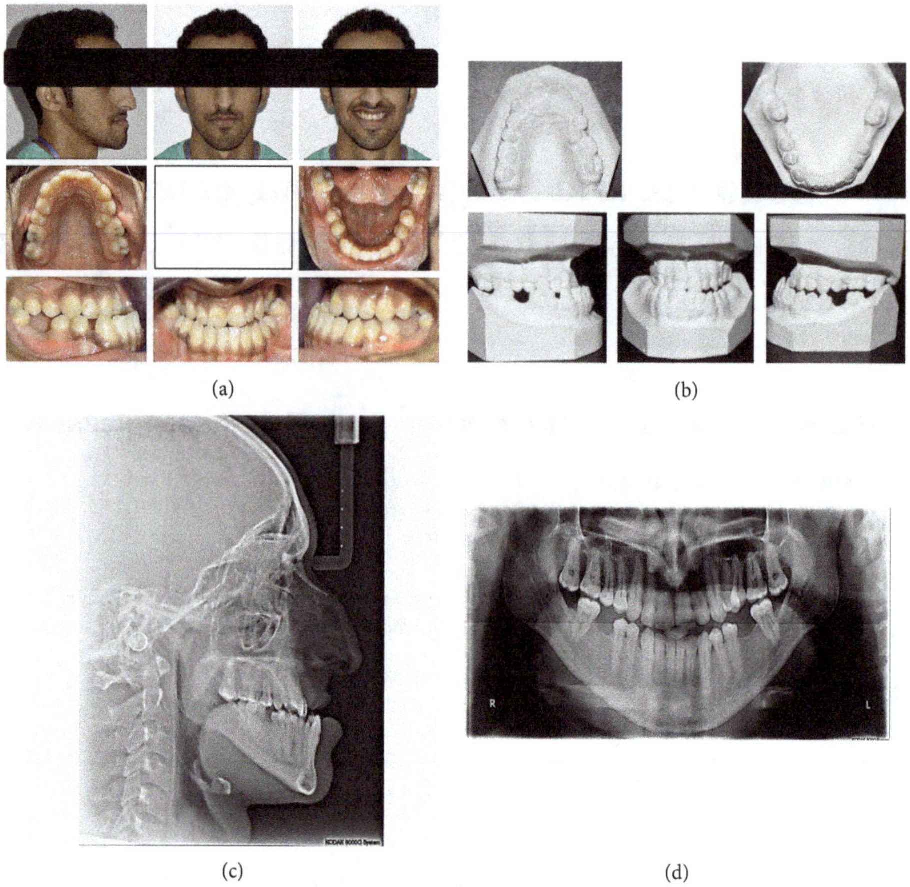

FIGURE 1: Pretreatment extraoral and intraoral photographs, study models cephalometric radiograph, and panoramic radiographs of the patient: (a) extraoral and intraoral photographs; (b) study models; (c) cephalometric radiograph; (d) panoramic radiograph.

percentage (<5%) had both maxillary deficiency and mandibular excess [6].

Surgical intervention in severe class III cases usually involves either maxillary advancement or mandibular setback. These procedures can be performed alone or in combination according to the case severity. Le Fort I osteotomy and/or bilateral sagittal split osteotomy (BSSO) are the most commonly used surgical procedures to treat severe class III malocclusion. In cases requiring orthognathic surgery, a proper treatment plan is required to achieve a good outcome for the treatment together with accurate identification of the patient's expectations [4, 7].

In this case report, we describe treatment of an adult patient with a severe skeletal class III malocclusion using a combination of orthodontic treatment and orthognathic surgery, and orthodontic expansion of the upper arch was performed followed by Le Fort I osteotomy and BSSO to correct this severe malocclusion.

2. Diagnosis

A 31-year-old male patient presented to the orthodontic clinic with a prominent lower jaw. Intraoral examination showed that his oral hygiene was fair, and his teeth showed areas of plaque accumulation and staining. The patient had a history of lower first molar extraction. Facial examination showed that the patient had the typical concave profile of skeletal class III with an increased mandibular plane angle and normal TMJ function. Additionally, intraoral examination revealed a shift in the upper midline to the left by 1.5 mm and a shift to the left of 3 mm in the lower midline in relation to the facial midline. The upper and lower arch relationship showed class III canines on both sides, anterior crossbite with a reverse overjet of −6 mm, and a bilateral posterior cross bite (Figures 1(a) and 1(b)).

Cephalometric analysis for this patient, as shown in Table 1, revealed some anteroposterior skeletal abnormalities including a skeletal class III jaw relationship that was caused by both maxillary deficiency and mandibular excess. Additionally, a normal anterior vertical relationship was found with decreased posterior facial height causing some degree of steepness in the mandibular plane angle. The upper dental arch showed crowding with a palatally erupted upper left second premolar. Upper and lower incisors showed compensatory mechanisms with mild proclination of the upper incisors and moderate retroclination of the lower incisors. Soft tissue analysis revealed the classical appearance of severe class III malocclusion with a retruded upper lip and protruded lower lip (Figure 1(c)). A panoramic radiograph showed condyles that were symmetrical in size and shape without any obvious pathology and missing lower first and third molars (Figure 1(d)).

Table 1: Cephalometric analysis.

	Measurement	Mean (±Sd)	Patient Initial	Patient Final
Ant-posterior	SNA (°)	82° (±3.3)	76.2	80
	SNB (°)	80° (±3.1)	82.1	79
	ANB (°)	2° (±1.7)	-5.9	1
	Wits (mm)	$M = -1.17$ (±1.9) $F = -0.10$ (±1.77)	-16.1 mm	-2
	Angle of convexity NA-APg (°)	0° (±5.1)	-11	-1
	A-B plane AB : NPg (°)	-4.6° (±3.7)	10	-2
Vertical	MP (Go-Gn) : SN (°)	32° (±3.5)	44	43
	MP (tangent lower border) : FH (°)	21.9° (±3.2)	31	31
	Pg : NB (mm)	4 (±2)	-1.5 mm	3.6 mm
	Y-axis (SGn : FH)	59.4° (±3.8)	69	70
	LAFH (ANS to Gn ÷ N to Gn)	.57 (±0.02)	56%	56
	OP : SN (°)	14° (±4.1)	21.8	21.1
Dental	U1 to palatal plane (°)	109° (±6)	102.6	105.9
	U1 to NA (°)	22° (±6.1)	26.4	27.2
	U1 to NA (mm)	4 (±1.2)	5 mm	6 mm
	L1 to NB (°)	25° (±4.5)	15.1	15.1
	L1 to NB (mm)	4 (±1.5)	2 mm	3 mm
	U1 to L1 (°) (Avg. Downs and Steiner)	131.7° (±6.5)	144	137
	L1 : APg (mm)	1 (±2)	7 mm	1 mm
	FMA (°)	25° (16-35)	31	31
	FMIA (°)	65° (60-75)	80	75
	IMPA (°)	90° (85-95)	69	74
Soft tissue	Facial angle (FH : N'Pg') (°)	90-92°	94	92
	Nasolabial angle (°)	90-110°	113	88
	Esthetic plane (E-line)–upper lip	-4 mm	-13 mm	-6 mm
	Esthetic plane (E-line)–lower lip	-2 mm	0 mm	-3 mm

3. Treatment

3.1. Treatment Objectives. The proposed treatment objectives were to reinforce and improve oral hygiene, improve the lip position, surgically advance the maxillary basal bone, surgically set back the mandibular basal bone, expand the maxillary arch, correct the anterior and posterior crossbites, correct the midline shifts in the upper and lower jaw, and achieve class I molar and canine relationships and suitable prosthesis for the missing teeth.

3.2. Treatment Plan. Surgical and nonsurgical treatment options were discussed with the patient. The nonsurgical approach was based on orthodontic camouflage by extraction of lower premolars followed by retraction with miniscrews combined with upper arch expansion.

Another treatment option was orthodontic decompensation with upper arch expansion followed by double jaw surgery including Le Fort I osteotomy in the maxilla and BSSO in the mandible.

After discussing these treatment alternatives with the patient and explaining the advantages and disadvantages of each option, taking into account both esthetic and functional demands, the second option for treatment was approved.

3.3. Treatment Progress. The treatment was initiated by banding the upper and lower molars together by bonding the other teeth using preadjusted 0.022 × 0.030 inch edgewise Roth prescription brackets. A quad helix was inserted to expand the upper arch. Leveling and alignment to decompensate the upper and lower arches was performed using a progressive increase in wire thickness in the upper and lower arches with Ni-Ti arch wires with bend-back in the lower arch, starting with 0.014″ and reaching 0.019 × 0.025″ (Figures 2(a) and 2(b)).

Open coil springs were inserted into the space from the extracted lower first molars to close the spacing anteriorly and to orient the lower second molars in an upright manner. Rigid stainless steel wires (0.019 × 0.025″) were used to prepare the patient for surgery. BSSO was performed in the mandible with a setback of 6.9 mm. This was combined with Le Fort I osteotomy in the maxilla with an advancement of 8.5 mm. The patient had also undergone a rhinoplasty procedure 2 months before the orthognathic surgery.

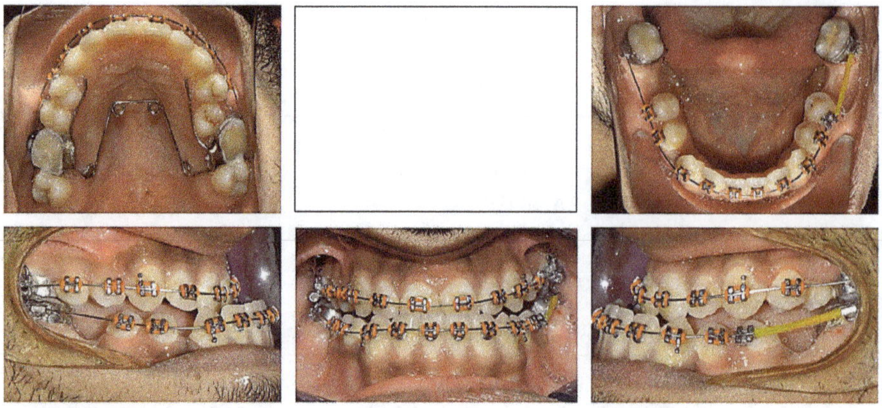

(a)

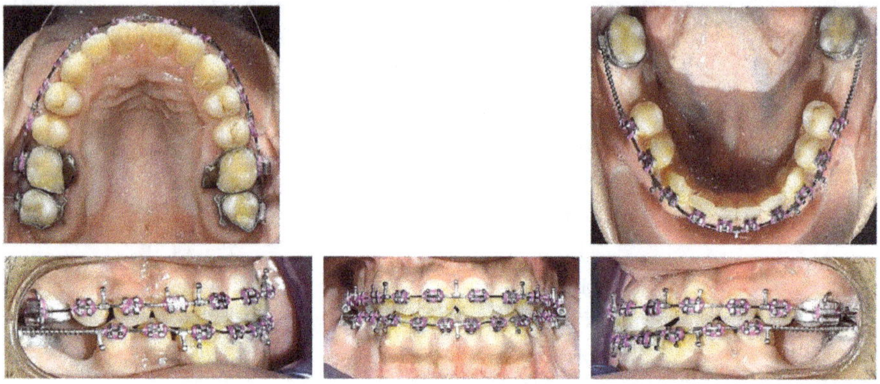

(b)

FIGURE 2: (a, b) Multiple progress photographs.

After surgery, finishing procedures were performed to obtain better interdigitation between the teeth. Vertical elastics were applied for 20 hours/day, and they were then reduced gradually until stable occlusal contacts were achieved. A maxillary wrap-around retainer and a fixed canine-to-canine with a wrap-around mandibular retainer were placed. Total treatment time was 2 years and 7 months.

3.4. Treatment Results. The extraoral posttreatment photographs showed marked improvement in the facial profile. Chin position was set backward, and the naso-labial angle was decreased to the normal values. The buccal corridors during smiling were reduced with pleasing smile characteristics. The midline shifts in both the upper and lower jaws were corrected together with class I skeletal and dental relationships. Both the posterior and anterior crossbites were eliminated, and normal overjet and overbite were reached (Figures 3(a) and 3(b)).

The cephalometric analysis showed favorable skeletal and dental changes in anteroposterior measurements with minimal changes in vertical proportions. All the teeth showed a normal level of bone with no evidence of root resorption when examined in the panoramic radiograph (Table 1; Figures 3(c)–3(e)).

4. Discussion

Combined orthodontic and orthognathic surgical treatment may be required in some cases to achieve the required esthetic and functional results [8]. If there is any skeletal problem that is beyond the limits of camouflage treatment according to the envelope of discrepancy, any trial on dental compensation may reach a reasonably acceptable occlusion using miniscrews as methods of absolute anchorage. However, this requires compromising facial aesthetics because it is not possible to achieve satisfactory facial esthetics using this method. This approach is no longer accepted in modern orthodontics because facial esthetics should never be compromised to reach ideal occlusion [9, 10].

This was why the orthognathic surgical treatment approach was chosen over the camouflage method. Additionally, it is well known that when starting a camouflage treatment approach, it is nearly impossible to go back to a surgical option of treatment using orthognathic surgery because both options are opposite to each other regarding teeth movements and extraction choices. Moreover, surgical correction of skeletal class III malocclusion after combined maxillary and mandibular strategies shows up to be stable for maxillary advancements up to 5 mm and for the correction of presurgical sagittal intermaxillary discrepancies smaller than 7 mm [2, 5, 11, 12].

Orthodontic expansion of the upper arch was performed because the amount of crowding and maxillary constriction was not severe. Although the bilateral posterior crossbite was obvious, this crossbite was partially caused by the backward position of the maxilla and the forward position of

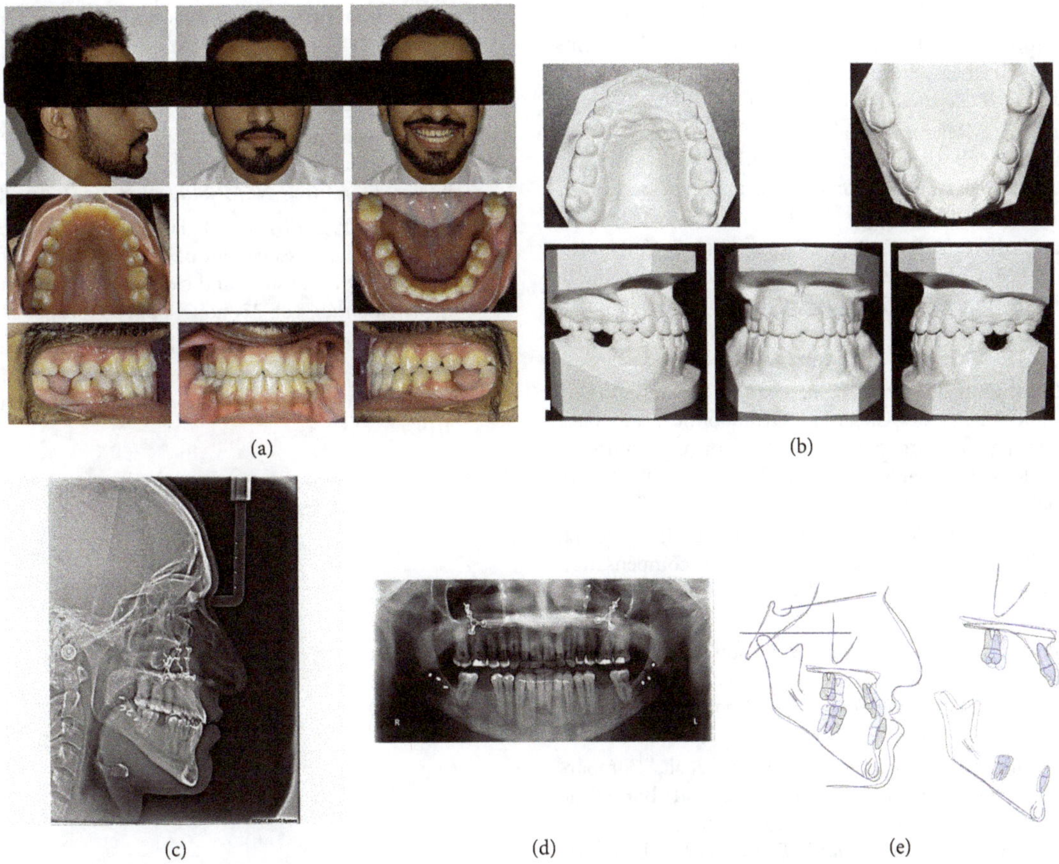

FIGURE 3: Posttreatment extraoral and intraoral photographs, study models cephalometric radiograph, and panoramic radiographs of the patient: (a) extraoral and intraoral photographs; (b) study models; (c) cephalometric radiograph; (d) panoramic radiograph; (e) cephalometric superimposition.

the mandible, which caused a wider molar area of the mandible to be occluded with the narrower premolar area of the maxilla, which suggests a severe maxillary deficiency. Moreover, by calculation of the needed space to relieve the crowding in the upper arch [13, 14], we found that expanding the upper arch from both the intercanine and intermolar area was sufficient to relieve the crowding without requiring extraction.

The most suitable appliance that was found to achieve a differential expansion at the intercanine and intermolar area was the quad helix. Quad helix was selected as an effective expansion method for this patient because of its ability to deliver a constant physiologic force to achieve the required expansion and prevent buildup of excessive forces on the maxillary complex [15, 16].

Surgically assisted rapid maxillary expansion was another option for expanding the upper arch, which has the ability to produce more skeletal expansion in adult patients with a completely fused midpalatal suture. However, root resorption and possible trauma to the condyles was reported in some cases that used this expansion technique. A significant amount of relapse was also reported [17, 18].

Finally, the rationale for selecting an upper wraparound retainer was based on its ability to maintain the achieved transverse correction by expansion. However, fixed canine-to-canine with a wraparound mandibular retainer was used to retain the incisor position and to prevent loss of the space from the extracted first molars [19, 20].

5. Conclusion

Severe skeletal class III malocclusion cases can sometimes be impossible to handle with orthodontic treatment alone, especially in adult patients, because orthodontic camouflage can produce less than optimal results with inadequate patient satisfaction. Orthognathic surgery may be the only reliable and evidence-based approach to achieve stable esthetic results. However, applying conservative orthodontic solutions to relieve crowding with an effective decompensation of the arches should be considered as a first choice during treatment planning. This conservative approach can reduce the treatment time and minimize the possibility of patient burnout during the course of treatment.

References

[1] C. Szuhanek, S. Dumitrescu, E. Paraschivescu, and R. Nagib, "Interdisciplinary orthodontic and surgical management of class III malocclusion in adult patients," *Journal of Dentistry And Oral Implants*, vol. 2, no. 3, pp. 1–6, 2019.

[2] S. Eslami, A. Fateh, F. Sheikholaemmeh, V. Grassia, A. Jamilian, and J. Faber, "Treatment decision in adult patients with class III malocclusion: surgery versus orthodontics," *Progress in Orthodontics*, vol. 19, no. 1, p. 28, 2018.

[3] H. Behnia, H. Mohammad-Rahimi, and M. Behnaz, "Treatment of an adult skeletal class III patient with surgically assisted rapid palatal expansion and facemask," *Case Reports in Dentistry*, vol. 2019, 6 pages, 2019.

[4] D. A. A. Marlière, T. E. Costa, S. . M. Barbosa, R. A. Pereira, and H. D. . M. Chaves Netto, "Alteration of occlusal plane in orthognathic surgery: clinical features to help treatment planning on class III patients," *Case Reports in Dentistry*, vol. 2018, 9 pages, 2018.

[5] P. Martinez, C. Bellot-Arcís, J. M. Llamas, R. Cibrian, J. L. Gandia, and V. Paredes-Gallardo, "Orthodontic camouflage versus orthognathic surgery for class III deformity: comparative cephalometric analysis," *International Journal of Oral and Maxillofacial Surgery*, vol. 46, no. 4, pp. 490–495, 2017.

[6] S. Spalj, S. Mestrovic, M. Lapter Varga, and M. Slaj, "Skeletal components of class III malocclusions and compensation mechanisms," *Journal of Oral Rehabilitation*, vol. 35, no. 8, pp. 629–637, 2008.

[7] B. A. Furquim, K. M. de Freitas, G. Janson, L. F. Simoneti, M. R. de Freitas, and D. S. de Freitas, "Class III malocclusion surgical-orthodontic treatment," *Case Reports in Dentistry*, vol. 2014, pp. 9–75, 2014.

[8] J. H. M. Watanabe, F. Fitarelli, D.-S. de Freitas et al., "Comparison of the facial profile attractiveness in class III borderline patients after surgical or compensatory orthodontic treatment," *Journal of Clinical and Experimental Dentistry*, vol. 12, no. 4, article e348, 2020.

[9] V. Krishnan, "Orthodontics: newer challenges, modern solutions," *Journal of the World Federation of Orthodontists*, vol. 6, no. 4, p. 141, 2017.

[10] K. Klaus, T. S. P. Serbesis, H. Pancherz, S. Ruf, and P. Stark, "Excellent versus unacceptable orthodontic results: influencing factors," *European Journal of Orthodontics*, vol. 39, no. 6, pp. 615–621, 2017.

[11] Z. Hakami, P. J. Chen, A. Ahmida, N. Janakiraman, and F. Uribe, "Miniplate-aided mandibular dentition distalization as a camouflage treatment of a class III malocclusion in an adult," *Case Reports in Dentistry*, vol. 2018, 9 pages, 2018.

[12] M. Mucedero, A. Coviello, T. Baccetti, L. Franchi, and P. Cozza, "Stability factors after double-jaw surgery in class III malocclusion. A systematic review," *The Angle Orthodontist*, vol. 78, no. 6, pp. 1141–1152, 2008.

[13] N. Germane, L. K. Rubenstein, J. H. Revere Jr., R. J. Isaacson, and S. J. Lindauer, "Increase in arch perimeter due to orthodontic expansion," *American Journal of Orthodontics and Dentofacial Orthopedics*, vol. 100, no. 5, pp. 421–427, 1991.

[14] C. A. Claro, J. Abrão, S. A. B. Reis, and S. M. . Fantini, "Correlation between transverse expansion and increase in the upper arch perimeter after rapid maxillary expansion," *Brazilian Oral Research*, vol. 20, no. 1, pp. 76–81, 2006.

[15] R. Njie, *Skeletal, Dental, and Nasal Airway Changes after Treatment with Quad-Helix Appliance as Evaluated by CBCT*, Medical Sciences-Dentistry, 2019.

[16] M. Fouda, A. Hafez, and H. Shoaib, "Effect of quad helix appliance on maxillary constriction (holdway measurements)," *Indian Journal of Orthodontics and Dentofacial Research*, vol. 3, no. 3, pp. 172–175, 2017.

[17] N. Taylor and P. Johnson, "Surgically assisted rapid maxillary expansion," in *Orthognathic Surgery: Principles, Planning and Practice, First Edition*, pp. 620–629, John Wiley & Sons Ltd., 2016.

[18] R. Olszewski and M. Wisniewski, "Complications in surgically assisted rapid maxillary expansion: a systematic review of the medical literature," *NEMESIS*, vol. 8, no. 1, pp. 20–20, 2019.

[19] J. R. Lustig, P. E. Rossouw, P. H. Buschang, R. G. Behrents, and R. D. Woody, "Assessment of post-orthodontic occlusal contacts with wrap-around and clear overlay retainers," *Seminars in Orthodontics*, vol. 23, no. 2, pp. 166–177, 2017.

[20] A. Malandkar, N. G. Toshniwal, N. Mote, S. Das, and N. Singh, "An Overview of Current Trends in Retention," *International Journal of Applied Dental Sciences*, vol. 5, no. 3, pp. 240–245, 2019.

6

Nonsurgical Orthodontic Intervention of a Severe Class II Case Accompanied by Posterior Crossbite using a Miniscrew-Assisted Straight Wire Technique

Abdulkarim A. Hatrom,[1] **Ahmed R. Afify**,[2,3] **and Ali H. Hassan**[2,4]

[1]*Ministry of Health, Makkah, Saudi Arabia. P.O. Box 4137, Makkah 24359, Saudi Arabia*
[2]*Orthodontic Department, Faculty of Dentistry, King Abdulaziz University, P.O. Box 80209, Jeddah 21589, Saudi Arabia*
[3]*Orthodontic Department, Faculty of Dentistry, Mansoura University, Mansoura, Egypt*
[4]*Alfarabi Private College for Dentistry and Nursing, P.O. Box 23643, Jeddah 21589, Saudi Arabia*

Correspondence should be addressed to Abdulkarim A. Hatrom; dr.hatrom@gmail.com

Academic Editor: Giuseppe Alessandro Scardina

Class II malocclusion in nongrowing patients is a great challenge in treatment especially if the degree of malocclusion is severe. In such cases, the use of miniscrews for orthodontic camouflage can produce results comparable to that of orthognathic surgery. This case report presents an adult patient with severe Class II malocclusion combined with bilateral posterior crossbite, deep bite, a crowded lower arch, and a history of extraction of the lower right first molar. The treatment involved upper arch expansion by a quad helix appliance followed by the extraction of the right and left upper 1st premolars. A miniscrew-assisted straight wire technique was used to close the extraction space and reduce the overjet. Lower molar protraction was done to close the previous extraction space in the lower arch. At the end of treatment, overjet was reduced, lower arch crowding was relieved, lip competency was established, and the wide buccal corridor was reduced with a pleasing smile and normal facial proportions.

1. Introduction

Patients suffering from Class II malocclusion are usually affected by their problems which make them the most common cases that seek orthodontic treatment [1]. Angle Class II Division 1 is usually characterized by maxillary protrusion and/or mandibular retrusion. This is usually accompanied by protrusion of the upper anterior teeth, narrow upper arch, and incompetent upper lip [1, 2]. The presence of such problems in adult patients is challenging because these patients usually have high expectations regarding the results of treatment [3].

In nongrowing patients, this malocclusion can only be treated by one of two methods; orthodontic camouflage which usually involves the extraction of two upper premolars [4] or even upper and lower premolars or orthognathic surgery to reposition the mandible and/or the maxilla in a normal position. It was shown that patient satisfaction and perception of outcome with camouflage treatment are nearly the same to those achieved by orthognathic surgery and that orthodontic camouflage showed fewer functional and temporomandibular joint problems [5].

With the recent advancement in anchorage devices and the introduction of miniscrews in orthodontics, orthognathic-like results can be achieved by utilizing such devices [6]. In patients with Class II malocclusion, it was shown that a maxillary incisors retraction of 8.2-9.3 mm can be achieved by using miniscrews [7, 8].

The following case had severe Class II malocclusion with bilateral posterior crossbite, deep bite, a crowded lower arch, and a history of extraction of the lower right first molar which was managed by orthodontic camouflage instead of orthognathic surgery.

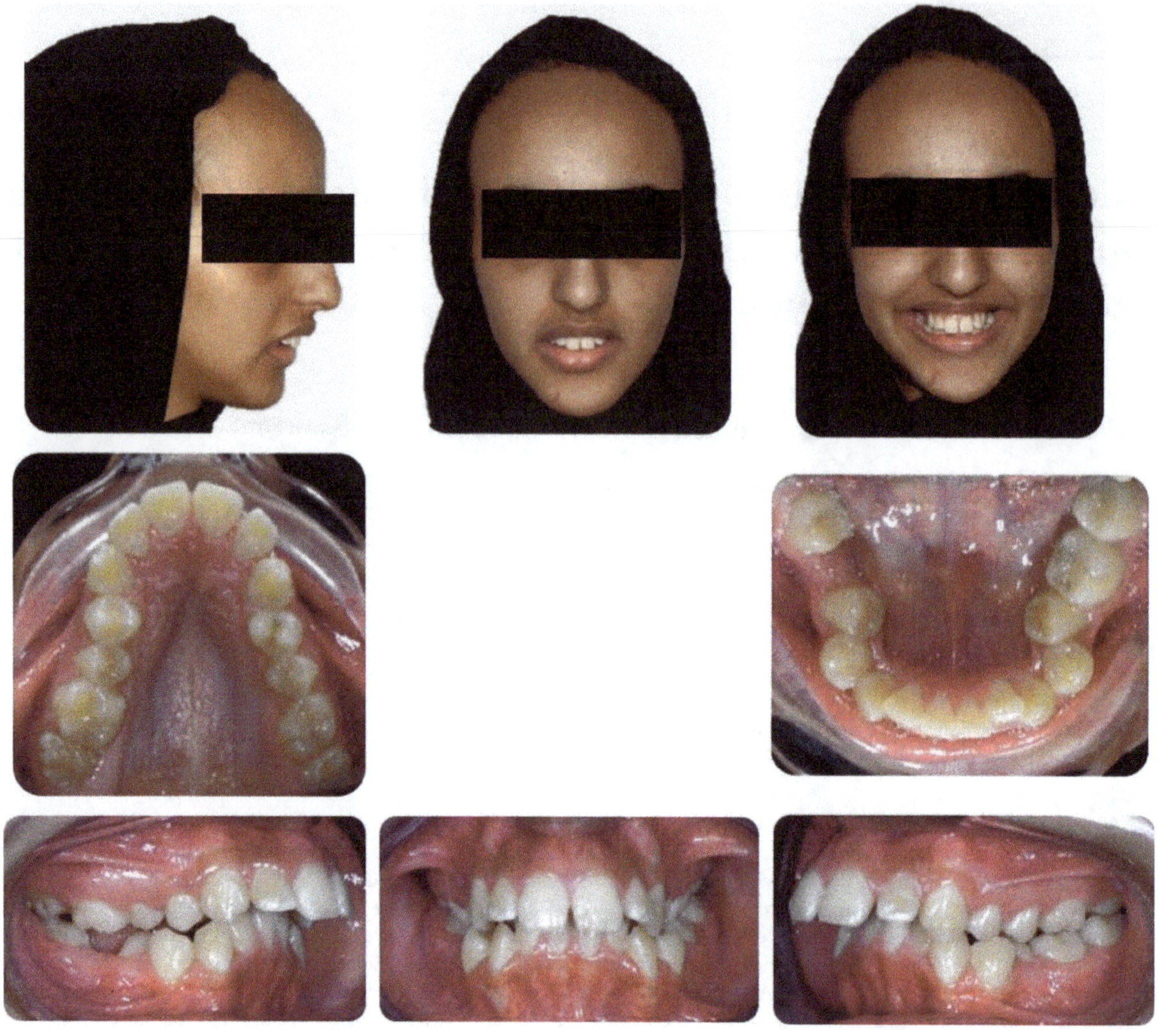

Figure 1: Pretreatment extraoral and intraoral photographs of the patient.

2. Diagnosis and Treatment Planning

A female patient aged 18 years presented to the Orthodontic Department of King Abdulaziz University with a chief complaint of sticking out front teeth. She had no significant medical history while her dental history showed extraction of the lower right first molar 1 year ago. Clinical extraoral examination showed a dolichocephalic facial type, convex profile with proclined upper incisors, and incompetent lips. Intraoral examination revealed Class II malocclusion with bilateral posterior crossbite, deep bite, and increased overjet. Both the upper and lower arches were narrow while the lower arch showed a moderate amount of crowding. Smile analysis showed that she had a very wide buccal corridor due to narrow arches and slight gingival display which is acceptable at this age (Figures 1 and 2).

Cephalometric analysis revealed a Class II skeletal relationship (ANB angle = 6.4°) and a steep mandibular plane angle (36.2°). Regarding dental measurement, it was found that she had proclined upper incisors (U1-PP = 116.6°) and retroclined lower incisors (L1-MP = 82°) (Figure 3).

A panoramic radiograph revealed a missing lower right first molar, an upper left first molar, and no sign of root resorption. The upper and lower third molars were still in the stages of root formation. No caries or periapical lesion was seen (Figure 3).

2.1. Treatment Objectives. In order to obtain a well-balanced facial esthetics, adequate smile parameters and good stable occlusion of the following treatment objectives were planned: (1) correcting the proclination of the upper incisors which in turn will reestablish the correct position of the relatively short and incompetent upper lip, (2) widening the upper arch to close the wide buccal corridor and enhance the smile esthetics, and (3) closing the extraction space of the lower right first molar to establish a stable occlusion.

2.2. Treatment Plan. First, it is necessary to expand the upper arch preferably by utilizing quad helix. Then, extraction of the upper right and left first premolars after completion of arch expansion and alignment of teeth was done. Protraction of lower right second molar was done to close the space of the

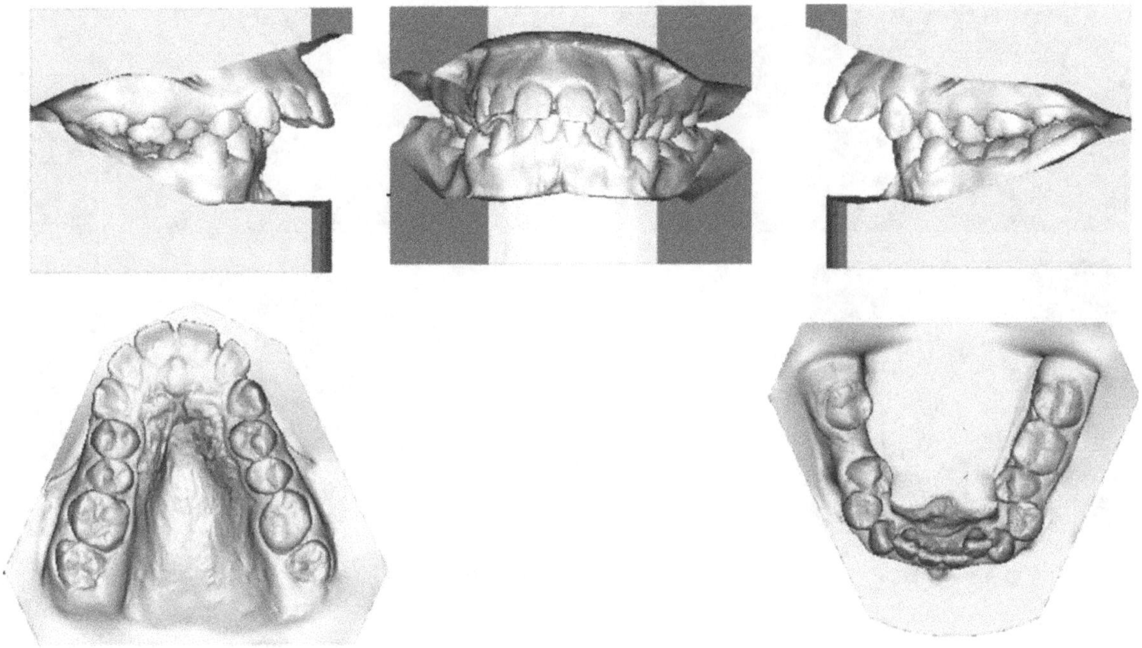

FIGURE 2: Pretreatment models.

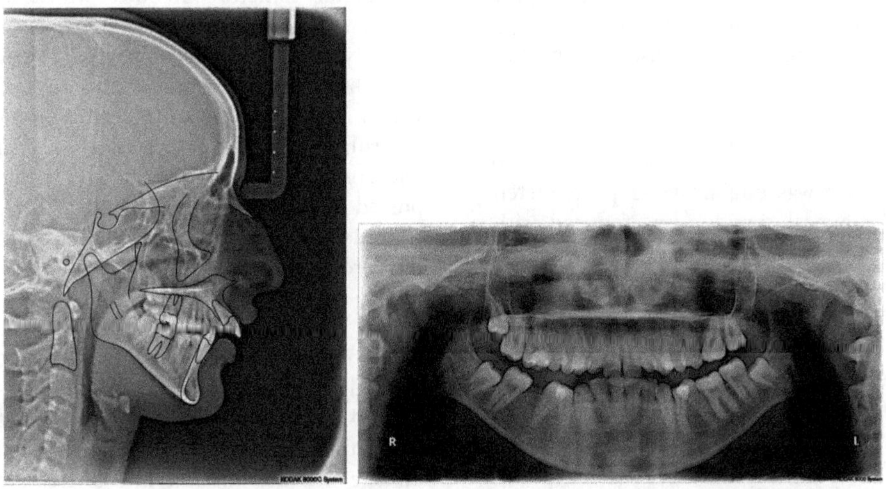

FIGURE 3: Pretreatment cephalometric and panoramic radiograph.

lower right first molar and allow the eruption of the third molar in its place. And finally, upper removable wraparound retainers and lower fixed retainer were used to retain the established results.

2.3. Treatment Progress. The treatment was initiated with a banding and bonding procedure using modified bidimensional preadjusted edgewise brackets, 0.018-inch slots in the incisors and canines, and 0.022-inch slots in the premolars and molars (3M Unitek, Monrovia, CA, USA). Roth prescription was combined with cementation of the quad helix appliance. Leveling and alignment were achieved with a straight wire technique which was used in the following sequence: 0.012″ Niti, 0.014″ Niti, 0.016″ Niti, and 0.016 × 0.025″ Niti followed by 0.018 × 0.022″ SS wire.

After finishing arch expansion in the upper arch, extraction of the upper right and left 1st premolars was done. Under local anesthesia, insertion of two miniscrews 1.6 mm in diameter and 8 mm in length (3 M Unitek, Monrovia, CA, USA) between the upper 2nd premolar and the first molar on both sides was done. An en-masse anterior tooth retraction by using a nickel-titanium closed coil spring with a force value of 250 gram force was performed on each side, and the nickel-titanium closed coil spring was attached to a power arm 5 mm in length positioned mesial to the canine. A rigid stainless steel wire (0.018 × 0.022″) was inserted during retraction. The force was repeated every 3 weeks until the overjet was reduced, and extraction spaces were completely closed. Finishing was done utilizing intermaxillary elastics until

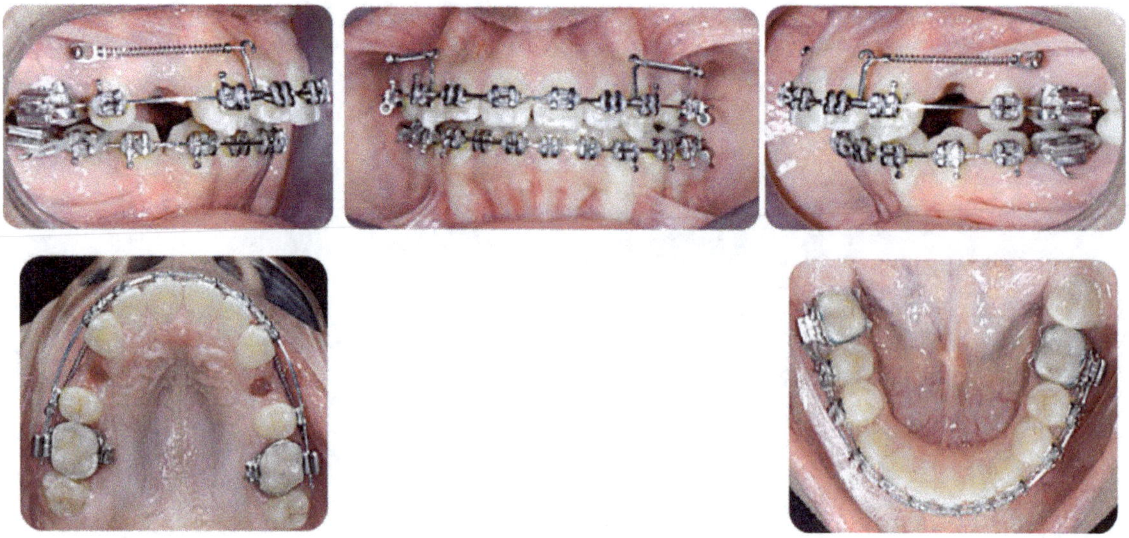

FIGURE 4: Progress photographs.

satisfactory functional and static occlusion were achieved. Active treatment time was 28 months, and the patient was instructed to wear the acrylic retainer in the upper arch, and a fixed bonded retainer was used in the lower arch (Figure 4).

2.4. Treatment Results. Amazing enhancement in both facial and smile esthetics was established. Lip competency was reached, and the buccal corridor was reduced with a pleasing smile and normal facial proportions (Figures 5 and 6). Regarding cephalometric analysis, mainly dental changes were observed after the end of treatment. Upper incisors became more retroclined (U1-PP = 93°) while the lower incisors became more proclined (L1-MP = 95°) making all the dental measurements within the normal range. The surrounding bone and periodontal tissues were found to be healthy during and after the treatment without any evidence pocket formation or bone loss. The teeth remained caries free with no signs of root resorption when viewed on the panoramic radiograph (Figures 7 and 8).

3. Discussion

Adult patients with severe Class II malocclusion may be treated by camouflage or a combination of orthodontic and orthognathic surgeries depending on the severity of malocclusion [9]. The main goal of treatment by orthodontic camouflage is to mask the marked skeletal discrepancy by dental compensations. In Class II malocclusion when extractions are needed, they are usually done in the maxillary first premolars to correct the proclination of the upper incisors [5]. This is usually followed by en-masse retraction of the upper incisor with absolute or maximum anchorage to close the extraction space and reduce overjet. This will lead to flattening of the nasolabial angle improvement lip position [10].

However, it was suggested that orthognathic surgery has better esthetic outcomes which are observed in the marked improvement of the soft tissue profile and high stability or the results obtained [11]. On the other hand, other studies proved that the amount of incisor retractions which are depending on the type of anchorage used is the determining factor for the resultant changes in lip position and soft tissue profile [4, 12]. This opinion was also supported with a study by Mihalik et al. that showed that orthodontic camouflage by extraction of the upper premolars produced stable results comparable to that of orthognathic surgery [5].

Orthognathic surgery is barely accepted by patients for many reasons such as high cost, risk of infection, fear of general anesthesia, and the risk of this invasive procedure [13, 14]. This patient refused orthognathic surgery due to all of the abovementioned reasons, and orthodontic camouflage was the possible line of treatment.

In this case, the expansion of the upper arch was done utilizing the quad helix appliance to gain more space and to close the wide buccal corridor seen during smiling. The choice of the quad helix appliance was due to its effect in decreasing the mandibular plane angle in hyperdivergent patients [15].

The extraction of the upper right and left first premolars was done to allow for the retraction of the proclined upper incisors and to reduce the overjet with concomitant restoration of lip competency. This was done by using miniscrews with en-masse anterior tooth retraction utilizing nickel-titanium closed coil springs on each side with a force value of 150 gram force as recommended by Upadhyay et al. [16]. The power chain was attached to a power arm 5 mm in length positioned mesial to the canine to apply the force directly at the center of resistance and to avoid tipping [17]. A rigid stainless steel wire ($0.018 \times 0.022''$) was utilized to control the torque of incisors during retraction.

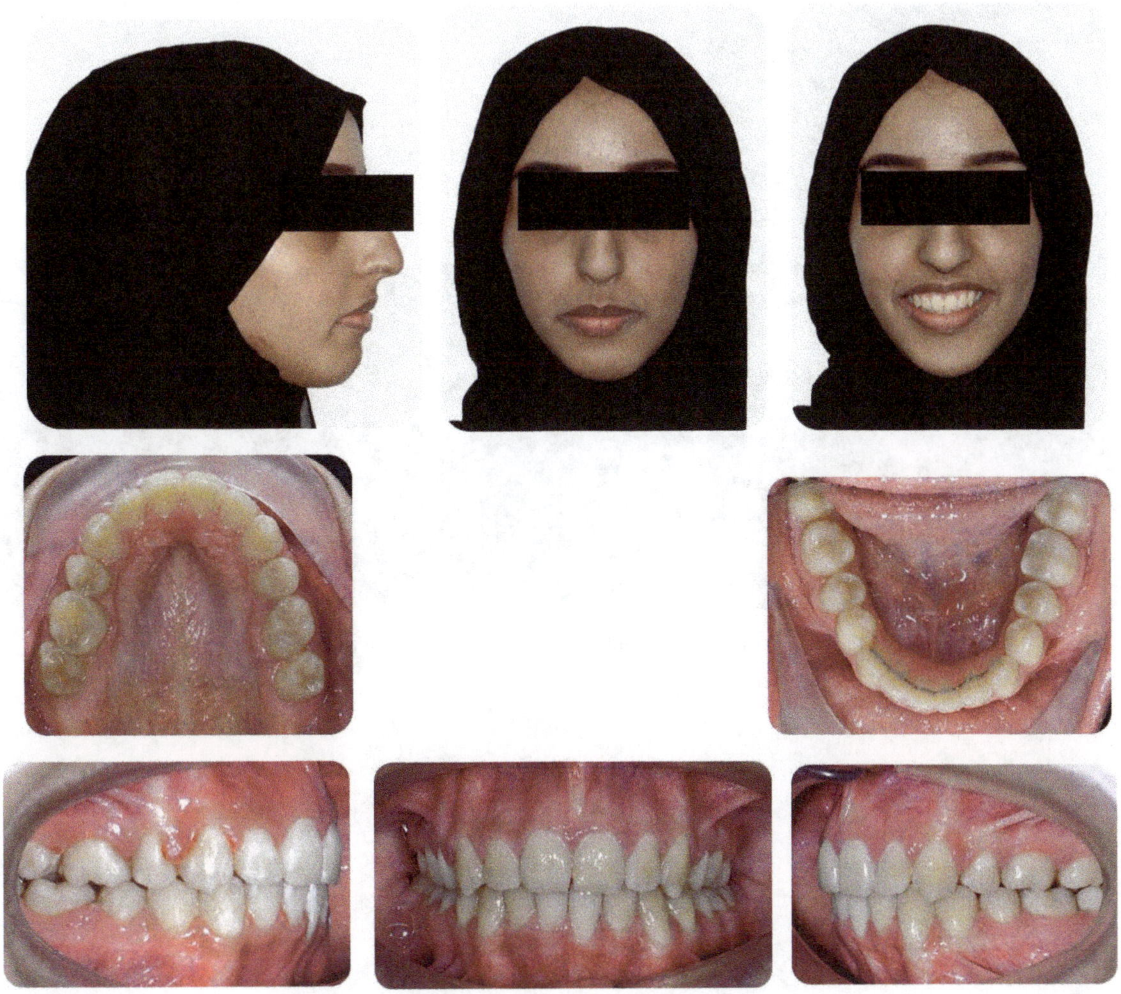

FIGURE 5: Posttreatment photographs of the patient.

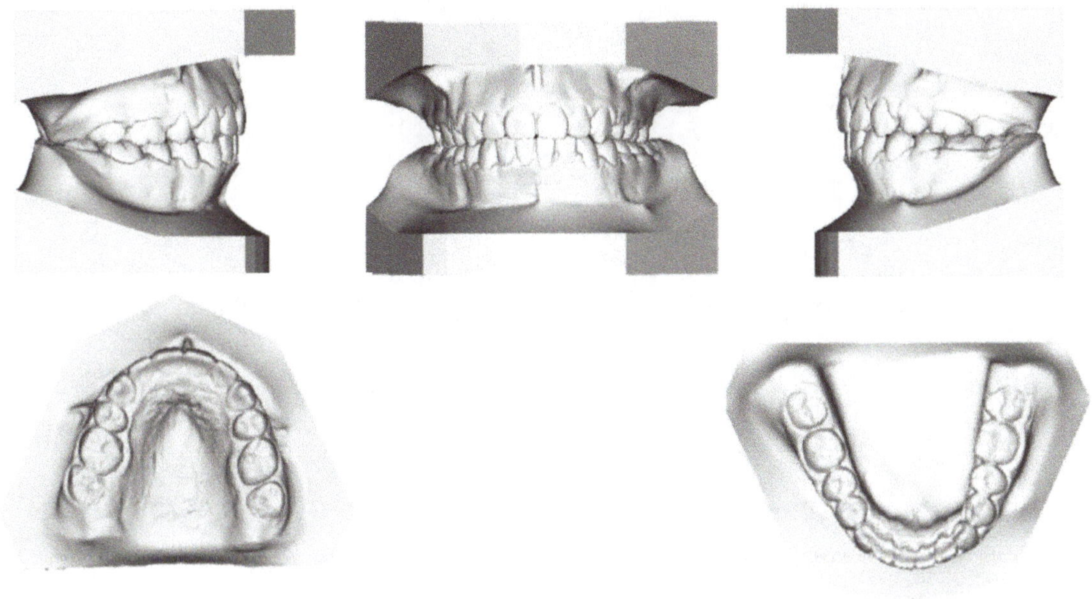

FIGURE 6: Posttreatment models.

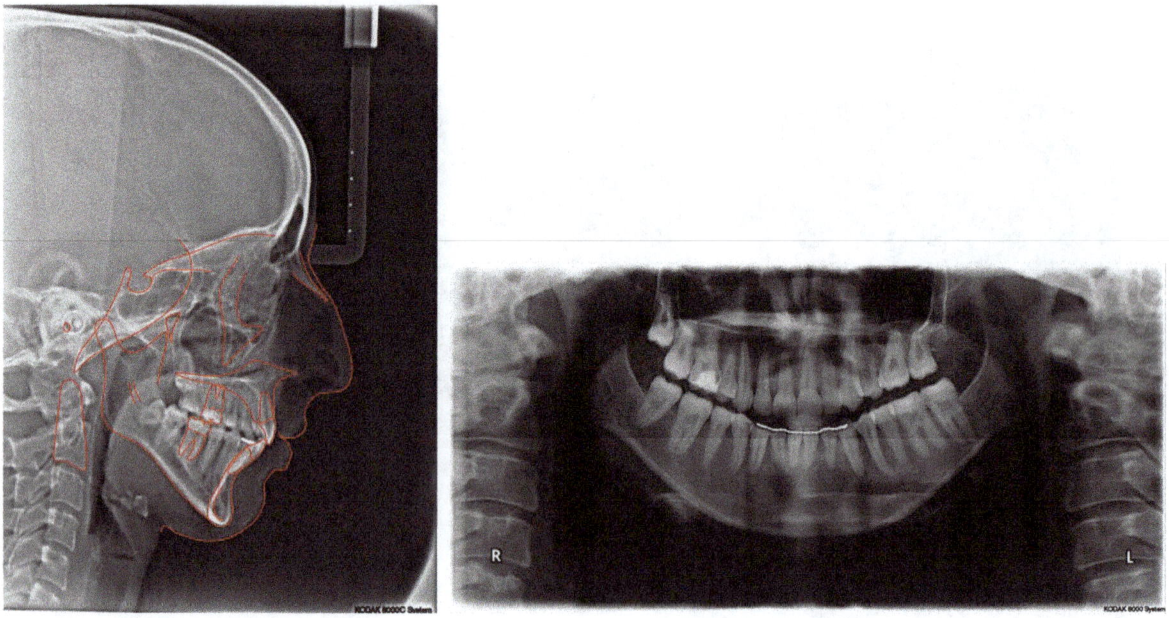

FIGURE 7: Posttreatment cephalometric and panoramic radiograph.

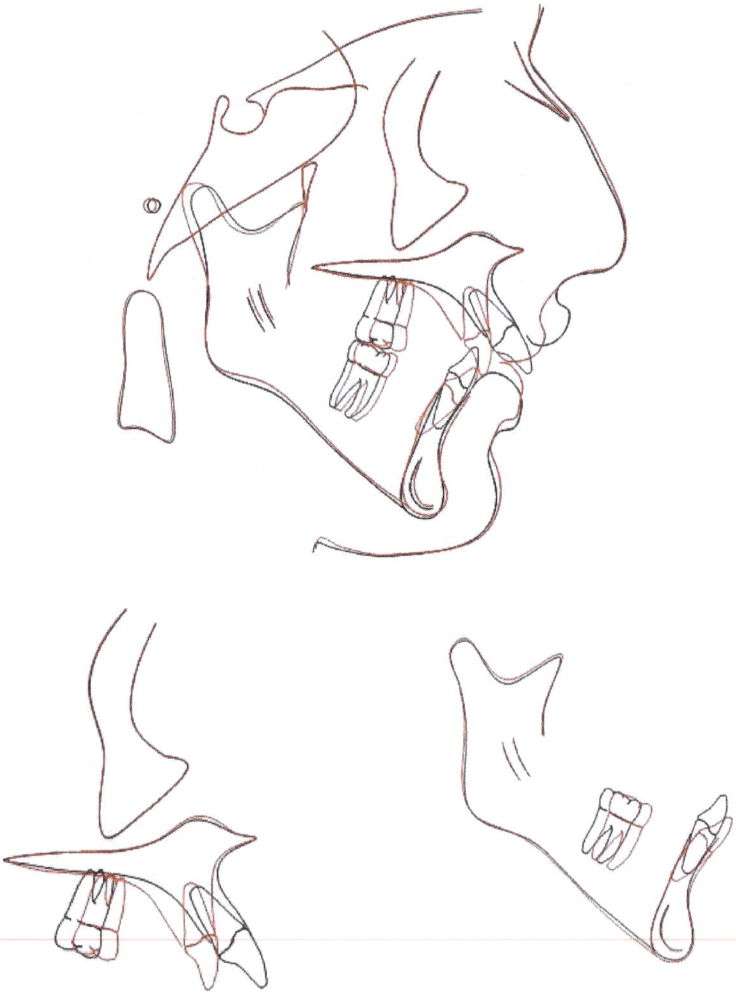

FIGURE 8: Posttreatment cephalometric superimposition.

The protraction of the lower right second molar was done to close the space of the lower right first molar and allow the eruption of the third molar in its place. Molar protraction has the advantage of preservation of the tooth structure when compared with a fixed bridge and reduced cost when compared with dental implants. Also, this method reduces the risk of impaction of the third molar.

References

[1] F. P. Carvalho Ferreira, A. P. Barbosa Lima, E. . C. M. de Paula, A. C. . C. Ferreira Conti, D. P. Valarelli, and R. R. de Almeida-Pedrin, "Orthodontic protocol using mini-implant for class II treatment in patient with special needs," *Case Reports in Dentistry*, vol. 2016, Article ID 1057263, 12 pages, 2016.

[2] S. Shioya and K. Arai, "Dentoskeletal morphology of adult class II division 1 and 2 severe deep overbite malocclusions," *Orthodontic Waves*, vol. 76, no. 2, pp. 97–104, 2017.

[3] N. A. van Wezel, A. Bos, and C. Prahl, "Expectations of treatment and satisfaction with dentofacial appearance in patients applying for orthodontic treatment," *American Journal of Orthodontics and Dentofacial Orthopedics*, vol. 147, no. 6, pp. 698–703, 2015.

[4] I. Qamruddin, F. Shahid, M. K. Alam, and W. Zehra Jamal, "Camouflage of severe skeletal class II gummy smile patient treated nonsurgically with mini implants," *Case Reports in Dentistry*, vol. 2014, Article ID 382367, 7 pages, 2014.

[5] C. A. Mihalik, W. R. Proffit, and C. Phillips, "Long-term follow-up of class II adults treated with orthodontic camouflage: a comparison with orthognathic surgery outcomes," *American Journal of Orthodontics and Dentofacial Orthopedics*, vol. 123, no. 3, pp. 266–278, 2003.

[6] R. Raposo, B. Peleteiro, M. Paço, and T. Pinho, "Orthodontic camouflage versus orthodontic-orthognathic surgical treatment in class II malocclusion: a systematic review and meta-analysis," *International Journal of Oral and Maxillofacial Surgery*, vol. 47, no. 4, pp. 445–455, 2018.

[7] S. Kuroda, K. Yamada, T. Deguchi, H. M. Kyung, and T. Takano-Yamamoto, "Class II malocclusion treated with miniscrew anchorage: comparison with traditional orthodontic mechanics outcomes," *American Journal of Orthodontics and Dentofacial Orthopedics*, vol. 135, no. 3, pp. 302–309, 2009.

[8] K. Kim, S. H. Choi, E. H. Choi, Y. J. Choi, C. J. Hwang, and J. Y. Cha, "Unpredictability of soft tissue changes after camouflage treatment of class II division 1 malocclusion with maximum anterior retraction using miniscrews," *The Angle Orthodontist*, vol. 87, no. 2, pp. 230–238, 2017.

[9] W. R. Proffit, C. Phillips, and N. Douvartzidis, "A comparison of outcomes of orthodontic and surgical-orthodontic treatment of class II malocclusion in adults," *American Journal of Orthodontics and Dentofacial Orthopedics*, vol. 101, no. 6, pp. 556–565, 1992.

[10] M. Upadhyay, S. Yadav, and R. Nanda, "Vertical-dimension control during en-masse retraction with mini-implant anchorage," *American Journal of Orthodontics and Dentofacial Orthopedics*, vol. 138, no. 1, pp. 96–108, 2010.

[11] M. R. Tucker, "Orthognathic surgery versus orthodontic camouflage in the treatment of mandibular deficiency," *Journal of Oral and Maxillofacial Surgery*, vol. 53, no. 5, pp. 572–578, 1995.

[12] R. Scott Conley and C. Jernigan, "Soft tissue changes after upper premolar extraction in class II camouflage therapy," *The Angle Orthodontist*, vol. 76, no. 1, pp. 59–65, 2006.

[13] S. Cunningham, N. Hunt, and C. Feinmann, "Psychological aspects of orthognathic surgery: a review of the literature," *The International Journal of Adult Orthodontics and Orthognathic Surgery*, vol. 10, no. 3, pp. 159–172, 1995.

[14] S. M. Rivera, J. P. Hatch, C. Dolce, R. A. Bays, J. E. van Sickels, and J. D. Rugh, "Patients' own reasons and patient-perceived recommendations for orthognathic surgery," *American Journal of Orthodontics and Dentofacial Orthopedics*, vol. 118, no. 2, pp. 134–140, 2000.

[15] S. Endo, W. Yamada, I. Shundo, Y. Kobayashi, A. Komatsuzakit, and T. Endo, "Short-term treatment effects of the quad-helix appliance on dentofacial morphology of hyperdivergent patients," *Australian Orthodontic Journal*, vol. 32, no. 2, pp. 211–220, 2016.

[16] M. Upadhyay, S. Yadav, and S. Patil, "Mini-implant anchorage for en-masse retraction of maxillary anterior teeth: a clinical cephalometric study," *American Journal of Orthodontics and Dentofacial Orthopedics*, vol. 134, no. 6, pp. 803–810, 2008.

[17] J.-y. Tominaga, M. Tanaka, Y. Koga, C. Gonzales, M. Kobayashi, and N. Yoshida, "Optimal loading conditions for controlled movement of anterior teeth in sliding mechanics: a 3D finite element study," *The Angle Orthodontist*, vol. 79, no. 6, pp. 1102–1107, 2009.

7

Patient with Crouzon Syndrome Treated with Modified Le Fort III Osteotomy without Previous Orthodontic Treatment: Case Report and a Review of the Literature

Farnoosh Mohammadi,[1] Afrooz Javanmard,[2] and Hamid Mojtahedi[1]

[1]*Craniomaxillofacial Research Center, Oral and Maxillofacial Surgery Department, Shariati Hospital, Tehran University of Medical Sciences, Tehran, Iran*
[2]*Department of Prosthodontics and Dental Research Center, Faculty of Dentistry, Tehran University of Medical Sciences, Tehran, Iran*

Correspondence should be addressed to Hamid Mojtahedi; hamid.mojtahedi91@yahoo.com

Academic Editor: John H. Campbell

Crouzon syndrome is the most common type of craniofacial dysostosis anomaly which presents a great challenge for clinicians since birth. Multiple synostoses in the sutures of the cranial base in this syndrome result in the hypoplasia of the midface, shallow orbits, a short nasal dorsum, maxillary hypoplasia, and, in severe cases, obstruction of the upper airways. Apart from esthetic and functional problems, these patients suffer from various psychological problems which mandate correction of midface deformities at younger ages. The aim of this report is to describe the case of a 26-year-old female patient with Crouzon syndrome displaying severe midface hypoplasia and proptosis with no history of orthodontic treatment, who was treated with modified Le Fort III osteotomy with a coronal and intraoral approach without periocular incisions.

1. Introduction

In 2012, Crouzon described the triad of skeletal deformity, facial anomalies, and exophthalmos as hereditary craniofacial dysostosis [1]. Crouzon syndrome is known as an autosomal dominant disorder with complete penetration and varying expression [2]. The prevalence of this syndrome is approximately 1 : 25000 births [3]. Premature closure of the coronal and sagittal sutures of the cranium in this syndrome results in the abnormal growth of the skull base, orbits, and maxillary complex [4]. Despite other autosomal dominant craniosynostosis syndromes, no digital anomalies are seen in the Crouzon syndrome [5]. Patients with Crouzon syndrome have normal mental development. However, in a small number of cases, there is a delay in cognitive development, which might be attributed to an increase in intracranial pressure during infancy [6].

Crouzon syndrome is due to a mutation in the FGFR-2 (fibroblast growth factor receptor-2) gene. It has been reported that in 50% of cases, Crouzon syndrome is due to a new mutation without a hereditary pattern [7]. Multiple synostoses in the sutures of the cranial base in this syndrome result in the hypoplasia of the midface, shallow orbits, a short nasal dorsum, maxillary hypoplasia, and, in severe cases, obstruction of the upper airways [8]. The manifestations of Crouzon syndrome during infancy might vary from minor characteristics in association with minor defects in the midface to the involvement of several sutures in the skull and severe midface deficiency and visual problems [9]. An increase in intracranial pressure might result in optic nerve atrophy and loss of vision if no intervention is made [10]. These patients might have other concomitant skeletal problems such as mandibular prognathism and/or retrognathism, possibly in association with midface deformity [11].

Apart from systemic and dental problems, patients with craniofacial synostosis suffer from various psychological problems due to defects in their appearance. As a result, these patients have more limited social activities and problems

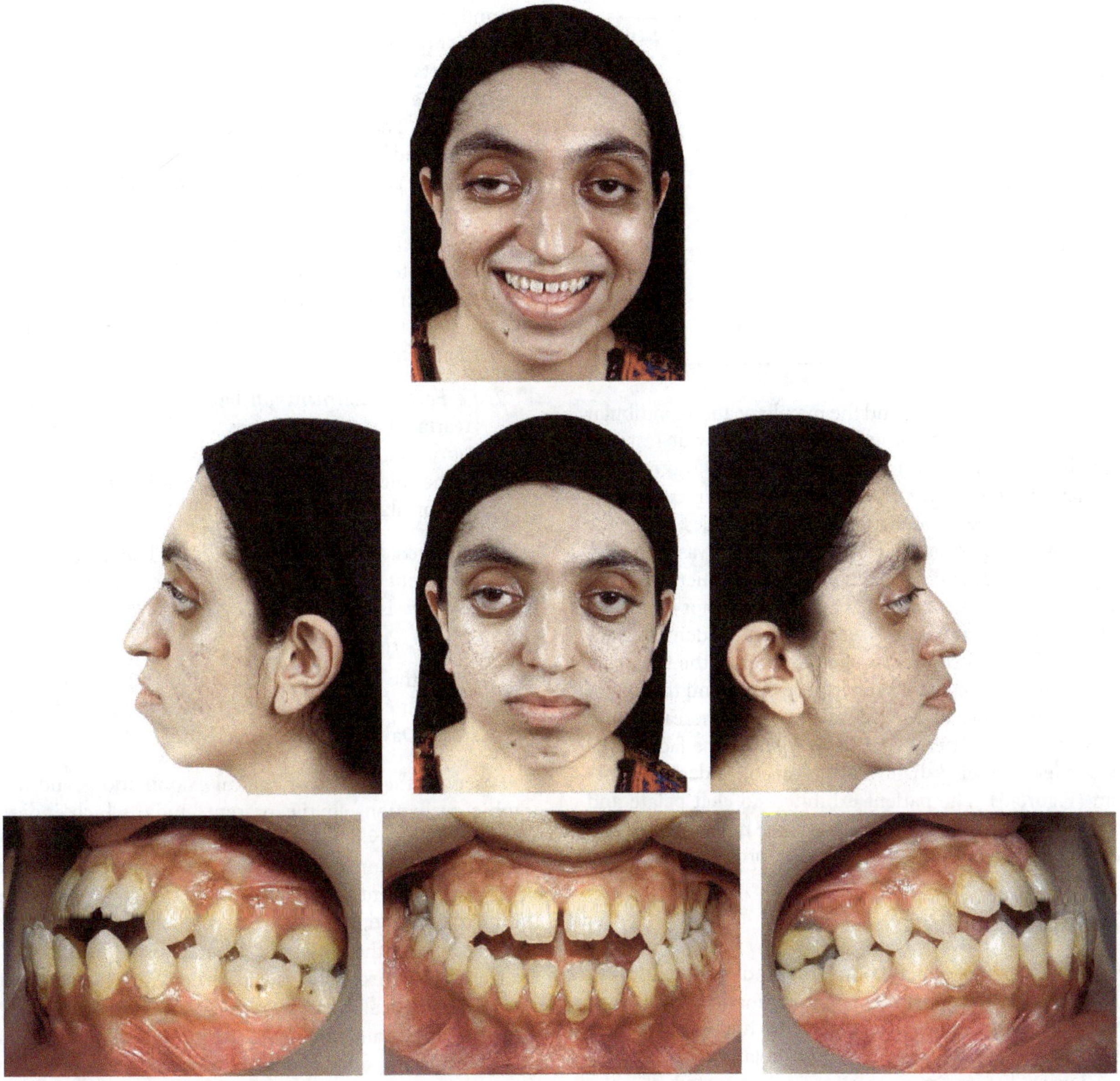

FIGURE 1: Pretreatment patient's extraoral and intraoral photographs.

with communication with their peers [12]. Correction of midface deformities at younger ages might have a significant role in decreasing the psychological problems of these patients [13]. The important role of the face in vision, respiration, speech, smelling, and hearing makes the defects that affect this area more important than the esthetic problems [11].

The aim of this report is to describe the case of a 26-year-old female patient with Crouzon syndrome displaying severe midface hypoplasia and proptosis with no history of orthodontic treatment, who was treated with modified Le Fort III osteotomy with a coronal and intraoral approach without periocular incisions.

2. Diagnosis and Patient History

The case described here is a 26-year-old female patient who referred to the Shariati Medical Center of Tehran, Iran, for treatment at this age. The chief complaint of the patient was facial abnormality and the inability to close the eyes. Clinical examinations revealed severe defects in the lower orbit area and the midface, moderate hypertelorism, and severe exophthalmos (Figure 1). The patient did not exhibit any signs of an increase in intracranial pressure and neurologic problems and had normal mental development. Consultation with an ophthalmologist revealed an approximately 30% decrease in visual acuity and amblyopia. Funduscopic examinations of the eye did not reveal any signs indicating papilledema. The patient did not complain of nocturnal apnea and respiratory obstruction. Intraoral examinations revealed a 5 mm anterior open bite and bilateral posterior crossbite. The molar and canine relationships were Cl III on both sides, and a reverse overjet of approximately 6 mm was measured (Figure 1). In cephalometric evaluations, she had retrusive maxilla with SNA angle of 80 (Table 1 and Figure 2). There

Table 1: Cephalometric analysis.

	Normal value	Pretreatment value	Posttreatment value
A point to N-P	1	-3	2
SNA	82	80	88
U1 to S-N	104	117	120
Nasolabial angle	102	58	65
Occlusal plane angle	17	7	19
Nasofrontal angle	120	120	119
Overjet	2-3	-6	3
Overbite	—	5	1
Molar discrepancy	0	-12	0

were no signs of crowding, and the maxillary and mandibular teeth had diastema. The amount of tooth show at rest and smiling had decreased, and paranasal deficiency was evident. Examinations showed that the upper and lower extremities were intact and there were no digital deformities. After the evaluations, a diagnosis of Crouzon syndrome was achieved. Owing to financial and social problems, the patient had not referred for treatment at younger ages and was not interested in orthodontic treatment in order to correct the dental status. Clinical evaluations showed proper contour of the forehead. The nasofrontal area had a proper projection, and the length of the nose was normal. The scleral show had increased, and the dystopia of the lateral canthus was seen. The facial axial CT scan views revealed shallow orbits on both sides and exorbitism (Figure 3). The patient exhibited no cleft palate and velopharyngeal insufficiency; however, the malocclusion and anterior open bite had resulted in speech problems.

3. Treatment Objectives

Given the patient's chief complaint and her refusal to undergo orthodontic treatment due to financial problems, the aim of treatment was to correct the hypoplasia of the midface and achieve a proper occlusal relationship. Due to minor hypertelorism, its correction was not included in the treatment plan. The objectives of the treatment in this patient were as follows based on the problems described above: (1) correction of the midface and infraorbital defects with midface advancement; (2) decreasing ocular proptosis; (3) no change in the nasal projection and contour of the forehead, considering their normality; (4) increasing maxillary tooth show at rest and smiling; and (5) closing the open bite and achieving maximum intercuspation at occlusion in the absence of orthodontic treatment.

4. Surgical Options for the Correction of Midface Deficiencies

The treatment options in patients with craniofacial dysostosis are very divergent, depending on the severity of skeletal and dental problems and the patients' psychosocial status. Facial skeletal deformities affect different structures in the form of repeated patterns; however, their expression and the severity of involvement are variable at different syndromic and nonsyndromic cases, affecting the treatment plans and the surgical correction of deformities [14]. Treatment of the sagittal midface deficiency in these patients consists of routine Le Fort osteotomies with or without distraction osteogenesis. The currently used osteotomy techniques to correct the midface deformities in patients with craniofacial dysostosis are generally divided into four categories:

1. *Subcranial Monoblock Advancement Osteotomy.* This is used to correct the general midface defects. It is the treatment of choice in cases in which the infraorbital, supraorbital, and the nasomaxillary complexes have a total defect
2. *Le Fort III Extracranial Osteotomy.* This is a proper treatment option in cases in which the frontal and supraorbital areas are normal and the defect is located in the middle third of the face, affecting the maxilla, infraorbital rim, and nasal unit
3. *Modified Le Fort III Osteotomy.* This is used in the treatment of midface defects when the nasomaxillary complex is not involved
4. *Le Fort II Osteotomy.* This treatment option is used when the extent of involvement of the orbital and zygomatic areas is less than that of the nasomaxillary areas (David, 2015).

Based on the results of clinical examinations and radiographic evaluations in the present study, which indicated the absence of any defects in the upper third of the face and the normal contour of supraorbital and frontal areas, monoblock advancement was not a proper choice in this patient. On the other hand, the patient did not exhibit nasomaxillary hypoplasia, and the classic Le Fort III osteotomy could be associated with excessive advancement of the nasal unit, which is esthetically inappropriate. Considering what was discussed above and the defect in the malar and maxillary areas, the anterior open bite, and the absence of proper dental arch, modified Le Fort III osteotomy in association with mandibular osteotomy after initial orthodontic treatment was suggested to the patient. The patient refused to undergo presurgical orthodontic treatment due to social and financial problems. Therefore, the modified Le Fort III osteotomy was decided, without orthodontic treatment, to correct the occlusion, the midface deficiency, and the exophthalmos.

Treatment of skeletal deformities and the midface defects has long been a great challenge for surgeons. In 1901, Le Fort and Tessier classified the different patterns of facial skeletal fractures for the first time [15]. Gillies and Harrison were the first to attempt to treat the facial defects of patients with craniofacial dysostosis by moving the midface in 1950. The advancement of the midface in association with external fixation did not result in favorable long-term stability [16]. Finally, in 1957, the efforts made by Tessier revolutionized the surgical treatment of the general midface defects by introducing intracranial and extracranial access to mobilize the midface. Tessier achieved stable long-term results in

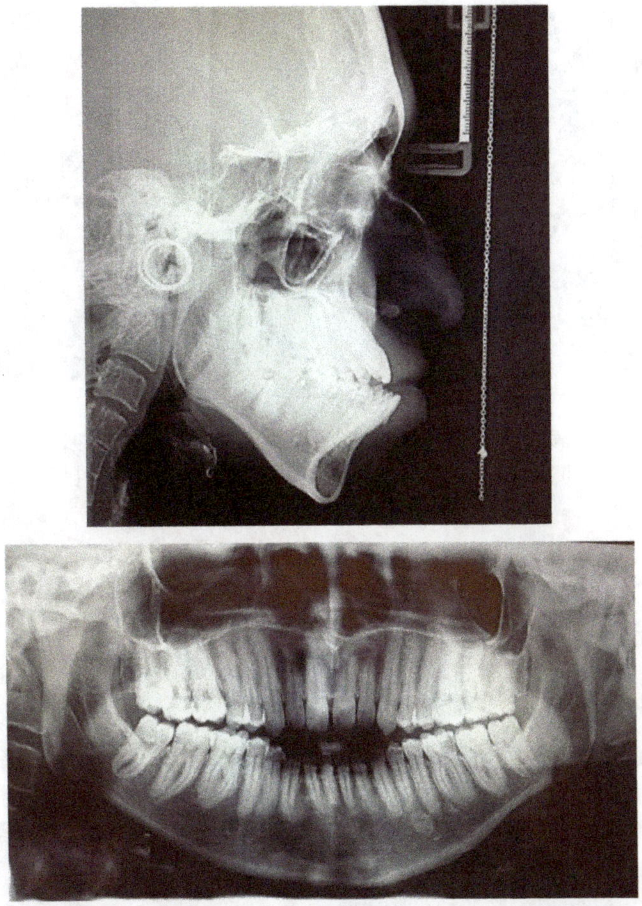

FIGURE 2: Pretreatment lateral cephalogram and panoramic views.

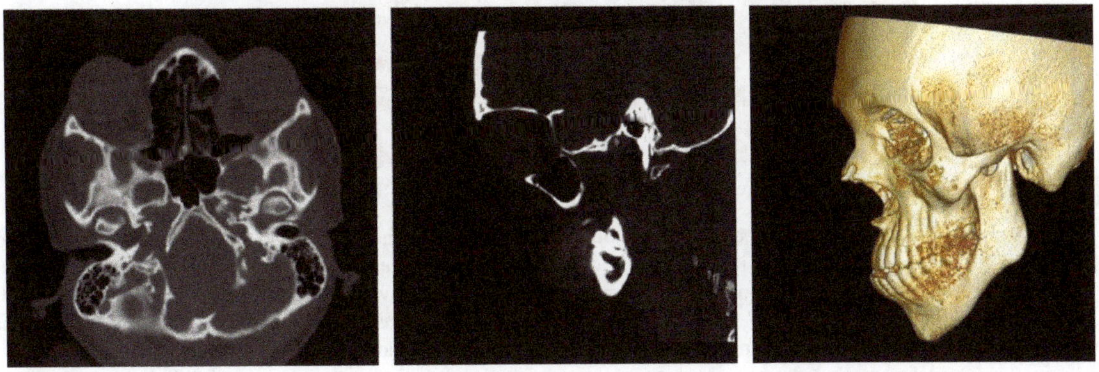

FIGURE 3: Pretreatment axial, sagittal, and three-dimensional computed tomographic views.

patients with craniofacial dysostosis by internal rigid fixation for the first time. Development of surgical techniques and the introduction of various modifications by Tessier and other surgeons resulted in improvements in the functional defects and facial appearance of patients with midface deficiencies [17].

5. Treatment

First, nasotracheal intubation was carried out by placing the tube inferiorly and moving it through the cheek. Oral intubation is not suggested in such cases because it is necessary to achieve occlusion and intermaxillary fixation during the surgical procedure. The tracheal tube was fixed to the membranous septum and columella, using sutures. Bilateral tarsorrhaphy suturing was carried out in order to protect the eye globe and the cornea. The coronal approach in association with intraoral approach was considered without access to periocular structures to make sure of the direct access to modified Le Fort III osteotomy field. Before draping the patient, the hairline was determined at a distance of 2 cm, and the hair anterior and posterior to the incision line was

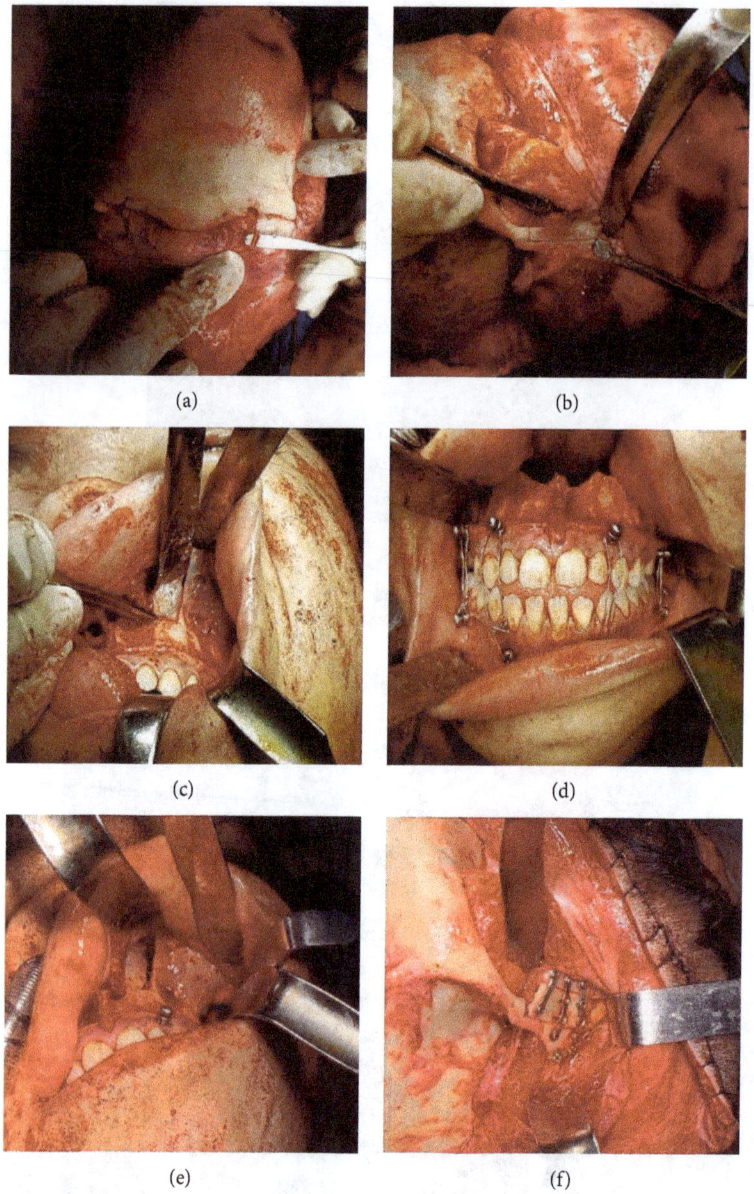

FIGURE 4: (a) The supraorbital nerve was released by a fissure bur and an osteotome and preserved above the eye globe afterward. (b) The vertical osteotomy line was initiated midway in this area and continued up to the lowest limit of the zygomatic buttress. (c) The osteotomy line which was extended vertically from the infraorbital rim from the relative site of orbital floor osteotomy termination up to the nasal cavity lower rim level and pyriform aperture. (d) The maxillary teeth were fixed in an edge-to-edge position with the mandibular teeth by IMF screws. (e) Amount of gap in the pyriform aperture area after disimpaction and advancement. (f) Rigid fixation was carried out in lateral orbital rim and zygomatic buttress areas by titanium microplates.

braided. 2% lidocaine with 1 : 100000 epinephrine was injected into the coronal incision line and the maxillary vestibular mucosa. Coronal approach was performed with a cutaneous incision in the midauricular area on one side ending on the midauricular area on the other side crossing the superior temporal line, approximately 2 cm behind the hairline on both sides. The cutaneous incision carried out to the depth of the galea layer on the pericranium, and then the supraperiosteal dissection in the avascular tissue plane continued up to approximately 2 cm above the superior rim of the orbit. In this area, a sharp incision was made using a scalpel on the pericranium, and the periosteum of the frontal area was elevated to gain full access to the upper rim and the lateral rim of the orbit. Electrocautery was used, and the coronal flap margins were sutured with 2-0 silk sutures to achieve hemostasis. The temporalis muscle was completely elevated in the subperiosteal plan superiorly from the superior temporal line on both sides up to the zygomatic arch area in order to gain access to the buttress and zygomatic arch. After completely releasing the periosteum from the superior orbital rim, the supraorbital nerve was released by a fissure bur and an osteotome and preserved above the eye globe afterward (Figure 4(a)). Next, complete periorbital dissection was carried out up to the infraorbital fissure from the lateral aspect, preserving the adhesion of the medial canthus. Dissection of 3/4 of the globe circumference prepared the lateral

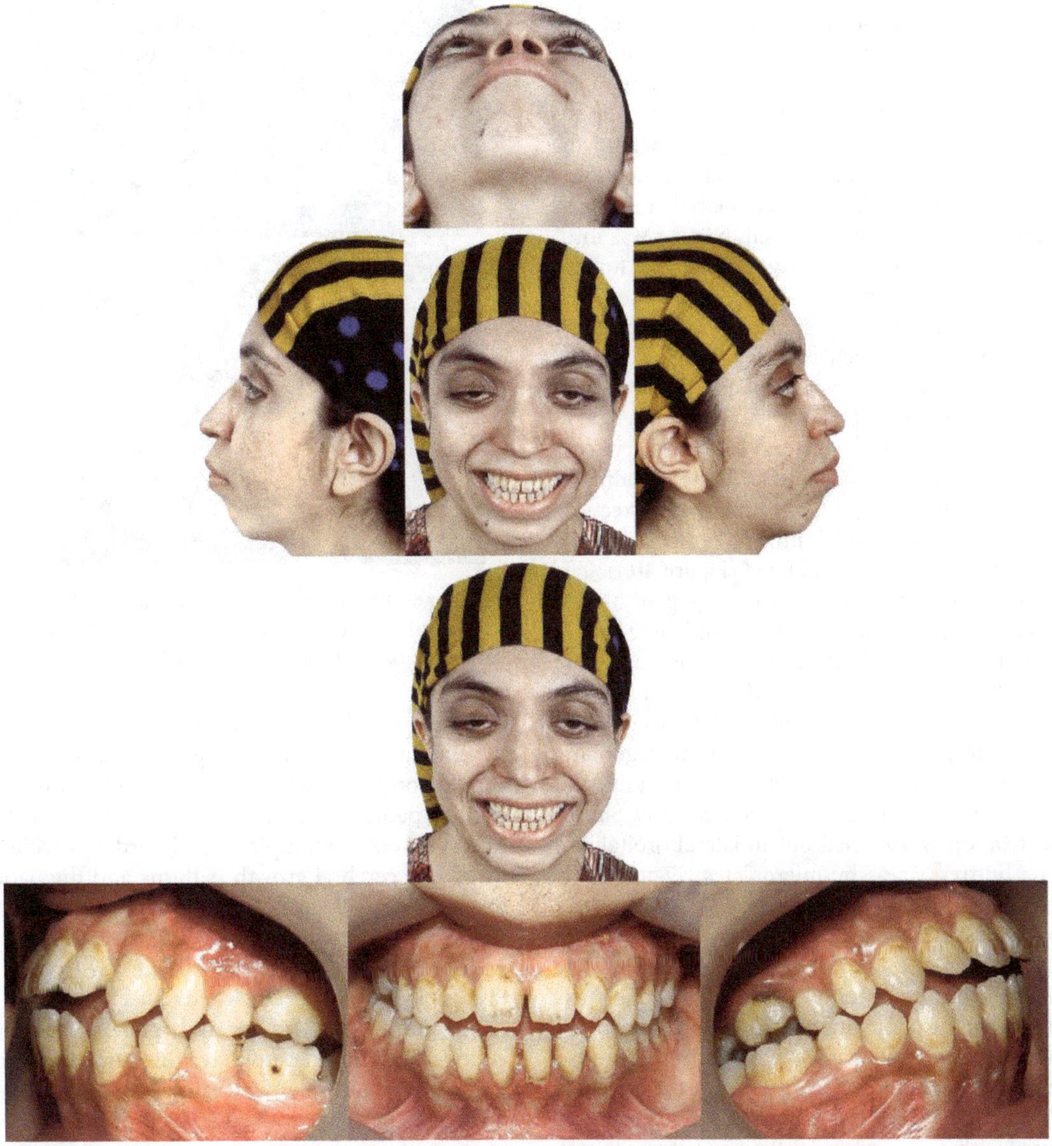

FIGURE 5: Postreatment patients extraoral and intraoral photographs.

and inferior rims and the floor of the orbit for osteotomy. A proper dissection was carried out in the subperiosteal plane to make sure of preservation of the facial nerve. Subsequently, access was provided to the piriform rim, zygomatic buttress, and pterygomaxillary areas on both sides by extending the circumvestibular incision between the first molar areas on both sides up to the midline. Keeping the dissection in the subperiosteal plane preserves the important arteries in this area, including the internal maxillary artery. After making sure of the complete release of the infraorbital nerve, the nasal cavity floor, and the anterior area of the nasal septum, dissection was terminated, and osteotomy was instituted.

First, the frontozygomatic suture was identified, and the osteotomy was initiated from the area superior to the suture with the use of a saw. Before terminating the transverse osteotomy line, the vertical osteotomy line was initiated midway in this area and continued up to the lowest limit of the zygomatic buttress (Figure 4(b)). Consideration should be given through the preservation of the globe soft tissue by malleable retractors, and the osteotomy of the lateral rim of the orbit continued from 1 cm posterior to the rim up to the infraorbital tissue with the use of a 2 mm osteotome. The bone at the floor of the orbit is paper-thin and can be osteotomized easily and with greater control, using an osteotome with no need for a saw and a fissure bur. Once the osteotomy of the infraorbital fissure and orbital floor had terminated, the Langenbeck retractor was fixed at the infraorbital rim and medial to infraorbital foramen through intraoral access, providing adequate space for osteotomy. The osteotomy line was extended vertically from the infraorbital rim from the relative site of orbital floor osteotomy termination up to the nasal cavity lower rim level (Figure 4(c)). Then, the direction of osteotomy was changed to continue horizontally to terminate at the piriform rim. Finally, similar to Le Fort I osteotomy, the vomer and nasal septum were completely tapped with the use of a nasal septum osteotome. To make sure of the osteotomy of the posterior wall of the maxilla and the pterygomaxillary area, the osteotomy of the pterygoid plates was completed through both extraoral access behind the zygomatic arch and intraoral access behind the maxillary tuberosity. Once we made sure that the osteotomy had been perfectly done, row forceps were placed at the nasal cavity floor and the hard palate, and disimpaction was initiated. After that, the midface is relatively released; row forceps were used to increase the range of midface mobilization. It is of paramount importance to make sure of complete mobility of the midface in order to achieve long-term and stable results. After that, the midface was advanced with the use of intermaxillary fixation screws which were placed at 8 points in the mandible, and maxilla and the maxillary teeth were fixed in an edge-to-edge position with the mandibular teeth (Figure 4(d)). The amount of exophthalmos correction, advancement of the inferior orbital rim, and projection of the malar and paranasal areas were evaluated (Figure 4(e)). The rigid fixation process was instituted with a gap of almost one cm in the frontozygomatic suture and one cm of advancement of the midface. Then, cortical monoblock bone graft was harvested paramedially from the parietal bone of one side with the use of a fissure bur and an osteotome. The harvested bone grafts were placed at frontozygomatic osteotomy site gaps in order to preserve the continuity of bone and decrease the chance of skeletal relapse. Subsequently, rigid fixation was carried out in lateral orbital rim and zygomatic buttress areas by microplates (Figure 4(f)). The tarsorrhaphy sutures were released on both sides, and force duction test was performed to make sure of the absence of any entrapment on the floor of the orbit and complete movement of the eye globe is restored. The temporalis muscle was suspended to the pericranium of the sculp in the overcorrected position, and hemostasis was ensured. Surgical field was debrided with copious irrigation, and the intraoral incision was sutured with 4-0 vicryl sutures; the coronal surface was sutured with 3-0 vicryl and 2-0 nylon sutures in two layers. A pressure pack was placed in the scalp area in order to redrape the soft tissue and to decrease the postoperative edema. The patient was extubated at the end of surgery for maintaining the airway condition; there was no reason to extend the patient's intubation period. Steroids and cephalosporins were prescribed before surgery and repeated every 4 hours during surgery. The steroids continued for 48 hours, and oral antibiotics were given for 10 days after surgery. In such surgeries, early ambulation and oral nutrition should be encouraged. Decongestant sprays were used for two weeks. A soft diet was continued for six weeks. Elastic guides were delivered to the patient for reducing the patient discomfort and control of occlusion.

6. Discussion

It is a challenge to treat patients with craniofacial dysostosis syndromes. Craniofacial teams consist of several specialists, including ophthalmologists, neurosurgeons, oral and maxillofacial surgeons, plastic surgeons, and orthodontists, who should contribute since birth in the diagnosis and treatment of these patients. The reconstruction in these patients should be carried out in multiple stages in order to accommodate the facial and cerebral growth patterns and the patients' cognitive and psychological statues. The patient described in this report was different from the routine treatment stages of such patients in many ways. The patient was from a family with low socioeconomic status and lived in one of the border towns in Iran. She had not undergone routine treatments at younger ages and did not have the required financial potential to accept orthodontic treatment. Preoperative orthodontic alignment of the teeth could have provided adequate space for correcting the occlusion in one step during the surgery in association with mandibular osteotomy.

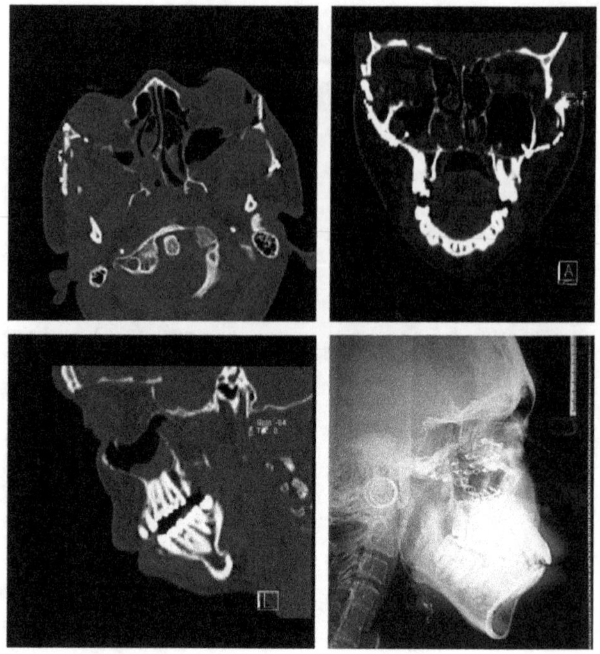

Figure 6: Postreatment axial, sagittal, and coronal computed tomographic views and lateral cephalogram demonstrated correction of orbital depth and exophthalmos.

Considering the proper contour of the forehead and the supraorbital area and absence of hypoplasia in the nasal unit, modified Le Fort III osteotomy procedure was planned for the patient in order to correct the malar and maxillary deficiency and proptosis. In 1971, Kufner modified the osteotomy plan of Gillis for the first time and made an attempt to advance the midface without disturbing the nasofrontal unit [18]. Kufner's efforts and others resulted in the introduction of the modified Le Fort III osteotomy [19]. In this case, by the modified Le Fort III osteotomy plan, a proper facial profile was achieved. The severity of proptosis and the scleral show were decreased, and the nasal dorsum and nasofrontal areas remained unchanged (Figures 5 and 6). Clockwise rotation of the maxilla resulted in anterior-superior autorotation of the mandible, decreasing the patient's open bite. A class I molar and canine relationship was achieved, and the patent's reverse jet decreased significantly (Figure 5). Comparison of

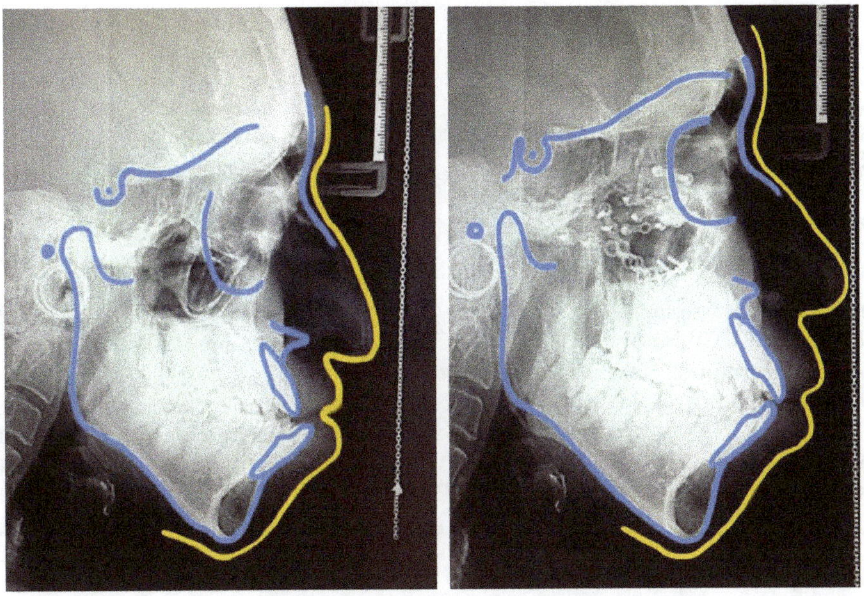

FIGURE 7: Pre- and posttreatment cephalometric tracings.

cephalometric analyses before and after surgery indicated the advancement of the maxilla and the lower orbital rim (Table 1 and Figure 7).

Intraoral and extraoral access is used to carry out modified Le Fort III osteotomy. Fariña et al. used a combination of intraoral and transconjunctival incisions in association with canthotomy to gain access to modified Le Fort III osteotomy areas and reported that the advantages of the above approach included less hemorrhage and shorter duration of surgery [20]. In the surgery of the patient reported here, a coronal and intraoral approach was used to gain access to the osteotomy sites. As reported by Tessier, after advancement of the midface, it is necessary to use bone grafts in the fixation areas in order to improve the stability of treatment and achieve proper bone healing [21]. Periorbital approach does not provide enough space for placement of grafts and fixation devices. The advantages of the coronal approach are an inconspicuous scar behind the hairline and the possibility of harvesting a calvarial graft without creating another donor site and its related morbidity. Ridgway studied the severity of lower lid malformation subsequent to periorbital incisions for the reconstruction of traumatic fractures of the face and reported that the highest risk of entropion was related to the transconjunctival approach; the highest risk of ectropion was related to the subciliary approach and the risk of a hypertrophic scar was related to the subtarsal approach [22]. Accessibility and visibility through the osteotomy sits of zygomaticofrontal, infraorbital rim and posterior maxillary walls are highly achieved by coronal approach. Through hypotensive anesthetic condition, proper surgical hemostasis, and oral and maxillofacial surgeons experienced in scalpel incision, the amount of bleeding and surgery time is controllable in the coronal approach.

Some researchers suggest distraction osteogenesis due to need for excessive advancements in patients with craniofacial dysostosis. This technique might result in better stability of the treatment outcomes and greater movement range with no need for bone grafts and no donor site morbidity [23]. On the other hand, this technique requires the patient's full compliance to activate the appliance regularly. The amount and direction of skeletal movements cannot be controlled in contrast to surgical advancements subsequent to osteotomy and the deformity remaining after it might require revision in some cases. The placed distractor appliances should be removed during a second surgery, and the appliances are very expensive in Iran and patients cannot afford it. Distraction treatment was initially considered for the patient reported here. However, due to lack of compliance by the patient and its high cost, it was excluded.

The patient was satisfied with the treatment and reported that it positively affected her social and occupational activities. The patient was followed for six months after treatment. The occlusion which was achieved during surgery had been maintained. The facial profile and the scleral show were favorable and the scar of the coronal approach was hidden behind the hairline, with no alopecia. The patient's visual acuity had improved compared to the preoperative period based on ophthalmologic examinations. In addition, the risk of injuries to the eye globe and corneal keratitis had decreased due to a decrease in proptosis.

7. Conclusion

This case report demonstrates that it is possible to treat patients with Crouzon syndrome with severe midface hypoplasia and proptosis by modified Le Fort III osteotomy, with a high success rate, in the absence of presurgical orthodontic treatment.

References

[1] O. Crouzon, "Dysostose cranio-faciale hereditair," *Bulletins et Mémoires de la Société Médicale des Hôpitaux de Paris*, vol. 33, pp. 545–555, 1912.

[2] P. Fogh-Andersen, "Craniofacial dysostosis (Crouzon's disease) as a dominant hereditary affection," *Nordisk Medicin*, vol. 18, pp. 993–996, 1943.

[3] M. M. Cohen, J. M. Opitz, J. F. Reynolds, and R. J. Gorlin, "Craniosynostosis update 1987," *American Journal of Medical Genetics*, vol. 31, Supplement 4, pp. 99–148, 1988.

[4] H. W. Dodge, M. W. Wood, and R. L. Kennedy, "Craniofacial dysostosis: Crouzon's disease," *Pediatrics*, vol. 23, no. 1, pp. 98–106, 1959.

[5] A. Franceschetti, "Cranial dysostosis with pronounced digital impressions (pseudo-crouzon dysostosis)," in *Congenital Anomalies of the Eye*, pp. 81–84, CV Mosby, St. Louis, 1968.

[6] T. Bertelsen, "The premature synostosis of the cranial sutures," *Acta Ophthalmologica Supplement*, vol. 36, Supplement 51, pp. 1–176, 1958.

[7] E. W. Jabs, X. Li, A. F. Scott et al., "Jackson-Weiss and Crouzon syndromes are allelic with mutations in fibroblast growth factor receptor 2," *Nature Genetics*, vol. 8, no. 3, pp. 275–279, 1994.

[8] E. L. Bowling and F. D. Burstein, "Crouzon syndrome," *Optometry - Journal of the American Optometric Association*, vol. 77, no. 5, pp. 217–222, 2006.

[9] M. Järund and C. Laurcitzen, "Craniofacial dysostosis: airway obstruction and craniofacial surgery," *Scandinavian Journal of Plastic and Reconstructive Surgery and Hand Surgery*, vol. 30, no. 4, pp. 275–279, 1996.

[10] O. Pinkerton and F. Pinkerton, "Hereditary craniofacial dysplasia," *American Journal of Ophthalmology*, vol. 35, no. 4, pp. 500–506, 1952.

[11] D. D. Vu and P. S. Tiwana, "Le Fort III and Le Fort II osteotomies," *Atlas of the Oral and Maxillofacial Surgery Clinics*, vol. 24, no. 1, pp. 15–25, 2016.

[12] K. A. Kapp-Simon, D. J. Simon, and S. Kristovich Ms., "Self-perception, social skills, adjustment, and inhibition in young adolescents with craniofacial anomalies," *The Cleft Palate-Craniofacial Journal*, vol. 29, no. 4, pp. 352–356, 1992.

[13] M. Pertschuk and L. Whitaker, "Social and psychological effects of craniofacial deformity and surgical reconstruction," *Clinics in Plastic Surgery*, vol. 9, no. 3, pp. 297–306, 1982.

[14] L. A. Whitaker, I. R. Munro, K. E. Salyer, I. T. Jackson, F. Ortiz-Monasterio, and D. Marchac, "Combined report of problems and complications in 793 craniofacial operations," *Plastic and Reconstructive Surgery*, vol. 64, no. 2, pp. 198–203, 1979.

[15] R. E. N. É. Fort and P. Tessier, "Experimental study of fractures of the upper jaw," *Plastic and Reconstructive Surgery*, vol. 50, no. 5, pp. 497–506, 1972.

[16] H. Gillies and S. H. Harrison, "Operative correction by osteotomy of recessed malar maxillary compound in a case of oxycephaly," *Plastic and Reconstructive Surgery*, vol. 6, no. 6, p. 486, 1950.

[17] P. Tessier, "Osteotomies totales de la face. Syndrome de Crouzon, syndrome d'Apert: oxycephalies, scaphocephalies, turricephalies," *Annales de Chirurgie Plastique*, vol. 12, pp. 273–275, 1967.

[18] J. Kufner, "Four-year experience with major maxillary osteotomy for retrusion," *Journal of oral surgery (American Dental Association : 1965)*, vol. 29, no. 8, pp. 549–553, 1971.

[19] B. N. Epker and L. M. Wolford, "Middle-third facial osteotomies: their use in the correction of acquired and developmental dentofacial and craniofacial deformities," *Journal of oral surgery (American Dental Association: 1965)*, vol. 33, no. 7, pp. 491–514, 1975.

[20] R. Fariña, S. Valladares, A. Raposo, and F. Silva, "Modified Le Fort III osteotomy: a simple solution to severe midfacial hypoplasia," *Journal of Cranio-Maxillofacial Surgery*, vol. 46, no. 5, pp. 837–843, 2018.

[21] P. Tessier, "The definitive plastic surgical treatment of the severe facial deformities of craniofacial dysostosis: Crouzon's and Apert's diseases," *Plastic and Reconstructive Surgery*, vol. 48, no. 5, pp. 419–442, 1971.

[22] E. B. Ridgway, C. Chen, S. Colakoglu, S. Gautam, and B. T. Lee, "The incidence of lower eyelid malposition after facial fracture repair: a retrospective study and meta-analysis comparing subtarsal, subciliary, and transconjunctival incisions," *Plastic and Reconstructive Surgery*, vol. 124, no. 5, pp. 1578–1586, 2009.

[23] E. Nout, E. Wolvius, L. van Adrichem, E. Ongkosuwito, and K. van der Wal, "Complications in maxillary distraction using the RED II device: a retrospective analysis of 21 patients," *International Journal of Oral and Maxillofacial Surgery*, vol. 35, no. 10, pp. 897–902, 2006.

8

A Prosthodontic Approach as a Complementary Solution for a Complicated Orthodontic Treatment of a Patient with Cleidocranial Dysplasia

Joanna Jasnoch, Maria Zielke, and Izabela Maciejewska

Department of Dental Prosthodontics, Medical University of Gdansk, Poland

Correspondence should be addressed to Izabela Maciejewska; izabelam@gumed.edu.pl

Academic Editor: Tatiana Pereira-Cenci

This clinical report describes a prosthodontic rehabilitation of a 29-year-old patient with cleidocranial dysplasia (CCD), who, after completing an orthodontic treatment, was not satisfied with the aesthetic outcome. Besides aesthetics, the patient complained about mastication muscles pain, and clicking while eating but was not aware about her unilateral open bite on the right side. The aim of this treatment was to improve smile appearance and patient's well-being, as well as to restore the proper occlusal vertical dimension (OVD) along with complete intercuspation and to establish masticatory function. The first phase of the treatment concentrated on eliminating the muscle pain and temporomandibular joint (TMJ) clicking with a repositioning splint. During the second phase, the functional and aesthetic rehabilitation was obtained using adhesive prosthesis overlays and veneers.

1. Introduction

Cleidocranial dysplasia (OMIM #119600; CCD) is a rare congenital autosomal disorder. Human genetics confirmed all kinds of mutations (dominant, recessive, and germ line mosaicism) in the RUNX2 sequence as the reason of the CCD [1–4]. Since RUNX2 (human 6p21) is a critical factor for both bone and cartilage development, the phenotype of CCD results from a disturbance in the intramembranous ossification, predominately, the skull and clavicles, but in severe cases, the entire skeleton might be affected [5, 6]. Individuals diagnosed with CCD are short and have either undeveloped or hypoplastic, thus hypermoving clavicles. The skull is brachycephalic with pronounced frontal and parietal bossing, midface hypoplasia, wide base of the nose, and depressed nasal bridge, coming in concert with the ocular hypertelorism. Severe dental abnormalities, which appear as a chaotic dentition, have been reported [7]. The most distinctive dental manifestations are the prolonged retention of deciduous teeth and delayed eruption of permanent teeth, which are impacted in the jaw bone next to the multiple supernumerary teeth [8]. The latter sporadically produce even a full set of additional dentition [7]. Due to the delayed eruption of permanent teeth and the limited space in the bone resulted from the existence of supernumerary teeth, the development of permanent teeth might be affected, reflecting ectopia and aberrant morphology especially in the roots, including taurodontism [9]. Thus, dental treatment of CCD positive patients is challenging and compels an interdisciplinary approach including surgery, orthodontics, conservative dentistry, and prosthodontics. It usually begins at youth, takes years, and beside an appropriate function, should address the patient's aesthetic expectations.

The aim of this paper was to present a prosthetic approach to the treatment of an adult patient with the CCD phenotype who suffered from the complicated outcome of the orthodontic treatment and was seeking the "profound improvement of her smile."

2. Case Presentation

A 29-year-old patient, clinically diagnosed with cleidocranial dysplasia, was searching for a "smile improvement." The patient was aware of all the limitations regarding the possible therapy due to her medical/dental condition, but still was determined to undergo any possible reconstruction to "make her smile visible". She presented short height and hypoplastic clavicles. Her head was slightly brachycephalic and exhibited frontal and parietal bossing. The nares were flared while the base of nose was depressed. Hypertelorism was also noted. The palate was gothic. At the time of appearance, the teeth were aligned but the crowns of the maxillary teeth were longer in width than height and completely invisible below the vermilion. Thus, the patient could have been mistaken as edentulous, even with the wide smile. The lower facial third was notably shorter than the middle and upper ones, respectively (Figures 1(a)–1(d)). Moreover, the patient complained about the pain and noise in the area of both temporomandibular joints (TMJ) while opening the mouth. TMJ reciprocal clicks were audible in both joints at the very beginning of mouth opening.

The patient's medical/dental history disclosed both orthodontic and surgical approaches, which began at the age of 16 due to the persistence of numerous deciduous teeth and unerupted permanent incisors, which significantly deteriorated her life quality. Panoramic radiographs revealed numerous imbedded permanent teeth in both arches and remaining deciduous teeth in the mandibular arch. In the maxilla, permanent teeth # 14, 13, 12, 11, 21, and 22 were imbedded, and both second premolars were lacking. In the mandible, there were persistent deciduous teeth # 75, 74, 73, 72, 82, 83, 84, and 85, imbedded permanent teeth #34, 33, 32, 42, 43, and 44, the lack of both second premolars, and all wisdom teeth. Despite the void of supernumerary teeth, the phenotype was specific for CCD (Figure 2) [8, 10]. According to the dental history, firstly, the embedded anterior permanent teeth were surgically exposed and orthodontically directed to the appropriate position in the maxilla. Fixed orthodontic appliance was used until the complete eruption, aligning, and leveling were achieved. Secondly, all primary lower teeth were extracted and the permanent teeth were exposed, followed by their alignment with the use of an orthodontic bracket. Although all permanent teeth were exposed in the mouth, lined, and set in the right position, the orthodontic treatment outcome did not meet the patient's aesthetic expectations.

The dental diagnosis was set after a comprehensive clinical and radiological examination (Figure 3) as well as extraoral picture analysis, which showed smile disharmony in accordance with both horizontal and midface axes. Specifically, the incisal plane was not parallel to the interpupillary line but ascended about 2 mm on the right. During the natural smile, the upper teeth were not exposed at all; the upper lip descended slightly on the right. The dental and facial midlines did not corelate, and the mandibular midline was deviated to the right side. The radiograph revealed absence of maxillary and mandibular second premolars, all wisdom teeth, and many abnormalities in the length and shape of roots, including taurodontism. A periapical lesion around the tooth # 36 was noticed as well as widening of the periodontal fissure around tooth #46 with unsatisfying root filling. We assumed the problems with the mandibular first molar periodontium might have been caused by excessive orthodontic forces and the occlusal overload.

The patient requested a reconstruction of the upper dental arch, exclusively. Since the patient's critical expectation was to make her smile visible, the reconstruction required an elongation of the upper incisors up to 10 mm, which at that time was twice as long as they were. Thus, the final treatment plan was divided into two phases.

2.1. Phase 1: Temporary Repositioning Occlusal Splint. In the first phase, which took over 11 months, the patient used the repositioning occlusal splint, with the recommendation to use it during the night and also during the day as often as possible. The main purpose of this treatment was to deprogram the muscles and rebuild the new occlusion including an increased occlusal vertical dimension (OVD). For the bite registration, we used the Arcus Digma II system by KaVo. Since our main concern was not to overcome the patent's physiological tolerance, initially, the lateral height of the splint was 3 mm, which allowed to keep the OVD in the envelope of function. The patient accepted the new vertical dimension very fast and reported an improvement in the masticatory muscles' relaxation. After each 4 months, the splint height was enlarged sequentially by 2 mm, up to 7 mm final increase of the initial OVD at the lateral parts of the splint (Figure 4).

2.2. Phase 2: Mock-up and Definitive Restoration. After over 11 months of preliminary treatment, the patient reported a complete subside of the TMJ pain and full acceptance of the new OVD. Hence, the final treatment was initiated on the wax-up formation, and the mock-up was set on the upper dental arch (Figure 5). The patient did not consent to surgical crown lengthening to harmonise the gingival margins of central incisors (black bars in Figure 5 indicate disharmony). For over a month, the patient used the mock-up, which increased the OVD about 7 mm and elongated the anterior teeth up to about 10 mm without any complains. Thus, after the next 4 weeks, the occlusal situation was checked with the Arcus Digma II system, and the final restorations were prepared. The posterior teeth (17, 16, 14, 24, 26, and 27) were prepared for the composite overlays, while the anterior teeth (13, 12, 11, 21, 22, and 23) for the ceramic veneers (Figures 6(a)–6(d)). Since the elongation of the incisors' crowns might have jeopardized the crown-to-root ratio, to enhance the stabilization of the anterior teeth, the orthodontic retainer was placed along the palatal surfaces of the teeth: 13, 12, 11, 21, 22, and 23 (Figure 6(b)). The patient was provided with the relaxation splint of the minimal ≤2 mm thickness to prevent the lower teeth from potential abrasion until completion of the lower arch rehabilitation. Unfortunately, since the patient was almost completely satisfied with the treatment of the upper arch, she eventually refused the lower arch reconstruction, so was warned that lack of the lower arch rehabilitation might cause future complications such as wear of the lower teeth.

To our surprise, even though the anterior teeth were elongated up to 10 mm and protruded the upper lip by about 2 mm, the patient claimed she would ask for an additional treatment (hyaluronic acid injection) to lift the upper lip to make the anterior teeth even more visible.

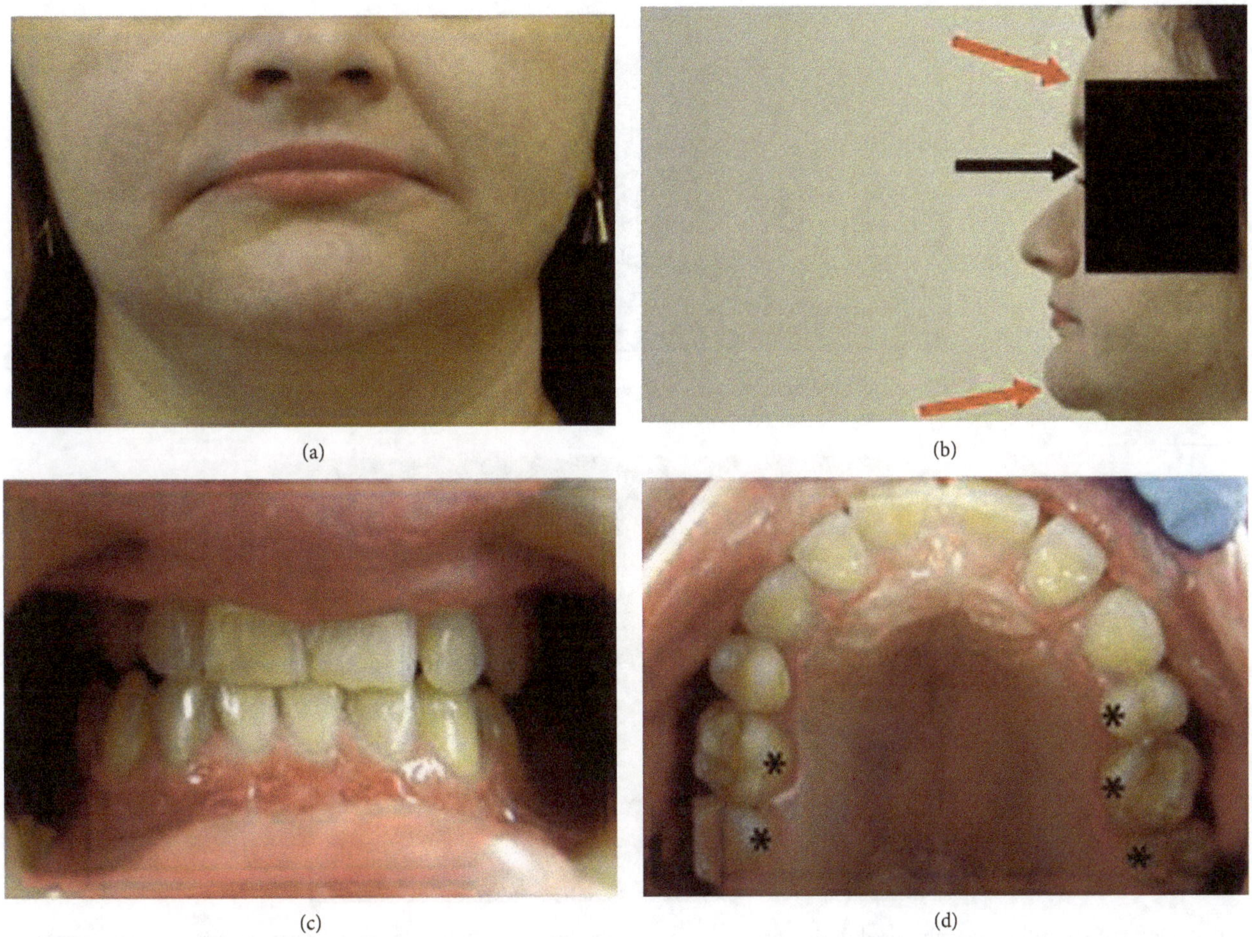

Figure 1: A 29-year-old patient with CCD. (a) Frontal view shows lowering corners of mouth and vermilion as well as deepening nasal-lip and chin wrinkles. (b) Profile view shows depressed nasal bridge (black arrow), frontal bossing, and prominent chin (red arrow). (c) Intraoral view before treatment shows disturbed proportions between height and width of maxillary anterior teeth with signs of tooth wear on incisal edges and posterior (right side) open bite. (d) Intraoral occlusal view of maxillary arch before treatment reveals gaps between teeth 21, 22, and 23. Tooth germs 15 and 25 are missing. Caries lesions in posterior teeth were noticed and had to be treated before placing overlays (asterisk).

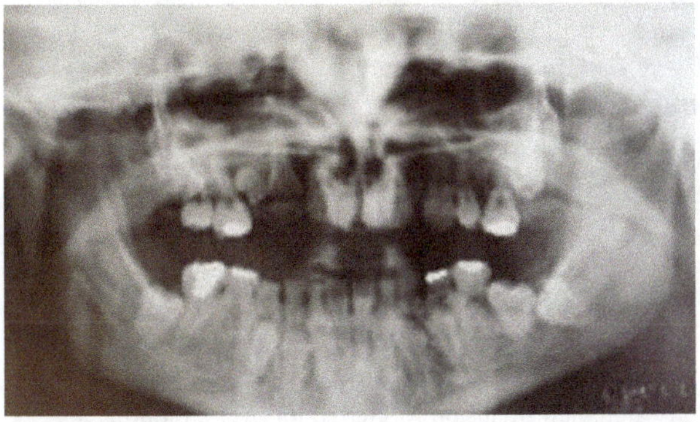

Figure 2: Panoramic radiograph taken at age of 16 before orthodontic treatment.

After 24-month observation, the entire reconstruction acted steadily (Figures 7(a) and 7(b)). A panoramic radiograph was taken for evaluation of periodontal soft and hard tissues and search of the potential periapical lesions (Figure 8). The tooth #36 had to be extracted due to a failed endodontic treatment, which the patient decided to conduct at her residence area due to pandemic reasons. At the same clinic, the patients underwent the conservative intervention in the cervical region of teeth # 24 and 26, which unfortunately exceeds the natural contour of the teeth. The patient request was to match the color of her restoration and natural tooth (Figure 6(d)). On the follow-up appointment, the elongated teeth showed neither hypermobilty nor hypersensitivity, and teeth vitality was followed with the ethylium chloride. The proper occlusal contacts (central and lateral) were checked with the 40 μm multicolor Bausch's articulation paper during every control appointment, and the ABC contacts were accepted as a reference point of the occlusion stability. From the patient's point of view, we followed any potential incidents of pain and/or muscle hypertension and TMJ clicking. During the observation time, none of the above was reported. The dental occlusion was stable and the patient did not report any muscle tension or TMJ clicking.

3. Discussion

Early diagnosis of the patients with CCD and subsequent surgical and orthodontic interventions lead to the best

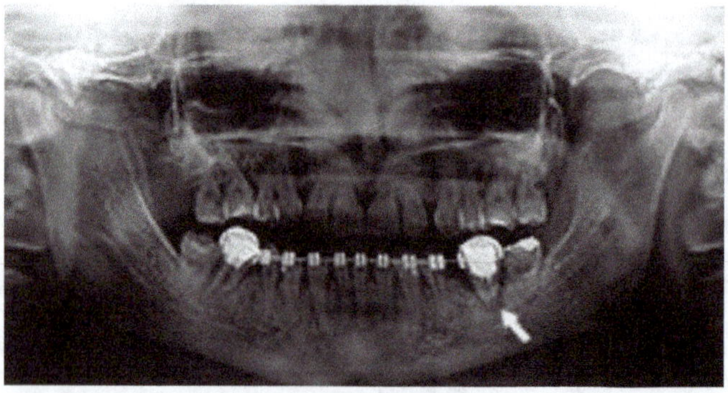

FIGURE 3: Panoramic radiograph taken at age of 29 right before prosthodontic treatment.

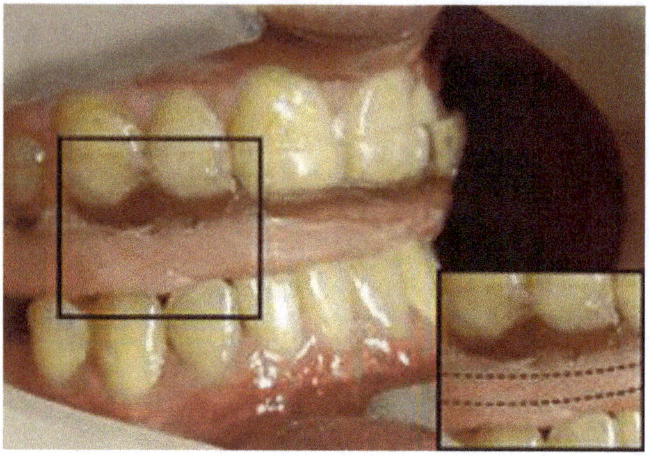

FIGURE 4: Occlusal repositioning splint used during first phase of prosthodontic treatment. In right corner, picture showing approximate thickness of each layer.

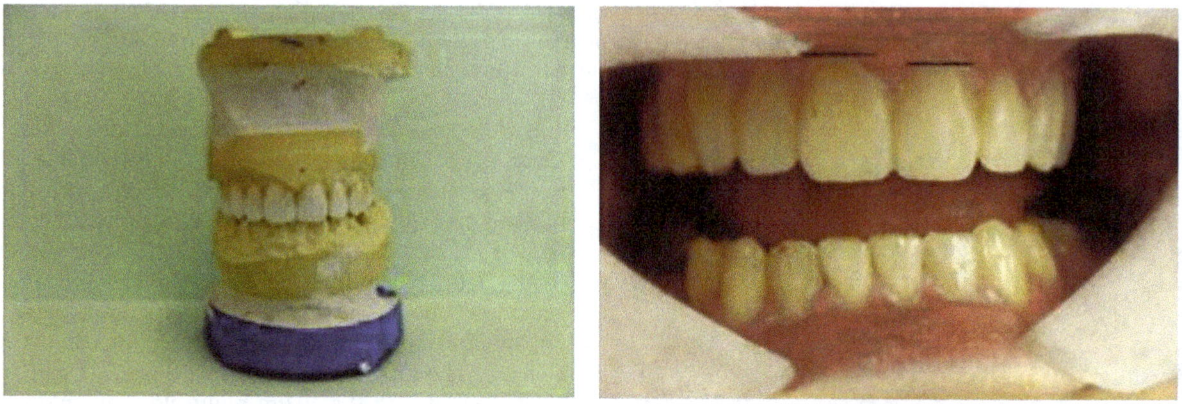

(a) (b)

FIGURE 5: (a) Wax-up of maxillary arch. (b) Mock-up of maxillary arch, new occlusion was tested for over a month.

orthognathic and orthodontic results. Sometimes, although delayed therapy and/or disrupted teeth development jeopardize the final outcome, thus, additional prosthetic intervention becomes indispensable. CCD, being a rare disorder, causes many uncertainties as no treatment guidelines are set. Thus far, the described approaches are concentrated on the close cooperation between a dental surgeon and an orthodontist and the suggestion that the treatment should start around the age of 9 [11, 12]. It is conceivable that the beginning of the therapy at the age of 16 limited only to surgery and orthodontics burdened the entire procedure with cardinal failure, which cost the patient a long-term struggle with masticatory disfunction, TMJs pathology, and unsatisfactory aesthetics. After thorough prosthetic evaluation, it was discovered that patent's complains arose from significantly diminished OVD and the unilateral open bite on the right

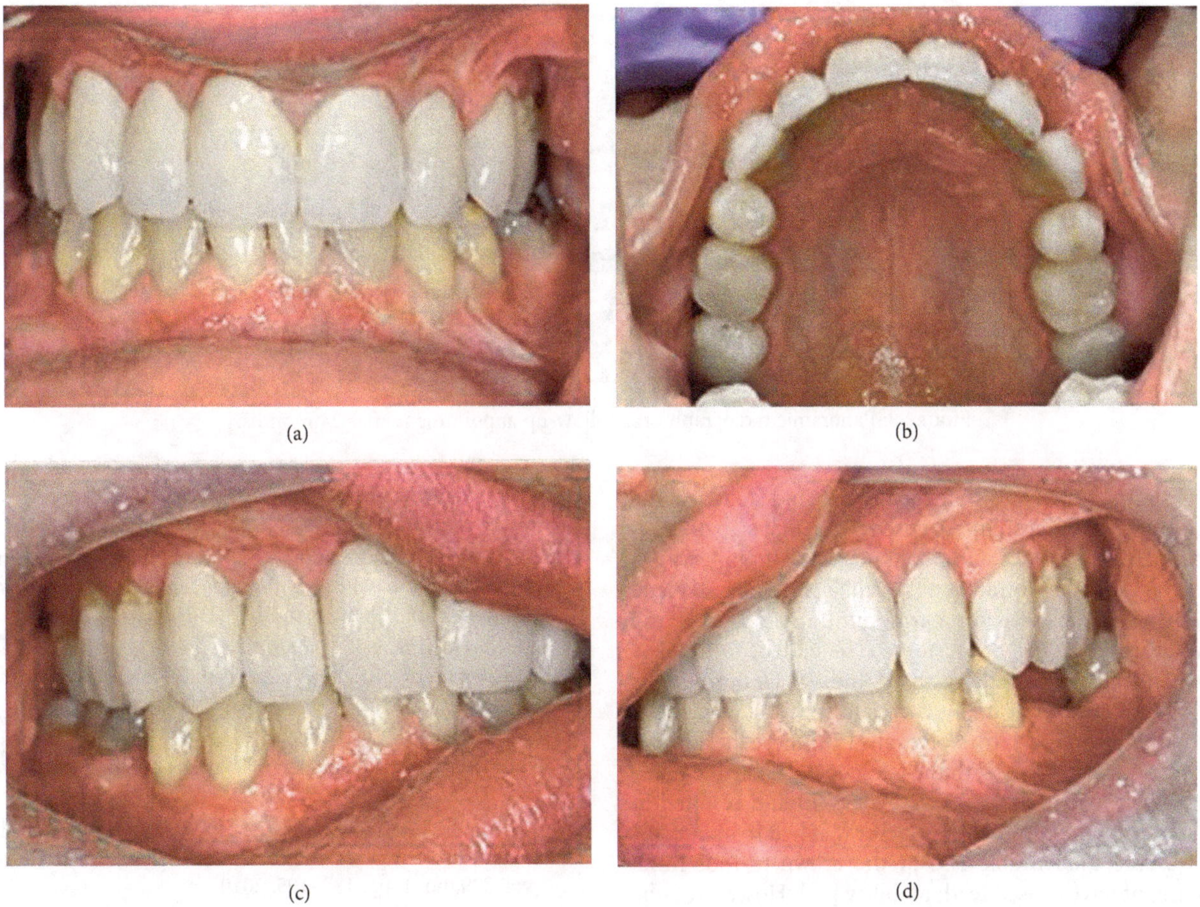

Figure 6: A 29-year-old patient with CCD. (a) Intraoral view of final restoration. It was patient's strong wish for restorations to be this bright, even though it did not match her natural teeth. (b) Intraoral occlusal view of maxillary arch after accomplished prosthodontic treatment. (c) Lateral view of the right side after 24 months follow-up. (d) Lateral view of the left side after 24 months follow-up.

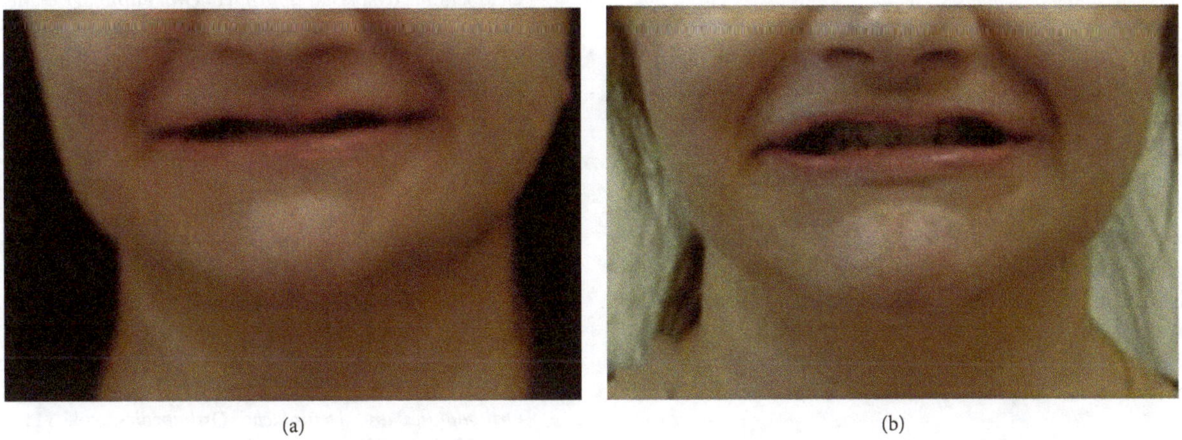

Figure 7: Comparison of facial appearance before (a) and after (b) treatment. (a) While smiling, maxillary teeth are not visible, giving impression that patient is edentulous. (b) Anterior teeth are visible during smile and dental midline correlates with facial midline.

side. Thus, the treatment plan focused on achieving maximum aesthetics but with the appropriate reestablishment of the OVD.

It is commonly known that patients adapt relatively easy towards an increased OVD when it is risen in the in the physiological range [13, 14]. However, even in such cases, muscle adaptation requires an appropriate period of time. Weinberg [15], stated that masticatory muscles showed minimal activity while remaining in the rest position and concluded that increasing the OVD to this point might relieve a patient from pain. To meet our patient's needs, the OVD had to not only be elevated up to 7 mm but also the madibule had to be

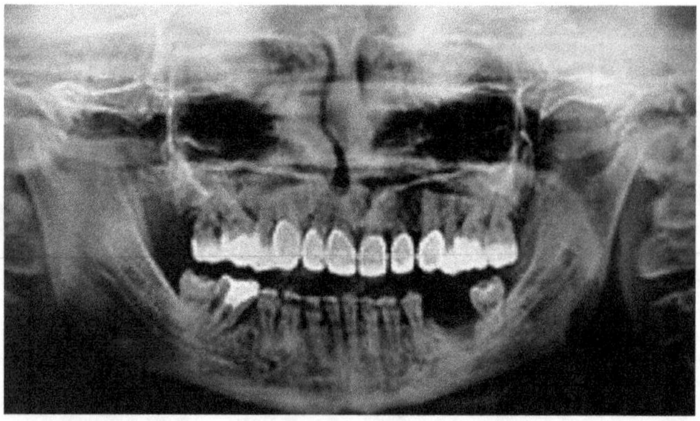

FIGURE 8: Panoramic radiograph on a follow-up appointment after 24 months.

slightly shifted to the left, so following the gold standard, the repositioning occlusal splint was used as the first step of prosthetic rehabilitation [16]. Our main goal at that point was to precisely guide the condyles to a stable muscular-skeletal position, which allowed for harmonic muscle stretch and relaxation and gradually accustomed the patient to the new OVD. The atraumatic increase of the OVD during our CCD patient treatment might correlate with the alternative prosthodontic approach by Noh et al. [17], where the authors treated the CCD patient with the telescopic detachable prosthesis, which increased the OVD by 11 mm and resulted in the stable outcome. Another risk factor that had to be considered was the unfavorable rise of the crown-to-root ratio, which might have caused teeth mobility [18]. However, Lulic et al. [19] claimed that even the severe loss of periodontium when maintained by meticulous oral hygiene and rigid splinting resulted in longtime survival.

4. Conclusions

This clinical report presents a prosthetic rehabilitation of a patient with CCD, who was unsatisfied with her smile and suffered from masticatory muscle pain after a long and demanding surgical and orthodontic treatment. Ultimately, the prosthetic treatment established the new occlusal plane and increased the OVD, which resulted in visibility of the anterior teeth while smiling and at rest. Moreover, bilateral stabilization of the posterior occlusion with the composite overlays relieved the pain, thus restoring the proper function and creating a pleasing facial appearance according to the patient's expectations.

Acknowledgments

The authors direct their appreciation to Mr. Piotr Stawowy for his assistance with language corrections.

References

[1] E. Hordyjewska-Kowalczyk, A. Sowińska-Seidler, E. M. Olech et al., "Functional analysis of novel RUNX2 mutations identified in patients with cleidocranial dysplasia," *Clinical Genetics*, vol. 96, no. 5, pp. 429–438, 2019.

[2] F. Otto, H. Kanegane, and S. Mundlos, "Mutations in the RUNX2 gene in patients with cleidocranial dysplasia," *Human Mutation*, vol. 19, no. 3, pp. 209–216, 2002.

[3] R. M. Goodman, R. Tadmor, A. Zaritsky, and S. A. Becker, "Evidence for an autosomal recessive form of cleidocranial dysostosis," *Clinical Genetics*, vol. 8, no. 1, pp. 20–29, 1975.

[4] T. Pal, D. Napierala, T. A. Becker et al., "The presence of germ line mosaicism in cleidocranial dysplasia," *Clinical Genetics*, vol. 71, no. 6, pp. 589–591, 2007.

[5] T. Komori, "Regulation of bone development and extracellular matrix protein genes by RUNX2," *Cell and Tissue Research*, vol. 339, no. 1, pp. 189–195, 2010.

[6] S. Mundlos, "Cleidocranial dysplasia: clinical and molecular genetics," *Journal of Medical Genetics*, vol. 36, no. 3, pp. 177–182, 1999.

[7] B. L. Jensen and S. Kreiborg, "Development of the dentition in cleidocranial dysplasia," *Journal of Oral Pathology & Medicine*, vol. 19, no. 2, pp. 89–93, 1990.

[8] S. Camilleri and F. McDonald, "Runx2 and dental development," *European Journal of Oral Sciences*, vol. 114, no. 5, pp. 361–373, 2006.

[9] J. L. Jarvis and T. E. Keats, "Cleidocranial DYSOSTOSIS," *American Journal of Roentgenology*, vol. 121, no. 1, pp. 5–16, 1974.

[10] A. Richardson and F. F. Deussen, "Facial and dental anomalies in cleidocranial dysplasia: a study of 17 cases," *International Journal of Paediatric Dentistry*, vol. 4, no. 4, pp. 225–231, 1994.

[11] A. Becker, A. Shteyer, E. Bimstein, and J. Lustmann, "Cleidocranial dysplasia: part 2—treatment protocol for the orthodontic and surgical modality," *American Journal of Orthodontics and Dentofacial Orthopedics*, vol. 111, no. 2, pp. 173–183, 1997.

[12] R. W. Berg, K. S. Kurtz, I. Watanabe, and I. Lambrakos, "Interim prosthetic phase of multidisciplinary management of cleidocranial dysplasia: "the Bronx approach"," *Journal of Prosthodontics*, vol. 20, pp. S20–S25, 2011.

[13] J. Abduo and K. Lyons, "Clinical considerations for increasing occlusal vertical dimension: a review," *Australian Dental Journal*, vol. 57, no. 1, pp. 2–10, 2012.

[14] E. J. Muts, H. van Pelt, D. Edelhoff, I. Krejci, and M. Cune, "Tooth wear: a systematic review of treatment options," *The*

Journal of Prosthetic Dentistry, vol. 112, no. 4, pp. 752–759, 2014.

[15] L. A. Weinberg, "Vertical dimension: a research and clinical analysis," *The Journal of Prosthetic Dentistry*, vol. 47, no. 3, pp. 290–302, 1982.

[16] J. A. De Boever, G. E. Carlsson, and I. J. Klineberg, "Need for occlusal therapy and prosthodontic treatment in the management of temporomandibular disorders. Part II: tooth loss and prosthodontic treatment," *Journal of Oral Rehabilitation*, vol. 27, no. 8, pp. 647–659, 2000.

[17] K. Noh, K. R. Kwon, H. Ahn, J. Paek, and A. Pae, "Prosthetic rehabilitation of a cleidocranial dysplasia patient with vertical maxillofacial deficiency: a clinical report," *Journal of Prosthodontics*, vol. 23, no. 1, pp. 64–70, 2014.

[18] Y. Grossmann and A. Sadan, "The prosthodontic concept of crown-to-root ratio: a review of the literature," *The Journal of Prosthetic Dentistry*, vol. 93, no. 6, pp. 559–562, 2005.

[19] M. Lulic, U. Bragger, N. P. Lang, M. Zwahlen, and G. E. Salvi, "Ante's (1926) law revisited: a systematic review on survival rates and complications of fixed dental prostheses (FDPs) on severely reduced periodontal tissue support," *Clinical Oral Implants Research*, vol. 18, pp. 63–72, 2007.

9

Effective and Efficient Correction of Severe Skeletal Class II Division 1 Malocclusion with Intermaxillary Elastics

Mohammed K. Badri

Department of Pedodontics & Orthodontics, College of Dentistry, Taibah University, Madinah, Saudi Arabia

Correspondence should be addressed to Mohammed K. Badri; mbadri@taibahu.edu.sa

Academic Editor: Khalid Zawawi

Treatment of Class II malocclusion accompanied with a skeletal discrepancy is challenging. The approach of correction depends on several factors such as the status and pattern of growth, severity of the malocclusion, and patient cooperation. This case report describes a successful management of a 12-year-old young adolescent boy that was presented with a Class II division 1 malocclusion with an underlying skeletal discrepancy in horizontal and vertical dimensions. Growth modification was achieved by means of bite opening and unlocking the mandible together with Class II elastics and mechanics. Treatment was highly effective and efficient by achieving all treatment goals within a period of 18 months.

1. Introduction

Class II dental malocclusion considered as the second most prevalent malocclusion after Class I, with a prevalence range of 13%-24% [1–5]. As described and categorized by Edward Angle more than a century ago, Class II division 1 malocclusion is characterized by distal occlusion of the lower first molars by at least a half cusp width in relation to upper first molars resulting in locking of the mandible in a distal position. Moreover, specific traits of this division were the protrusion of the upper incisors and interruption of the relation of upper and lower incisors by the lower lip [6, 7]. Nevertheless, Class II malocclusion often accompanied by a skeletal discrepancy that could be caused by either a deficient mandible, excessive growth of maxilla, or a combination of both [8, 9].

Treatment approach and modality for Class II division 1 with an underlying skeletal problem depend on several factors that should be considered by the clinicians such as chronological age, growth potential, skeletal maturity, severity of the condition, and patient motivation and cooperation [10, 11]. The treatment options for growing patients with such malocclusion mainly based on growth modification on an exact time-frame taking advantage of the adolescent growth spurt. Failure to initiate proper treatment within the proper timing will lead to deviation of treatment option towards camouflage or even orthognathic surgery. Treating growing adolescents could involve the use of Class II elastics, headgear, or functional appliances in order to restrain further maxillary growth and promote favorable mandibular growth.

Several studies showed that over the long-term treatment results achieved with Class II elastics are similar or comparable to those achieved with functional appliances, given that treatment started at an appropriate timing [12–17]. Both Class II elastics and functional appliances contributed to correction of the malocclusion by skeletal and dental changes, but Class II elastics resulted in a more dentoalveolar modification [17–19]. Several dentofacial changes are associated with the use of Class II elastics such as maxillary retraction, mandibular protraction, increase of lower anterior facial height, clockwise rotation of the occlusal plane, retroclination of maxillary incisors, proclination of mandibular incisors, and forward movement and extrusion of mandibular molars [16–22]. Most of the effects of Class II elastics are favorable, but in order to control any unwanted side effects, a good case selection and application of appropriate biomechanics should be considered by the orthodontist.

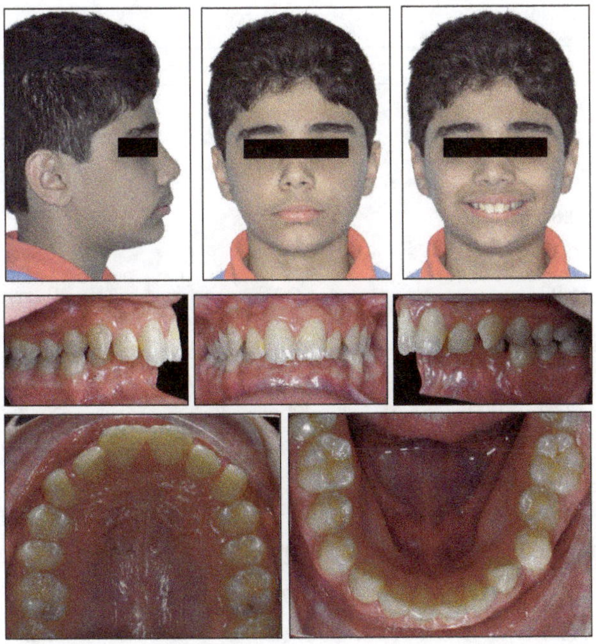

FIGURE 1: Pretreatment facial and intraoral photographs.

In the current case report, we discuss the treatment of a Class II division 1 malocclusion accompanied with a severe Class II skeletal discrepancy and hypodivergent growth pattern in a growing adolescent.

2. Diagnosis and Etiology

12 years and 8 months young boy referred to the orthodontic specialty clinic with a chief complaint of "protruded front teeth". Medical and dental history indicated no significant findings. Extraoral clinical examination revealed a symmetrical euryprosopic face type, convex soft tissue profile, retruded mandible, deep mentolabial sulcus, decreased lower facial third, and on smiling lower lip was trapped by the upper central incisors (Figure 1).

Intraoral and dental cast examination showed Class II division 1 malocclusion with full-step molars and canines bilaterally, severe overjet of 9 mm, overerupted lower incisors with deep (100%) impinging overbite, deep curve of Spee (COS) of 3 mm, and unilateral posterior cross-bite on the upper left 1st and 2nd molars. Mild anterior crowding with rotated canines (uppers rotated disto-palatal and lowers rotated mesio-lingual). Patient had poor oral hygiene, plaque accumulation, and mild gingival inflammation. All permanent teeth are erupted while the 3rd molars are still developing (Figures 1–3).

Cephalometric analysis revealed a severe skeletal Class II relationship (ANB = 7.8°) with horizontal growth pattern tendency (hypodivergent mandibular plane angle, MPA = 28.1°, FMA = 19.6°), and anterior facial height is markedly reduced. Cervical vertebral maturation (CVM) indicates cervical stage 1 (CS1). Lower incisors are proclined (L1 – MP = 99.3°), and both lips are anterior to the E-line by 1 mm (Figure 3 and Table 1).

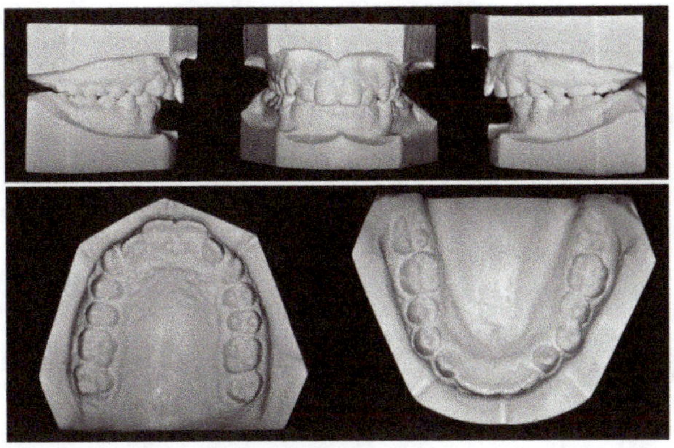

FIGURE 2: Pretreatment orthodontic study models.

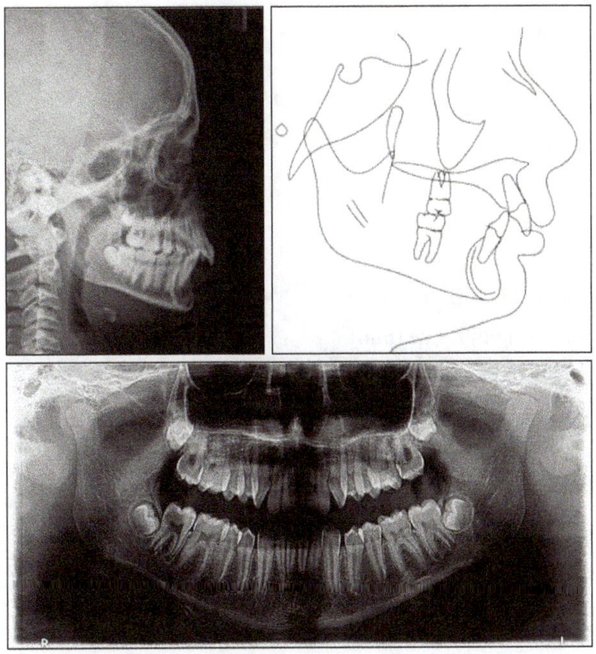

FIGURE 3: Pretreatment radiographs and tracing.

3. Treatment Objectives

The following were the list of treatment objectives: (1) improve the sagittal and vertical skeletal relationships; (2) enhance and guide mandibular growth; (3) resolve increased overjet; (4) establish Class I canine and molar relationship; (5) resolve the impinging overbite, deep COS, and traumatic occlusion; (6) resolve the left posterior cross bite; (7) resolve crowding and rotations; and (8) improve facial profile and smile esthetics.

4. Treatment Alternatives

Given the patient's age and problem list, a nonsurgical and nonextraction treatment plan based on growth modification to enhance mandibular growth was developed. The primary plan presented to the patient and his family was to start with growth modification using a removable Class II functional appliance or cervical pull headgear with anterior bite plane

Table 1: Cephalometric measurements.

Measurement	Pretreatment	Posttreatment	1-year follow-up	Norm
Skeletal (sagittal)				
SNA (°)	85.8	81.5	82	82 ± 3.5
SNB (°)	78	76.7	77.5	80 ± 3.5
ANB (°)	7.8	4.8	4.5	2 ± 2
Wits (mm)	5.6	0.4	1	5
Convexity (NA-APg) (°)	12.9	6.9	6.2	0 ± 5
Skeletal (vertical)				
SN-MP (°)	28.1	31	30.8	32 ± 5
FMA (°)	19.6	21.4	21.2	24 ± 4.5
Y-axis (SGn/SN) (°)	64.7	68.1	68	67 ± 5.5
Dental				
U1-SN (°)	101.5	93.6	96.2	103 ± 5.5
U1-NA (mm)	2.8	0.7	2	4.3 ± 2.7
Interincisal angle (°)	132	123.6	127.6	130 ± 6
L1-MP (°)	99.3	111.5	105.8	95 ± 7
L1-NB (mm)	4.1	5.6	5.5	4 ± 1.8
Soft tissue				
Nasolabial angle (°)	118.2	111.7	116.6	102 ± 8
Upper lip to E-line (mm)	0.8	-1.8	-1.2	−4 ± 2
Lower lip to E-line (mm)	1.3	-1.2	-2.4	−2 ± 2

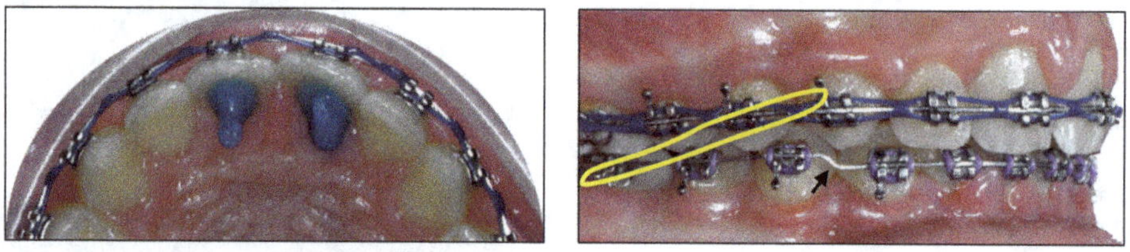

(a) (b)

Figure 4: (a) Anterior bite turbo cemented on palatal of maxillary central incisors. (b) The use of reverse COS in the lower arch wire, step down bends (black arrow) for lower anterior teeth, and Class II elastic bands (yellow imaginary band).

followed by leveling and aligning with a fixed edgewise appliance. The option was not considered by the family due to increased cost from the use of additional device. In addition, the treatment duration could be prolonged especially if it was divided into two phases. Therefore, an alternative plan addressing those concerns was presented which involved bonding a fixed edgewise appliance, anterior bite turbo, and simultaneous growth modification using intermaxillary elastics taking advantage of the patient's early adolescence and prepubertal stage of development.

5. Treatment Progress

The patient demonstrated a poor oral hygiene and few carious lesions, so before starting orthodontic treatment, oral hygiene instructions were given, and patient was referred for periodontal and restorative clearance.

Once cleared, a full-fixed straight wire appliance of slot size $0.022'' \times 0.028''$ MBT was bonded in both arches. Leveling and aligning lasted for 6 months, which were achieved by the following NiTi wire sequence ($0.014''$, $0.016''$, $0.018''$, $0.016'' \times 0.022''$) then followed by stainless steel (SS) working wires ($0.016'' \times 0.022''$, $0.018'' \times 0.025''$, and $0.019'' \times 0.025''$). SS arch wire expansion and criss-cross elastic from palatal of upper left first molar to buccal of lower left molar were used to correct the unilateral posterior cross bite on left molars.

In addition, to address the vertical and sagittal skeletal problems, anterior bite turbos palatal to upper central incisors were cemented (Figure 4(a)); gradual step-down of lower anterior teeth (total of 3 mm) and reverse curve of Spee were implemented by the lower SS arch wires (Figure 4(b)). Moreover, Class II intermaxillary elastics were started using light forces then replaced by medium force elastics as we progressed in treatment (Figure 4(b)).

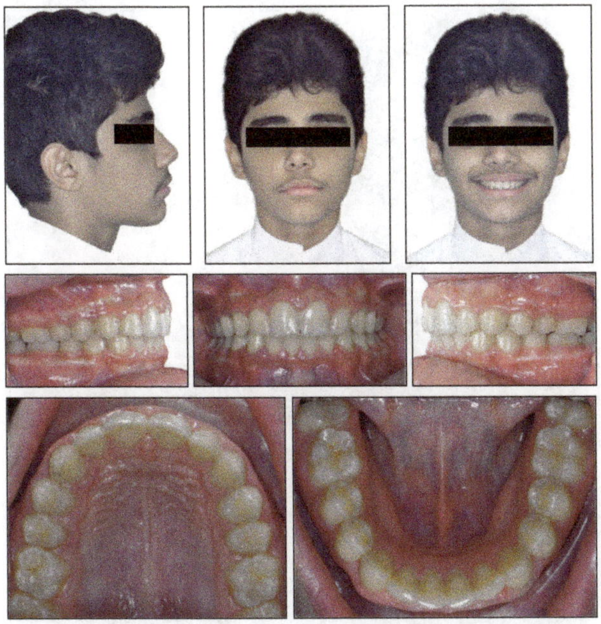

FIGURE 5: Posttreatment facial and intraoral photographs.

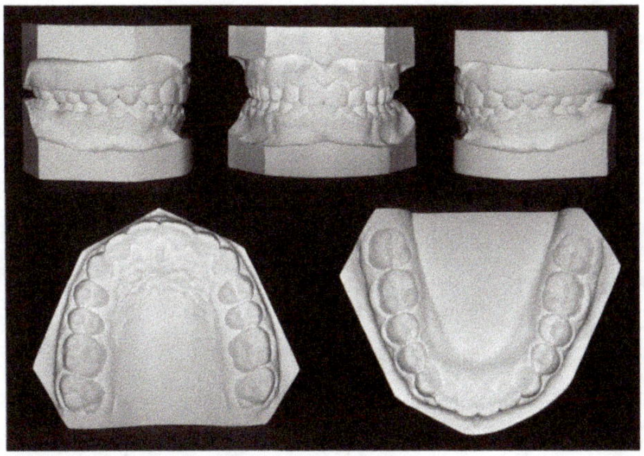

FIGURE 6: Posttreatment orthodontic study models.

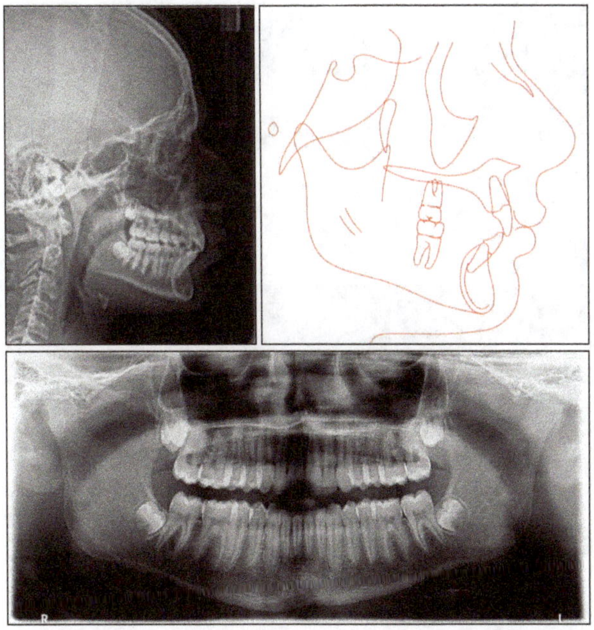

FIGURE 7: Posttreatment radiographs and tracing.

After 10 months in treatment, the antro-posterior canines and molars relationships were corrected. Final detailing and finishing included arch wire adjustments and power chain use for some remaining spaces closure. The fixed appliance was debonded after 18 months of active treatment. Clear vacuum retainers were delivered, and after 1 month, they were replaced by Hawley retainers with anterior bite plate on the upper appliance.

6. Treatment Results

The overall outcome of treatment was successful, and the patient's chief complaint was addressed. Treatment objectives were achieved in an efficient treatment duration (18 months and 14 visits). The skeletal and dental relationships were significantly improved. Facial profile showed great improvement as facial proportions were restored, mandible was advanced, convexity was reduced, and restored normal mentolabial sulcus. Moreover, smile esthetics were improved, and lip position was corrected with no entrapment (Figure 5). Intraoral photographs and dental models showed that Class I canine and molar were established both sides, normal overjet and overbite were achieved, and correction of deep COS and overerupted lower incisors. The unilateral posterior cross bite on left side molars was corrected with resulted increase in intermolar width of upper arch (Figures 5 and 6).

Lateral cephalometric analysis and superimposition showed significant skeletal improvement in sagittal and vertical dimensions with clockwise rotation of the mandible. Antro-posterior skeletal relationship changed from pretreatment (ANB 7.8°, Wits 5.6 mm) to posttreatment (ANB 4.8°, Wits 0.4 mm), facial convexity decreased from 12.9° to 6.9°, mandibular plane angle increased from (SN-MP 28.1°, FMA 19.6°) to (SN-MP 31°, FMA 21.4°), total face height (Na-Gn) increased from 105.2 mm to 116.9 mm, lower face height (ANS-Gn) increased from 59.7 mm to 65.5 mm, and the hypodivergent growth pattern improved from (y-axis 64.7°) to (y-axis 68.1°). Maxillary incisors were retroclined, and the deep bite was corrected by relative intrusion of a combination of molar extrusion and mandibular incisors intrusion and proclination. In addition, mandibular molars moved mesially while maxillary molars slightly distalized (Figures 7 and 8, Table 1).

At 1-year follow-up, the occlusion was stable with no significant relapse, and the patient demonstrated poor oral hygiene with mild gingival inflammation (Figure 9). Lateral cephalometric superimposition showed that both maxilla and mandible still growing in a favorable downward and forward direction and sagittal and vertical relations are maintained. Maxillary incisors slightly proclined while mandibular incisors slightly extruded, and its inclination to mandibular plane was improved (Figures 8 and 10, Table 1).

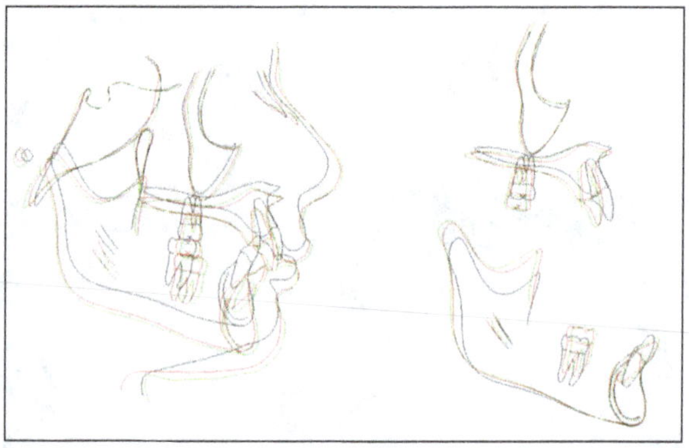

FIGURE 8: Superimposition of pretreatment (black), posttreatment (red), and follow up (green) lateral cephalograms.

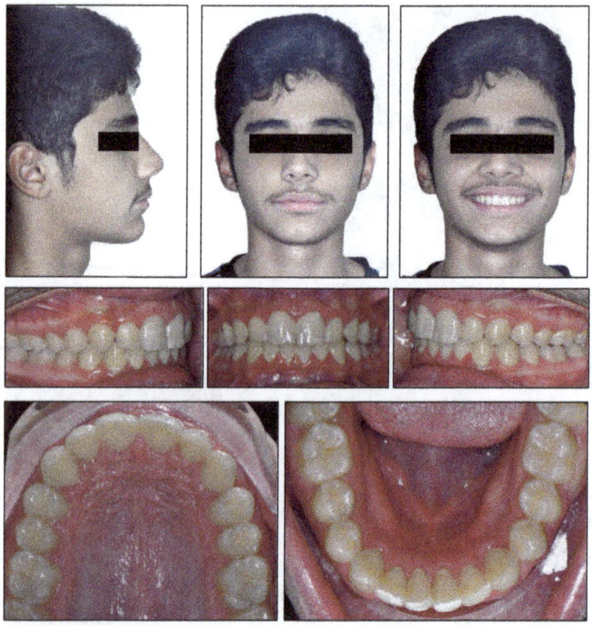

FIGURE 9: 1-year follow-up facial and intraoral photographs.

7. Discussion

This case report showed a successful management of a 12-year-old adolescent boy presented with a Class II division 1 malocclusion accompanied with a severe skeletal Class II discrepancy. Several key factors contributed to the success of this treatment mainly including early intervention at prepubertal stage, pattern of skeletal growth, patient's cooperation, and mechanics applied.

The time of intervention in this case was of great impact in correcting the skeletal discrepancy. The treatment started when the patient was in the prepubertal stage of growth. The patient was at early stage of CVM (CS1, Figure 3), secondary sexual characteristics did not appear, and no significant increase in patient's height during the last 2 years, indicating that the growth spurt was yet to be hit. At posttreatment time point, the patient was in the postpubertal stage of maturity marked by the CVM (early CS4, Figure 7), appearance of secondary sexual characteristics (such as facial hair and hoarse voice), and noticeable increase in height, thus indicating that growth spurt had hit during treatment. At the 1-year follow-up with a CVM of early CS5 (Figure 10), patient showed further mandibular growth with an increase of 2 mm in length; however, the mandibular growth spurt occurred during treatment with an increase of 6.7 mm (Co-Gn at pretreatment = 111.3 mm, Co-Gn at posttreatment = 118 mm, Co-Gn at follow – up = 120 mm). Cases of severe Class II skeletal problems are better to be treated as early as possible and to take advantage of the patient's growth spurt [9, 15]. Moreover, regardless the type of intervention, the earlier the treatment, the greater the impact on mandibular growth [23] and the more stable the results are on the long term [15].

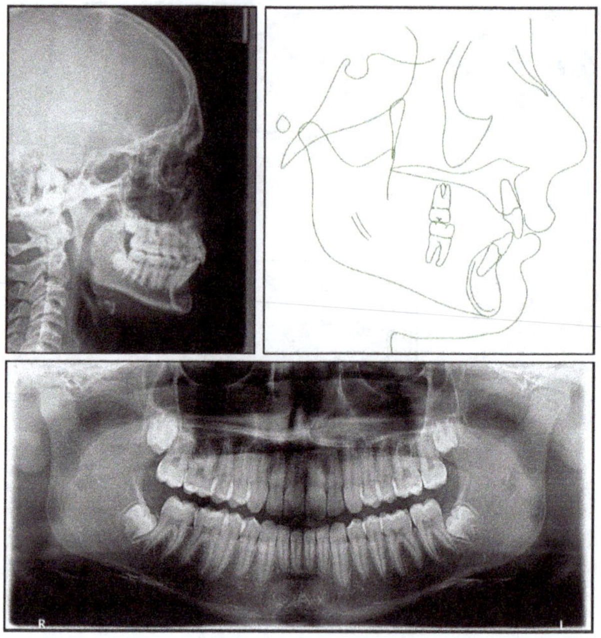

FIGURE 10: 1-year follow-up radiographs and tracing.

In the current case, upon opening the patient's bite and releasing the locked mandible from the impinging overbite, a great improvement in sagittal skeletal relation was achieved. Angle indicated that in Class II malocclusion, the lower dentition is locked in distal occlusion, and thereby, the mandible will be locked as well [6]. Several studies advocated that dental and occlusal interferences will restrict normal range of movement of the mandible by displacing it in a more posterior position and will hinder its normal growth [24–26]. Removal of such interferences by opening the bite will allow the mandible to shift forward, establish normal range of movement, reposition the condyles in the center of the fossae, and promote mandibular growth, thus reducing the sagittal skeletal discrepancy [9, 24–28]. In a study of 60 patients with Class II deep bite of hypodivergent and normodivergent vertical relations, they showed great forward movement of the mandible with normal growth after bite opening [28].

It was well noticed that most of the sagittal discrepancy was improved after removing the restriction from the impinging deep bite and unlocking the mandible, while the use of Class II intermaxillary elastics was for a short period still effective to add to the final sagittal correction. Class II elastics carried out further guidance and enhancement of mandibular growth toward normal skeletal relation, added considerable restriction to the growth of the maxilla, and improved the vertical skeletal relationship (Table 1). Despite the correction of the sagittal skeletal problem and the increase in the mandibular body and ramus size, the patient did not show increase in the SNB angle (Table 1). This could be explained by the backward rotation of the occlusal plane and mandible from Class II elastics and mechanics used [18, 20, 22]. In hypodivergent growing patients, bite opening is achieved by incisors intrusion, molars eruption, or a combination of both. If the amount of molar extrusion overcame the amount of vertical condylar growth, a backward mandibular rotation will occur [27]. Therefore, a better reflection of the sagittal results will be using the Wits appraisal [29], and in this study, Wits improved significantly from 5.4 mm at pretreatment to 0.4 mm at posttreatment indicating Class I skeletal relationship (Table 1).

The vertical skeletal relationship improved significantly from the correction of the deep bite by use of reverse COS wires, Class II elastics, and bite turbos. Those mechanics helped to extrude the molars, intrude and procline the incisors, and facilitate further mandibular growth. As mentioned earlier, with Class II elastics, there is a clockwise rotation of the occlusal plane and mandible with a final outcome of increase in lower anterior face height [18, 20, 22]. Such changes considered to be highly favorable in the current case which helped improve the hypodivergent vertical relationship.

The skeletal growth pattern of the patient was a favorable adjunct in the management of his case and helped in accommodating the current treatment plan. The vertically hypodivergent mandibular plane angle, the forward rotation of the mandible, and the underdeveloped anterior face height facilitated in toleration of the applied extrusive mechanics and the resulted backward rotation of the mandible. On the opposite, cases of vertical growth pattern with high mandibular plane angle are challenging and difficult to treat, and applying such extrusive mechanics should be avoided as they would deteriorate the final results and will not work in favor of the patients while more control of the vertical dimension should be considered [30].

Among the challenges that were faced in this case was to maximize the orthopedic changes using Class II elastics while minimizing elastics possible side effects. Proclination of lower incisors was significantly increased (Table 1) from Class II elastics, reserve wires use, and correction of deep COS. Such side effect could have been minimized if strict anchorage preparation was applied. Tweed advocated for rigorous anchorage preparation prior to the application of Class II elastics and mechanics in order to avoid proclination of anterior teeth [31]. In addition, Class II skeletal cases with excellent anchorage preparation prior to treatment showed greater orthopedic effects (such as maxillary retraction and mandibular protraction) comparing to cases treated with no anchorage preparation [21].

8. Conclusion

Class II elastics considered a viable orthodontic option for correcting Class II skeletal discrepancy in growing patients, given the careful case selection based on timing of growth spurt, pattern of skeletal development, severity of the malocclusion, and patient's cooperation and motivation.

Moreover, orthodontists should consider the benefits and potential side effects of Class II elastics use, plan that in the treatment, and be able to handle and direct them to the patient's favor once executed in treatment.

References

[1] S. Al-Emran and P. J. Wisth, "Prevalence of malocclusion and need for orthodontic treatment in Saudi Arabia," *Community Dentistry and Oral Epidemiology*, vol. 18, no. 5, pp. 253–255, 1990.

[2] W. R. Proffit, H. W. Fields Jr., and L. J. Moray, "Prevalence of malocclusion and orthodontic treatment need in the United States: estimates from the NHANES III survey," *The International Journal of Adult Orthodontics and Orthognathic Surgery*, vol. 13, no. 2, pp. 97–106, 1998.

[3] C. O. Onyeaso, G. A. Aderinokun, and M. O. Arowojolu, "The pattern of malocclusion among orthodontic patients seen in Dental Centre, University College Hospital, Ibadan, Nigeria," *African Journal of Medicine and Medical Sciences*, vol. 31, no. 3, pp. 207–211, 2002.

[4] M. O. Sayin and H. Türkkahraman, "Malocclusion and crowding in an orthodontically referred Turkish population," *The Angle Orthodontist*, vol. 74, no. 5, pp. 635–639, 2004.

[5] M. A. AlQarni, A. H. Banihuwaiz, F. D. Alshehri, A. S. Alqarni, and D. S. Alasmari, "Evaluate the malocclusion in subjects reporting for orthodontic treatment among Saudi population in Asser region," *Journal of International Oral Health*, vol. 6, no. 4, pp. 42–46, 2014.

[6] E. H. Angle, *Treatment of Malocclusion of the Teeth: Angle's System*, S.S. White dental manufacturing Company, Philadelphia, PA, USA, 7th edition, 1907.

[7] W. R. Proffit, H. W. Fields, B. E. Larson, and D. M. Sarver, *Contemporary Orthodontics*, Mosby Elsevier, St. Louis, MO, USA, 2019.

[8] R. E. Moyers, M. L. Riolo, K. E. Guire, R. L. Wainright, and F. L. Bookstein, "Differential diagnosis of class II malocclusions," *American Journal of Orthodontics*, vol. 78, no. 5, pp. 477–494, 1980.

[9] S. E. Bishara, "Class II malocclusions: diagnostic and clinical considerations with and without treatment," *Seminars in Orthodontics*, vol. 12, no. 1, pp. 11–24, 2006.

[10] W. R. Proffit, C. Phillips, J. F. Tulloch, and P. H. Medland, "Surgical versus orthodontic correction of skeletal class II malocclusion in adolescents: effects and indications," *The International Journal of Adult Orthodontics and Orthognathic Surgery*, vol. 7, no. 4, pp. 209–220, 1992.

[11] J. F. Camilla Tulloch, B. E. Lenz, and C. Phillips, "Surgical versus orthodontic correction for class II patients: age and severity in treatment planning and treatment outcome," *Seminars in Orthodontics*, vol. 5, no. 4, pp. 231–240, 1999.

[12] A. A. Gianelly, S. A. Arena, and L. Bernstein, "A comparison of class II treatment changes noted with the light wire, edgewise,

and Fränkel appliances," *American Journal of Orthodontics*, vol. 86, no. 4, pp. 269–276, 1984.

[13] S. T. Adenwalla and J. H. Kronman, "Class II, division 1 treatment with Fränkel and Edgewise appliances-a comparative study of mandibular growth and facial esthetics," *The Angle Orthodontist*, vol. 55, no. 4, pp. 281–298, 1985.

[14] L. Weichbrodt and B. Ingervall, "Treatment of class II, div. 1 malocclusion with the activator and with the Begg technique," *Schweizer Monatsschrift fur Zahnmedizin*, vol. 102, no. 9, pp. 1037–1045, 1992.

[15] B. Nelson, U. Hägg, K. Hansen, and M. Bendeus, "A long-term follow-up study of class II malocclusion correction after treatment with class II elastics or fixed functional appliances," *American Journal of Orthodontics and Dentofacial Orthopedics*, vol. 132, no. 4, pp. 499–503, 2007.

[16] G. Jones, P. H. Buschang, K. B. Kim, and D. R. Oliver, "Class II non-extraction patients treated with the Forsus fatigue resistant device versus intermaxillary elastics," *The Angle Orthodontist*, vol. 78, no. 2, pp. 332–338, 2008.

[17] G. Janson, R. Sathler, T. M. F. Fernandes, N. C. C. Branco, and M. R. de Freitas, "Correction of class II malocclusion with class II elastics: a systematic review," *American Journal of Orthodontics and Dentofacial Orthopedics*, vol. 143, no. 3, pp. 383–392, 2013.

[18] B. Nelson, K. Hansen, and U. Hägg, "Class II correction in patients treated with class II elastics and with fixed functional appliances: a comparative study," *American Journal of Orthodontics and Dentofacial Orthopedics*, vol. 118, no. 2, pp. 142–149, 2000.

[19] S. Jayachandran, W. A. Wiltshire, S. M. Hayasaki, and F. H. S. L. Pinheiro, "Comparison of AdvanSync and intermaxillary elastics in the correction of class II malocclusions: a retrospective clinical study," *American Journal of Orthodontics and Dentofacial Orthopedics*, vol. 150, no. 6, pp. 979–988, 2016.

[20] C. M. Stewart, S. J. Chaconas, and A. A. Caputo, "Effects of intermaxillary elastic traction on orthodontic tooth movement," *Journal of Oral Rehabilitation*, vol. 5, no. 2, pp. 159–166, 1978.

[21] A. E. Phelps, "A comparison of lower face changes," *The Angle Orthodontist*, vol. 48, no. 4, pp. 283–290, 1978.

[22] B. Zimmer and D. Nischwitz, "Therapeutic changes in the occlusal plane inclination using intermaxillary elastics," *Journal of Orofacial Orthopedics*, vol. 73, no. 5, pp. 377–386, 2012.

[23] T. Baccetti, L. Franchi, and J. A. McNamara, "The cervical vertebral maturation (CVM) method for the assessment of optimal treatment timing in dentofacial orthopedics," *Seminars in Orthodontics*, vol. 11, no. 3, pp. 119–129, 2005.

[24] L. S. Timmons, "Induced change in the anteroposterior relationship of the jaws," *The Angle Orthodontist*, vol. 42, no. 3, pp. 245–251, 1972.

[25] C. F. Gugino and I. Dus, "Unlocking orthodontic malocclusions: an interplay between form and function," *Seminars in Orthodontics*, vol. 4, no. 4, pp. 246–255, 1998.

[26] T. A. Sellke, "Zero base bioprogressive: unlocking the door to the future," *Seminars in Orthodontics*, vol. 4, no. 4, pp. 210–218, 1998.

[27] R. I. Levin, "Deep bite treatment in relation to mandibular growth rotation," *European Journal of Orthodontics*, vol. 13, no. 2, pp. 86–94, 1991.

[28] M. G. Woods, "Sagittal mandibular changes with overbite correction in subjects with different mandibular growth directions: late mixed-dentition treatment effects," *American Journal of Orthodontics and Dentofacial Orthopedics*, vol. 133, no. 3, pp. 388–394, 2008.

[29] A. Jacobson, "The "Wits" appraisal of jaw disharmony. 1975," *American Journal of Orthodontics and Dentofacial Orthopedics*, vol. 124, no. 5, pp. 470–479, 2003.

[30] P. Cozza, A. Marino, and L. Franchi, "A nonsurgical approach to treatment of high-angle class II malocclusion," *The Angle Orthodontist*, vol. 78, no. 3, pp. 553–560, 2008.

[31] C. H. Tweed, "The application of the principles of the edgewise arch in the treatment of class II, division 1, malocclusion," *The Angle Orthodontist*, vol. 6, no. 3, pp. 198–208, 1936.

10

Comprehensive Management of Ectodermal Dysplasia with Interceptive Orthodontics in a Young Boy Who was Bullied at School

A. A. A. K. Wimalarathna,[1] **W. B. M. C. R. D. Weerasekara**,[2] **and E. M. U. C. K. Herath**[2]

[1]*Department of Prosthetic Dentistry, Faculty of Dental Sciences, University of Peradeniya, Sri Lanka*
[2]*Department of Community Dental Health, Faculty of Dental Sciences, University of Peradeniya, Sri Lanka*

Correspondence should be addressed to A. A. A. K. Wimalarathna; arunaw@dental.pdn.ac.lk

Academic Editor: Leandro Napier de Souza

Aim. The management of hypohidrotic ectodermal dysplasia with oligodontia in Class-I malocclusion in late mix dentition. *Case Report.* An 11-year-old boy with ED was treated and managed by means of interceptive orthodontic treatment accompanied by direct and indirect restorative methods in a successful manner. The patient was prepared to receive definitive oral rehabilitation with dental implants for the missing teeth when the patient reaches a suitable age. The patient was followed for 5 years from the beginning of treatment. *Conclusion.* Management of the child with ectodermal dysplasia with oligodontia was a real challenge. Early diagnosis, necessary investigation, and providing age-appropriate multidisciplinary treatment were key steps in successful outcomes. The objectives were not only just orthodontic or paedodontics but also prosthetic and psychological.

1. Introduction

The term ectodermal dysplasia (ED) is described as a rare heterogeneous group of congenital disorders which is characterized by defects of two or more ectodermaly derived tissues [1]. These are primarily the nails, skin, hair, sweat glands, and teeth [2]. Though only eight forms of ED were identified by 1971, currently, it comprises more than 200 different types; about 30% have been identified at the molecular level with identification of the causative genes [3].

According to the mode of inheritance, ED can be classified into autosomal dominant, autosomal recessive, or X-linked. Hypodontia, hypohidrosis, and hypotrichosis are a triad of clinical features characteristic of the hypohidrotic form [4]. Based on the function and number of sweat glands, ED can be broadly divided into two clinically distinguished forms: first, autosomal dominant hidrotic type (Clouston's syndrome) with normal sweat glands, and second, the X-linked recessive anhidrotic or hypohidrotic type (Christ-Siemens-Touraine Syndrome) with absent or diminished sweat glands. The X-linked trait is the most common phenotype with an incidence of 1-7 per 100,000 live births, with 28% of mortality rate in males up to 3 years of age [3].

Patients with ED can easily be recognized from normal individuals by their typical facial and clinical features such as frontal bossing, prominent supraorbital ridges, sunken cheeks, wrinkles and periorbital hyperpigmentation, saddle nose, everted lips, large low-set ears, dysplastic nails, and reduced lower facial height [2]. Occasionally some of them have asthma and eczema [5].

Dental manifestations include multiple congenitally missing teeth, conical- or pegged-shaped anterior teeth, ankylosed primary molars due to missing permanents, delayed eruption of permanent teeth, hypoplastic alveoli, xerostomia and thickened frena, macrodontia or microdontia, enamel hypoplasia, and taurodontism [2]. Normally, children with ED have normal psychological and social development [6].

Considering oral aesthetics, rehabilitation of a patient with ED has a big challenge due to missing teeth. According to the number of missing teeth, it can be classified into hypodontia (missing less than six teeth), oligodontia (six or more missing teeth), and anodontia (completely absence of teeth) [7]. The problems associated with missing teeth are directly proportionate to the number of missing teeth in both deciduous and permanent dentition. The most rarely missing teeth are maxillary central incisors, maxillary canines, and maxillary first molars [8]. Mostly, the presenting teeth are conical in shape, malformed, with restricted alveolar bone development, and often showing unaesthetic spacing.

A multidisciplinary approach is now recommended for managing ED patients. Early and extensive dental treatment is needed throughout childhood because of the absence of most of the deciduous and permanent teeth, and they are still in the developing stage. Therefore, the management basically consists of prevention of caries, restoration of malformed teeth, replacement of missing teeth, management of infraocclusion, and correction of malocclusions [7].

Therefore, in many cases of hypodontia, orthodontic treatment can greatly facilitate any restorative treatment or sometimes even eliminate the need for it [9]. Carrying out orthodontic treatment in order to eliminate or to simplify later orthodontic treatment in young patients is called "interceptive orthodontics" (IO) [10]. The main aims of IO treatments in hypodontia are management of available space, uprighting and alignment of teeth, and management of increased overbite, as well as interdisciplinary inputs of hypodontia management [9].

The presenting case shows the total care management of a paediatric patient with ED which is associated with oligodontia was managed by the means of interceptive orthodontic treatment accompanied by direct and indirect restorative methods in a successful manner.

2. Case Report

An 11-year-old schoolboy presented to the paedodontic clinic with the main complaint of having abnormal and uneven teeth and requesting treatments. The parents had noticed that the permanent teeth were abnormal in shape and malaligned. Most importantly, when the child was inquired about his concern, he said that his biggest problem was being teased and bullied by his peers at school.

There was no history of trauma related to the teeth. The child has had a history of asthma but is otherwise healthy. He had been brushing his teeth with fluoridated toothpaste twice daily, using a toothbrush. The child's dietary habits did not show a high consumption of sugar. There was no history of parafunctional habits. Parents have no consanguineous marriage (Figure 1).

On examination, it was observed that the overall development was appropriate for his chronological age. On extraoral examination, he was noticed to have fine sparse hair, scanty eyelashes and eyebrows, protruding lips with reduced lower facial height, periorbital pigmentation, and protruding low set of ears (Figure 2). His palms and soles showed hyperkeratosis.

Intraoral examination showed normal soft tissues and no signs of periodontal disease. The lower anterior teeth were stained and showed crowding with overretained 81 and 62. There was a superficial dentinal caries on 73 with slight

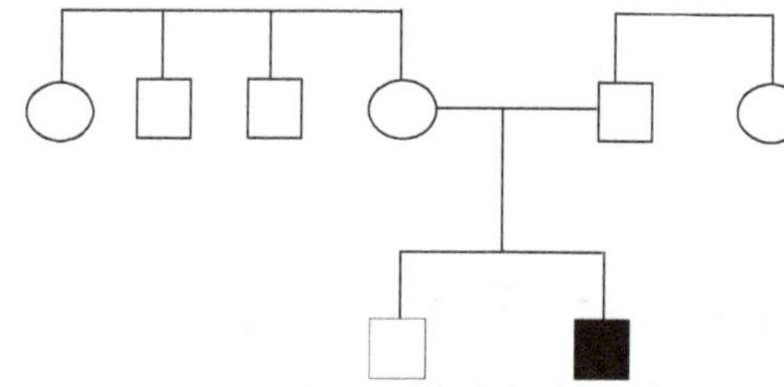

Figure 1: The genealogy of the presenting patient.

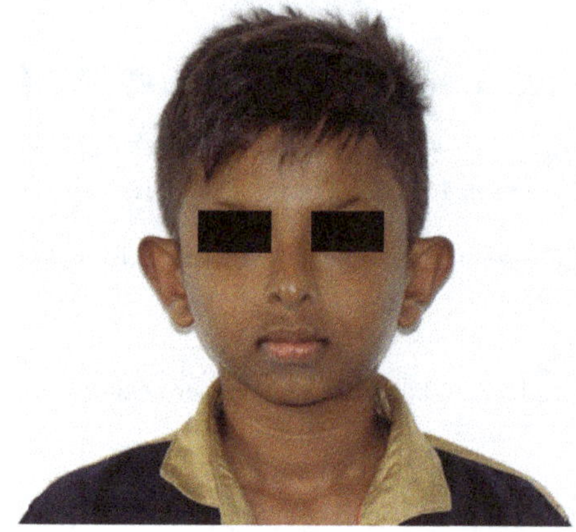

Figure 2: Facial image of the patient.

mobility. The lower permanent incisors (32 and 42) were conical in shape (Figure 3).

All four deciduous canines were slightly overretained with the canine bulges evident in relation to 13 and 43, whereas 33 had already erupted. There was a restoration on 55 with secondary caries. With mild attrited facets on 85, the occlusal surface showed slight mobility. 65 and 75 had been extracted due to caries, and 37 was erupting (Figures 3). His *dmft* index was 4. He had a Class-I skeletal pattern, with average "Frankfort mandibular plane angle" associated with incisor Class-I and bilateral molar Class-II 1/2 unit relationship. Lips were competent and everted. There was evidence of normal tongue and adaptive tongue thrust during the activity.

The radiographic investigation, sensibility tests, and basic periodontal examination (BPE) were performed to identify missing permanent teeth, pulp status, and periodontal health, respectively. All the teeth gave a vital response, and the plaque score was 29%. There was no evidence of deep pockets more than 3 mm. The radiological findings revealed 6 missing teeth: 12, 15, 22, 23, 31, and 41 while 25 was impacted due to space loss. There were anterior conical teeth and overretained 81 with resorbing root and taurodontic molar teeth (Figure 4).

With the information gathered from the history, examination, and investigations, this case was diagnosed as "a patient with hypohidrotic-type ectodermal dysplasia with oligodontia in Class-I malocclusion in late mix dentition on skeletal base Class-I.".

Written consent was obtained from the parents after explaining the proposed treatment plan. At the initial stage,

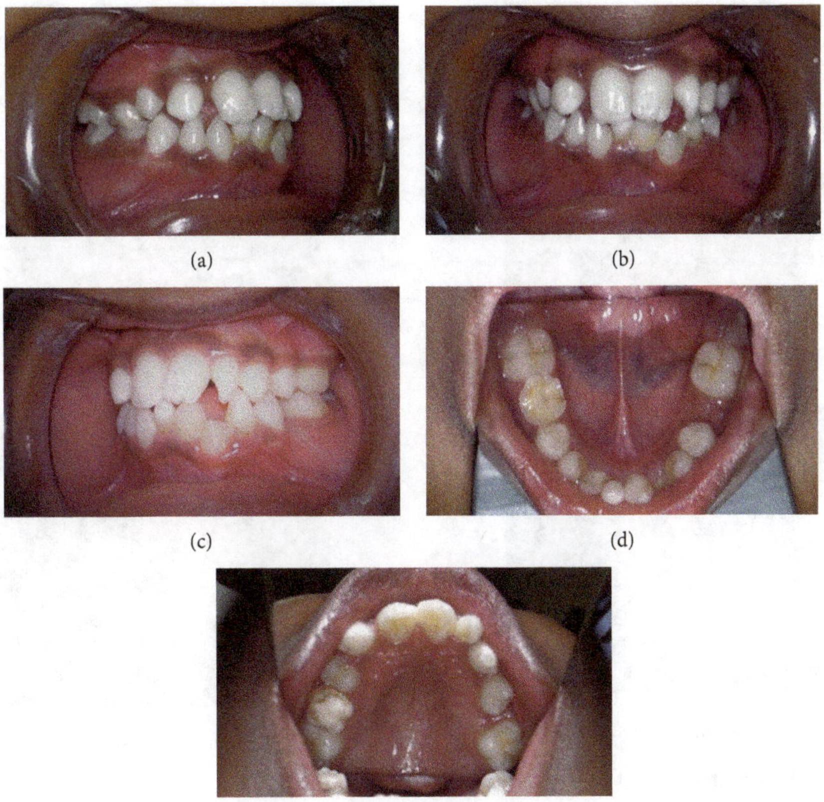

FIGURE 3: Preoperative intraoral images of (a) right buccal, (b) closed mouth, (c) left buccal, (d) lower arch, and (e) upper arch views.

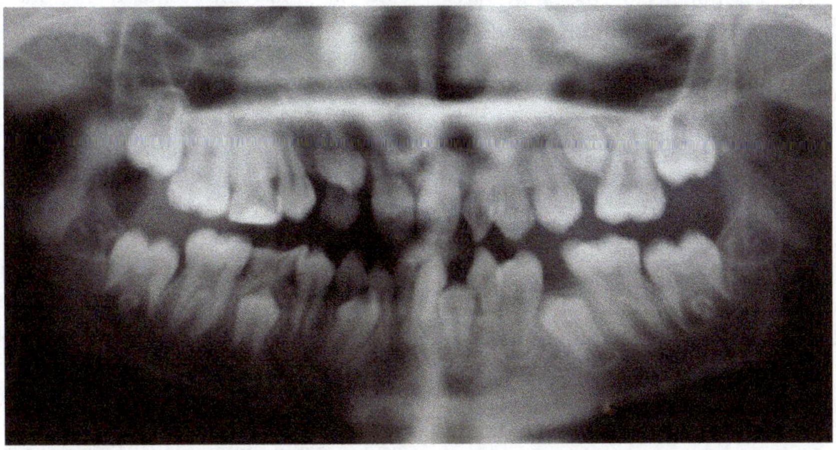

FIGURE 4: Preoperative photoimage of dental panoramic tomograph.

the routine preventive measures like the use of fluoridated toothpaste and correct brush instructions were introduced after plaque demonstration. At the second visit, dietary modification and counselling were done. Fluoride varnish was introduced for professional application. Further CPP-ACP containing GC tooth mousse plus was introduced to use at home on a daily basis.

During the third visit, the child demonstrated a good relationship with the dental team and seemed to have adapted well to the clinical environment. According to the treatment plan, 53, 73, and 83 were extracted after placing separators to facilitate molar bands and stainless steel crown on 55 in the next visit. At the fourth visit, fissure sealants on permanent molars and cementation of a stainless steel crown for 55 were done using luting GIC. The molar bands were cemented to all first molars (Figure 5).

During that period, the permanent canines erupted as expected after extraction of deciduous canines; the patient was reassessed at the ortho-paedodo joint clinic, and the following management steps were planned: derotation of 13 and 24, surgical exposure of 25, extraction of 81, uprighting and distalization of distally tilted 72, distalization of 26 to

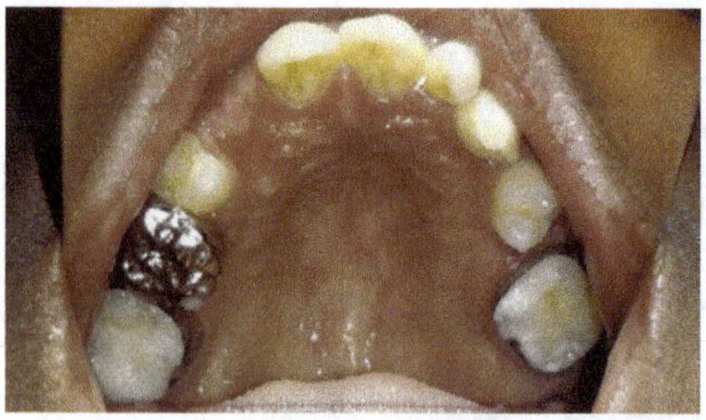

FIGURE 5: Intraoral photograph shows cemented crown and molar bands.

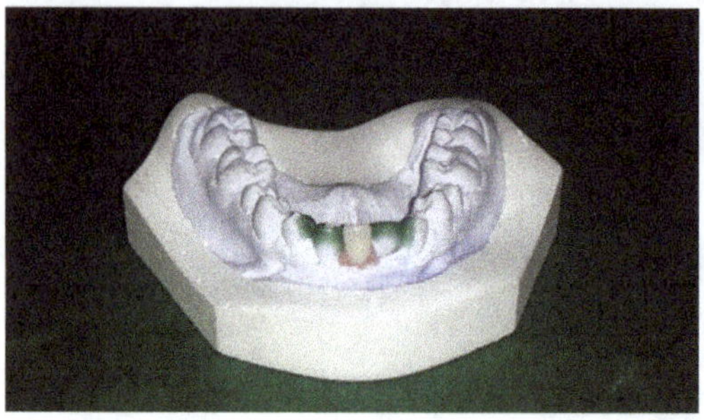

FIGURE 6: Lower arch "Kesling diagnostic setup."

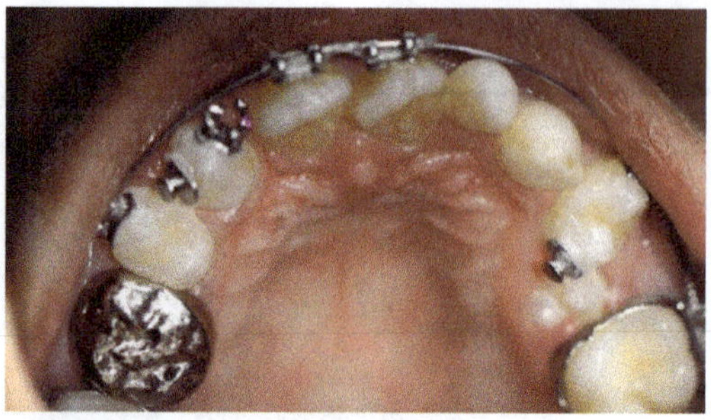

FIGURE 7: Intraoral photograph showing cemented palatal button on rotated 13 and 24.

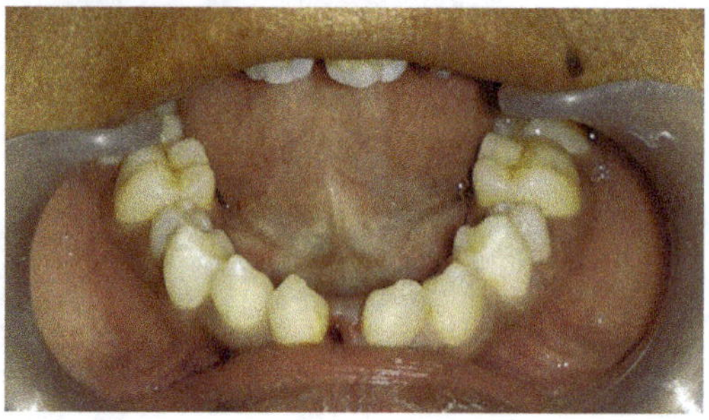

FIGURE 8: Intraoral photograph showing immediately after extraction of 81.

facilitate the eruption of 25, recontouring of upper and lower incisors with composites after completing orthodontic treatment, and replacement of missing 31 and 41 spaces with one tooth with a cantilevered resin-bonded bridge (RBB) from 32.

Before commencing the second half of the orthodontic treatment, the lower arch "Kesling diagnostic setup" was made (Figure 6). At the next visit, palatal buttons were fixed on rotated 13 and 24 in order to derotate (Figure 7). The overretained 81 was extracted prior to bond up of the lower arch (Figure 8).

In parallel to the orthodontic treatment, surgical exposure of 25 and distalization of 26 with a coiled spring was done to facilitate the eruption of 25 (Figure 9). Prior to debonding the fixed applications, a "near-end radiograph" was taken to observe the status of root resorption, teeth position, and the available spaces and root parallelism for future implant placement of the overretained teeth (Figure 10).

Immediately after debonding, all the conical incisors and canines were recontoured using composites (Figure 11). The missing upper laterals were managed by right-side canine lateralization and left-side overretained deciduous canine recontouring by selective grinding and composite buildups. The missing 41 was replaced by a cantilever RBB (Figure 12).

The total care rehabilitation, including aesthetic and preventive measures, seemed to be alright in our patient at the end of the 5-year follow-up period (Figure 13). He is still on review. Implant-supported crowns for the missing 15, 22, 23, 31, and 41 could be considered when the patient is at the age of 18 years.

3. Discussion

Ectodermal dysplasia associated with oligodontia is a complex dental condition that significantly effects on aesthetics and function. In order to provide aesthetically and functionally pleasing outcomes, a multidisciplinary management approach may be required. The aims of that approach should include improving aesthetics, maintaining the existing dentition, improving speech, enhancing the masticatory efficacy, improving acceptance by family and peers, and promoting psychological wellbeing [7]. Most of these requirements can be achieved by addressing the hypodontia by replacing missing teeth with recommended options such as removable prosthesis, conventional or resin adhesive bridgework, implant-supported prosthesis, or autotransplantation [11]. All the options have a common prerequisite in which they need space management before replacing the missing teeth.

Therefore, managing the child especially in mixed dentition with ED and interceptive orthodontics plays a major role. The patient is awaiting the orthodontic treatments which mean he/she became a candidate for the preventive care like plaque control, fissure sealant, dietary counselling, and fluoride therapy [12]. Therefore, our patient also underwent all the preventive measures. Even though we clinically diagnosed this case as hypohidrotic ED, the ideal way of confirming it is a skin biopsy that shows absent or hypoplastic sweat glands. Furthermore, to diagnose the subtypes of EDs, many ways of genetic tests are also available [13].

Currently, there is no causative treatment available [14]. ED-associated hypodontia can be affected by both deciduous and permanent dentition [15]. Most often, the permanent maxillary central incisors, maxillary first molars, mandibular first molars, and maxillary canines are present in hypohidrotic ED [16]. The most common concern of the children with ED is about the dental anomalies and facial appearance [17], and it was common for the present case study also.

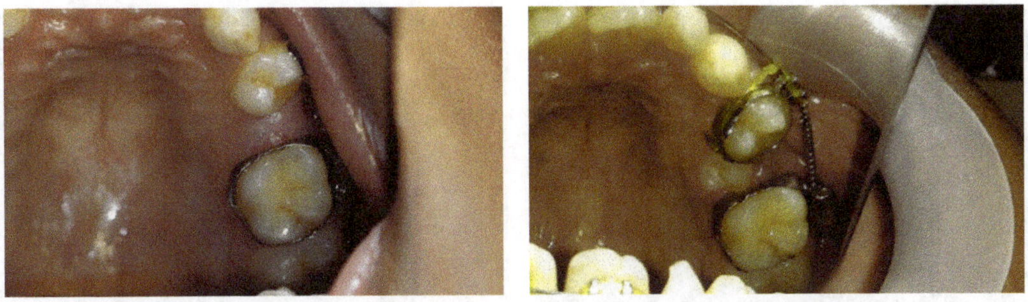

(a) (b)

Figure 9: Intraoral photographs of 25 (a) before and (b) after surgical exposure.

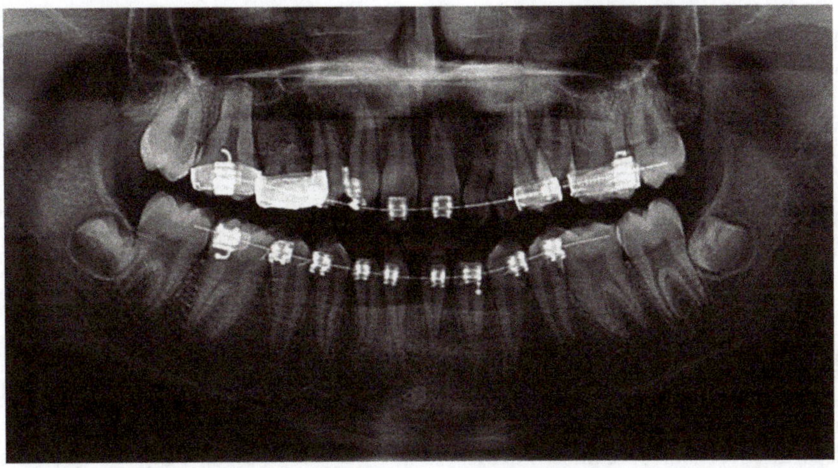

Figure 10: The "near-end radiograph" (digital dental panoramic tomograph).

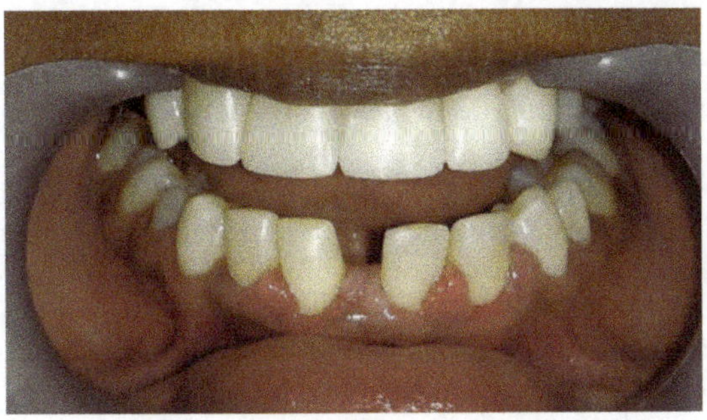

Figure 11: All conical incisors were recontoured with LCC.

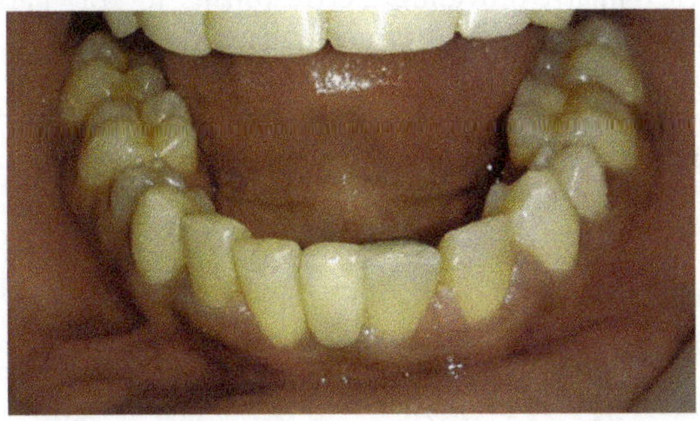

Figure 12: RBB was cemented to replace missing lower central incisors.

The main demand of these patients is replacing their missing teeth and recontouring of the malformed teeth to improve their aesthetics and functions. But the conventional prosthodontic treatments are considered problematic in severe hypodontic cases [18] that may be associated with underdeveloped alveolar ridges in edentulous areas and malformed or overretained deciduous abutment teeth which will lead to poor support, stability, and retention of the prosthesis.

The new trends of managing EDs are moving towards implant-supported rehabilitation [19]. Therefore, the introduction of interceptive orthodontics to the ED patients is of utmost importance to prepare them as candidates for future implant therapy. Interceptive orthodontic treatments are a method to restore a normal occlusion when a malocclusion has started to occur. Furthermore, the development of the dentoskeletal complex, possible discrepancies, and malposition are identified and removed throughout the interceptive orthodontic period. Applications undertaken in interceptive orthodontics are serial extraction, correction of developing crossbite, control of abnormal habits, space reclamation and distribution, extraction of supernumerary and retained primary teeth, root parallelism, and correction of possible predictable malocclusions [20, 21]. The main factors guiding the decision towards the orthodontic and prosthetic choice

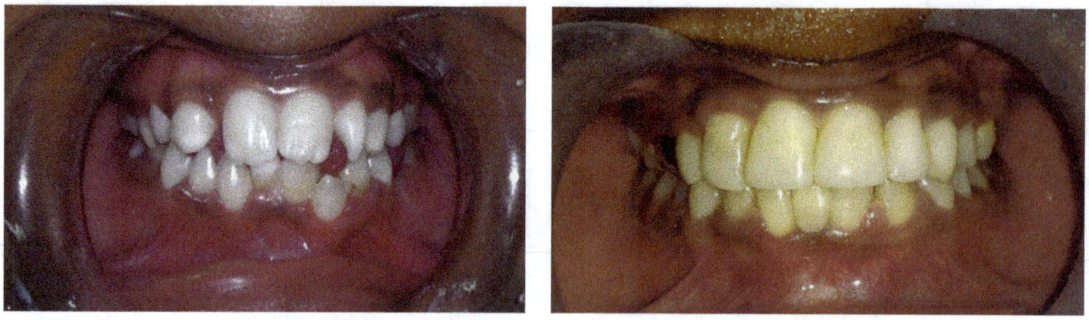

(a) (b)

Figure 13: Comparison of preoperative and postoperative aesthetic outcomes.

are the presence of posterior natural teeth, facial aesthetics, lip support, number and size of existing natural teeth, and the occlusal vertical dimension.

The successful outcomes of the patient presented in this case report are due to good understanding and the commitments of both clinicians and the child's parents, who always had positive attitudes towards the proposed multidisciplinary treatment plan.

4. Conclusion

Management of a child with ectodermal dysplasia with oligodontia was a real challenge. Early diagnosis, necessary investigation, and providing age-appropriate multidisciplinary treatment were key steps in successful outcomes. Furthermore, selecting the most suitable treatment option among a verity of modalities is of utmost importance to the long-term sustainability of both provided and future treatments as well. Finally, providing the treatments for ED patients while preparing them for future implant therapy is an added advantage for the patients. Most importantly, upliftment of the psychological wellbeing of the young children provided by proper management of ED is of utmost importance to improve their quality of life.

References

[1] S. Y. Chee, C. H. Wanga, W. D. Lina, and F. J. Tsaia, "Ectodermal dysplasia (ED) syndrome," *Biomedicine (Taipei)*, vol. 4, no. 4, p. 27, 2014.

[2] T. Halai and C. Stevens, "Ectodermal dysplasia: a clinical overview for the dental practitioner," *Dental Update*, vol. 42, no. 8, pp. 779–790, 2015.

[3] G. Rashu and M. Manjul, "Prosthodontic management of children with ectodermal dysplasia: review of literature," *Dentistry*, vol. 5, no. 11, 2015.

[4] I. Tarjan, K. Gabris, and N. Rozsa, "Early prosthetic treatment of patients with ectodermal dysplasia: a clinical report," *The Journal of Prosthetic Dentistry*, vol. 93, no. 5, pp. 419–424, 2005.

[5] K. Salem and F. Moazami, "Dental reconstruction in hypohydrotic ectodermal dysplasia: case report," *Iranian Journal of Pediatric Dentistry*, vol. 11, no. 2, pp. 77–82, 2016.

[6] M. A. Pigno, R. B. Blackman, R. J. Cronin Jr., and E. Cavazos, "Prosthodontic management of ectodermal dysplasia: a review of the literature," *The Journal of Prosthetic Dentistry*, vol. 76, no. 5, pp. 541–545, 1996.

[7] J. H. Nunn, N. E. Carter, T. J. Gillgrass et al., "The interdisciplinary management of hypodontia: background and role of paediatric dentistry," *British Dental Journal*, vol. 194, no. 5, pp. 245–251, 2003.

[8] L. Suri, E. Gagari, and H. Vastardis, "Delayed tooth eruption: pathogenesis, diagnosis, and treatment. A literature review," *American Journal of Orthodontics and Dentofacial Orthopedics*, vol. 126, no. 4, pp. 432–445, 2004.

[9] N. E. Carter, T. J. Gillgrass, R. S. Hobson et al., "The interdisciplinary management of hypodontia: orthodontics," *British Dental Journal*, vol. 194, no. 7, pp. 361–366, 2003.

[10] J. L. Ackerman and W. R. Proffit, "Preventive and interceptive orthodontics: a strong theory proves weak in practice," *The Angle Orthodontist*, vol. 50, no. 2, pp. 75–87, 1980.

[11] R. Holliday, N. Lush, J. Chapple, F. Nohl, and B. Cole, "Hypodontia: aesthetics and function part 2: management," *Dental update*, vol. 41, no. 10, pp. 891–898, 2014.

[12] R. Hawkins, D. Locker, J. Noble, and E. J. Kay, "Prevention. Part 7: professionally applied topical fluorides for caries prevention," *British Dental Journal*, vol. 195, no. 6, pp. 313–317, 2003.

[13] F. Clauss, M. C. Manière, F. Obry et al., "Dento-craniofacial phenotypes and underlying molecular mechanisms in hypohidrotic ectodermal dysplasia (HED): a review," *Journal of Dental Research*, vol. 87, no. 12, pp. 1089–1099, 2008.

[14] D. Celli, A. Manente, C. Grippaudo, and M. Cordaro, "Interceptive treatment in ectodermal dysplasia using an innovative orthodontic/prosthetic modular appliance A case report with 10- year follow-up," *European Journal of Paediatric Dentistry*, vol. 19, no. 4, pp. 307–312, 2018.

[15] R. S. Hobson, N. E. Carter, T. J. Gillgrass et al., "The interdisciplinary management of hypodontia: the relationship between an interdisciplinary team and the general dental practitioner," *British Dental Journal*, vol. 194, no. 9, pp. 479–482, 2003.

[16] A. D. Guckes, M. W. Roberts, and G. R. McCarthy, "Pattern of permanent teeth present in individuals with ectodermal dysplasia and severe hypodontia suggests treatment with dental implants," *Pediatric Dentistry*, vol. 20, no. 4, pp. 278–280, 1998.

[17] M. B. Siegel and W. P. Potsic, "Ectodermal dysplasia: the otolaryngologic manifestations and management," *International Journal of Pediatric Otorhinolaryngology*, vol. 19, no. 3, pp. 265–271, 1990.

[18] J. R. Boj, J. Duran von Arx, M. Cortada, A. Jimenez, and J. Golobart, "Dentures for a 3-yr-old child with ectodermal dysplasia: case report," *American Journal of Dentistry*, vol. 6, no. 3, pp. 165–167, 1993.

[19] I. P. Sweeney, J. W. Ferguson, A. A. Heggie, and J. O. Lucas, "Treatment outcomes for adolescent ectodermal dysplasia patients treated with dental implants," *International Journal of Paediatric Dentistry*, vol. 15, no. 4, pp. 241–248, 2005.

[20] R. M. Ricketts, "Dr. Robert M. Ricketts on early treatment (part 1)," *Journal of Clinical Orthodontics*, vol. 13, no. 1, pp. 23–38, 1979.

[21] N. Karaiskos, W. A. Wiltshire, O. Odlum, D. Brothwell, and T. H. Hassard, "Preventive and interceptive orthodontic treatment needs of an inner-city group of 6- and 9-year-old Canadian children," *Journal of the Canadian Dental Association*, vol. 71, no. 9, p. 649, 2005.

11

Digital Workflow for Indirect Bonding with 2D Lingual Brackets: A Case Report and Procedure Description

Federico Rosti,[1] **Maria Francesca Sfondrini**,[2] **Davide Bressani,**[3] **Marina Consuelo Vitale,**[2] **Paola Gandini,**[2] **and Andrea Scribante**[2]

[1]*Private Practice, Cesano Boscone, Italy*
[2]*Unit of Orthodontics and Paediatric Dentistry-Section of Dentistry-Department of Clinical, Surgical, Diagnostic and Paediatric Sciences, University of Pavia, Pavia, Italy*
[3]*Dental Technician, Pavia, Italy*

Correspondence should be addressed to Andrea Scribante; andrea.scribante@unipv.it

Academic Editor: Mine Dündar

Objective. During orthodontic therapy, accuracy in bonding procedures makes it easier to correct tooth alignment by decreasing the need for midcourse corrections by changing bracket positions. Indirect bonding allows the transfer of the appliance components from model casts to patient's teeth potentially meaning shorter appointments for bracket bonding and rebonding and best comfort during chairside practice. At the same time, there has been a steady increase in requests for invisible lingual orthodontic treatment. *Clinical Considerations.* Accordingly, the aim of the present report is to illustrate the workflow to realize a complete digital indirect bonding for lingual brackets (2D, Forestadent). The procedure starts with intraoral digital scans, digital 3D model, and virtual bracket positioning, ending with the realization of a CAD-CAM prototyped transfer tray. A 3D intraoral scanner (True Definition, 3M) is used to create digital scans and digital models. A virtual bracket positioning is performed using software (NemoCast, Dentaurum), and a prototyped transfer tray is created by a CAD-CAM device. 2D lingual brackets were positioned inside the tray, so the appliance was bonded to the dental surface using light curing adhesive resin. *Conclusions.* During orthodontic treatment, CAD/CAM technology could help clinicians. Computer-constructed transfer trays can reduce clinician error and improve the everyday workflow in the office.

1. Introduction

In straight-wire orthodontic devices, ideal bracket placement can correct tooth position in the three planes of space during treatment [1]. Accuracy in bracket placement allows an efficient orthodontic treatment [2, 3].

According to Carlson and Johnson [4], there are four elements necessary for ideal bracket placement: (1) bracket base adaptation to dental surface, (2) evaluation of the rotational bracket position in relation to the occlusal plane, (3) determination of vertical position of each bracket, and (4) determination of slot angulation according to the position of the roots.

Several studies claim that indirect bonding can be more accurate than direct bonding on labial appliances with a reduction in bracket position errors in each of the three orientations examined [5–7]. Accuracy in bracket placement can also reduce the need for repositioning and can then shorten treatment time [8, 9]. These studies were related to labial and not lingual appliances and results, however, are preliminary and inconclusive about precision of positioning and total treatment time. Therefore, the reduction of chairside time can be considered the main real advantage of indirect bracket placement.

Because of its outstanding aesthetic preconditions and its growing practicability, lingual orthodontics accounts for an ever-increasing percentage of orthodontic treatments and even more studies evaluated various aspects of this technique [10–14]. Although the lingual orthodontic treatment provides several aesthetic advantages, its use has been limited due to the increased chair time and more difficult mechanical control [15]. Placement of lingual orthodontic appliance can be made easier however with new technologies such as intraoral scanning, virtual positioning of brackets, and computer-aided transfer tray manufacturing [16, 17].

Advances in CAD/CAM technology are providing new possibilities in orthodontics: the application of CAD/CAM for establishing a virtual set-up or creating transfer trays/jig [16, 17] has improved the indirect bonding workflow.

The aim of this manuscript is to illustrate the workflow to realize a complete digital indirect bonding, after an intraoral scanning and construction of a prototyped transfer tray has been created for indirect bonding.

2. Case Report

2.1. Diagnosis and Aetiology. A male patient, aged 19 years old, was referred to a private orthodontic practice. He was diagnosed with a bilateral Class I canine relationship and left Class I molar relationship in the permanent dentition with a crossbite of tooth 12 (Figures 1–3). Patient chief complaint was to resolve the anterior crossbite with an invisible orthodontic appliance.

2.2. Treatment Objectives. A lingual orthodontic appliance has been projected using a CAD/CAM digital workflow. The objective of the treatment was the resolution of anterior crossbite and retention of the case over time [18].

2.3. Treatment Alternatives. As the patient wanted to avoid conventional vestibular orthodontic treatment, a lingual orthodontic appliance was chosen. Other alternatives to conventional visible metallic attachments would have been orthodontic treatment with ceramic brackets or aligners that are both effective to obtain tooth movement [19, 20]. The patient, however, wanted to avoid ceramic brackets because of the possibility of adverse staining midtreatment and refused aligners so as to avoid treatment with removable appliances.

2.4. Treatment Progress. Written informed consent was obtained by the patient to proceed with orthodontic diagnosis and treatment. The procedure for the virtual indirect bonding started with the polishing of all dental surfaces with pumice powder; then, intraoral scan (Figure 3) was performed by a 3D intraoral scanner (True Definition, 3M, US). NemoCast software (Dentaurum, Germany) acquired the 3D models and recognized the shape of each tooth and the gum. The software realized a virtual set-up, and then, the orthodontist placed the virtual brackets on 3D virtual models according to the lingual prescription (Figure 4). The bracket placement tool ensured the precise bracket positioning according to the virtual set-up using the virtual bracket's position on the screen. Once all brackets were positioned on the 3D models, the software allowed designing a virtual transfer tray for indirect bonding (Figure 5). A prototype of the digital transfer tray was manufactured using a rapid-prototyping machine (Figure 6). exocad software (exocad GmbH, Germany) was used to create bilateral posterior overlays to act as customized bite raisers (Figures 7 and 8).

The patient wore protective glasses to prevent eye damage [21], and the tooth surfaces were first etched with 37% orthophosphoric acid gel (3M, US) for 30 seconds (Figure 9) followed by washing and drying. A primer (Transbond XT, 3M, US) was applied in a thin film on the etched tooth surface (Figure 10). 2D lingual brackets (Forestadent, Germany) were positioned inside the prototyped transfer tray, and an adhesive resin (Transbond XT, 3M, US) was applied over the bracket bases [22]. The brackets were then positioned in the maxilla on the upper teeth (Figure 11), using the prototyped transfer

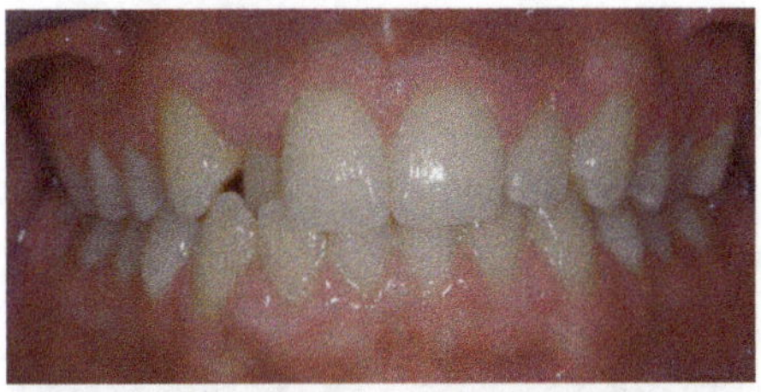

Figure 1: Front view of initial occlusion.

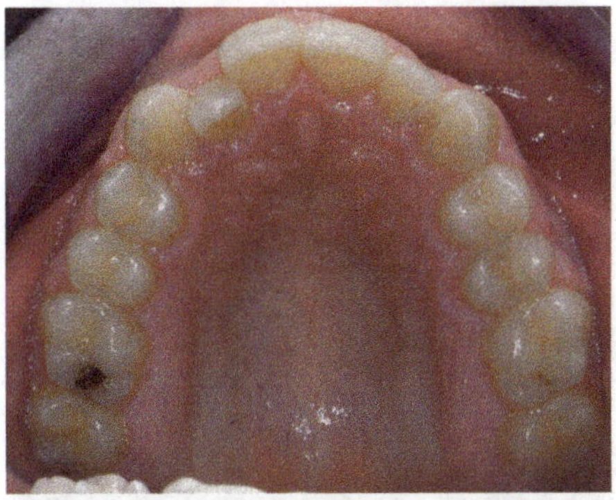

Figure 2: Occlusal view of initial occlusion.

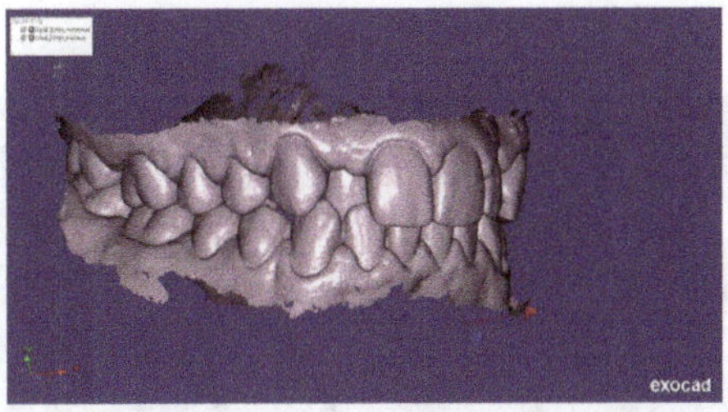

Figure 3: 3D intraoral scan view of initial occlusion.

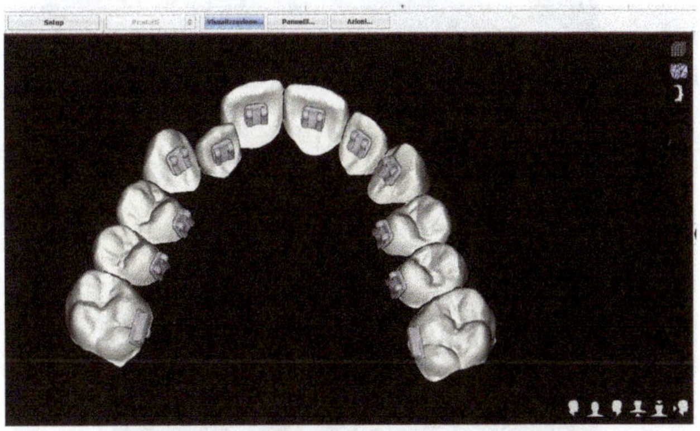

Figure 4: Case planning with virtual brackets.

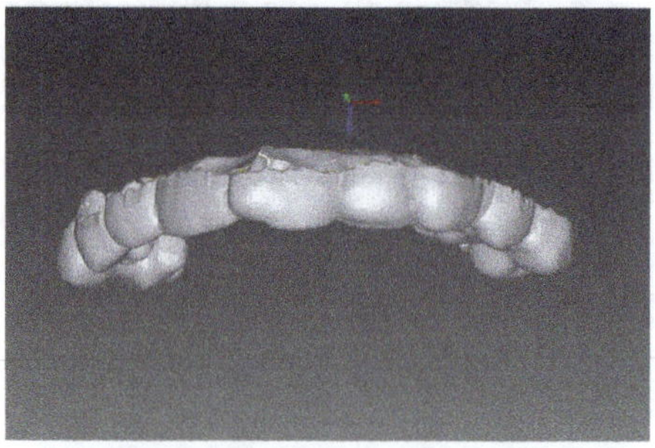

Figure 5: Virtual transfer tray.

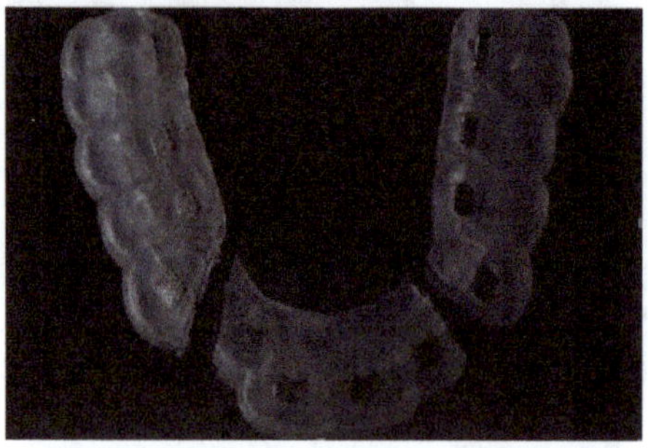

Figure 6: Prototype of digital transfer tray.

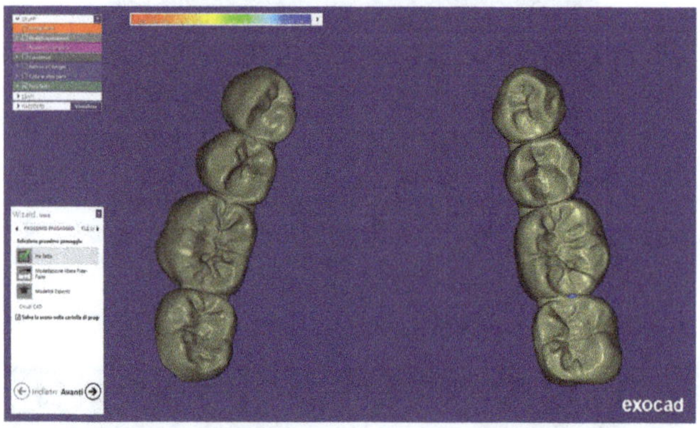

Figure 7: Virtual customized bite raisings.

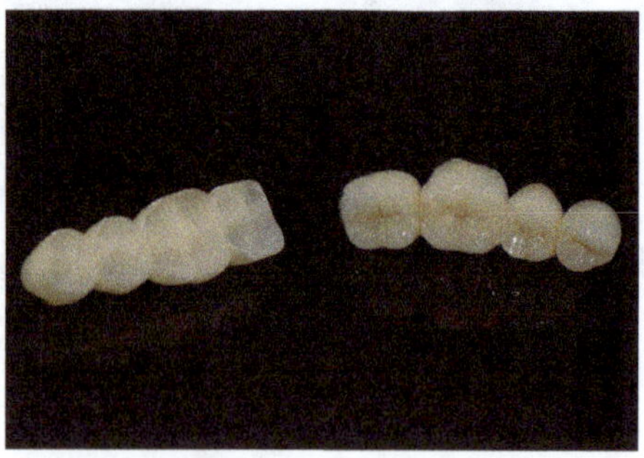

Figure 8: Customized bite raisings.

jig, and were light cured for 60 seconds each by an LED lamp (Elipar DeepCure, 3M, US). Subsequently, the transfer tray was removed by forcing a probe in the fracture line (Figures 12 and 13) and separating the jig in two halves. The

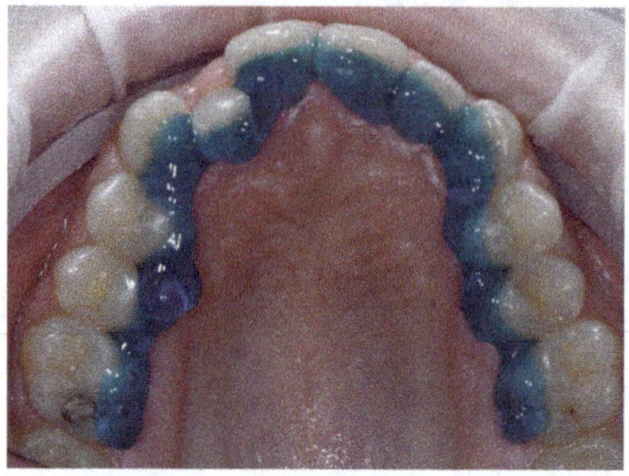

Figure 9: Etching procedure.

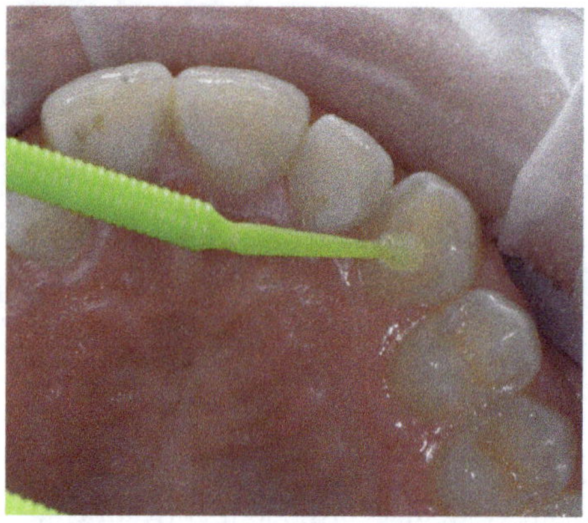

Figure 10: Adhesive application.

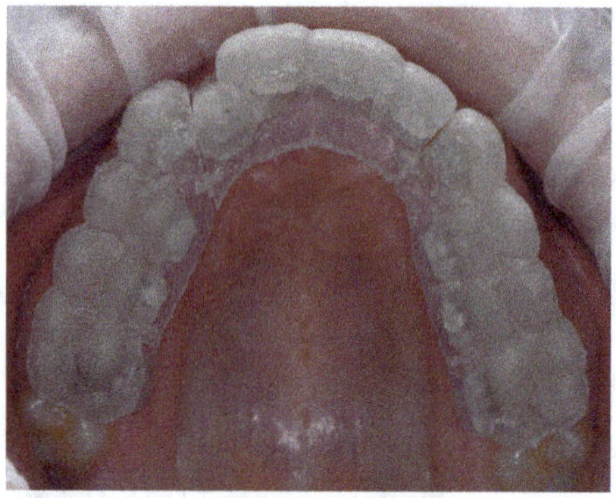

Figure 11: Device placement.

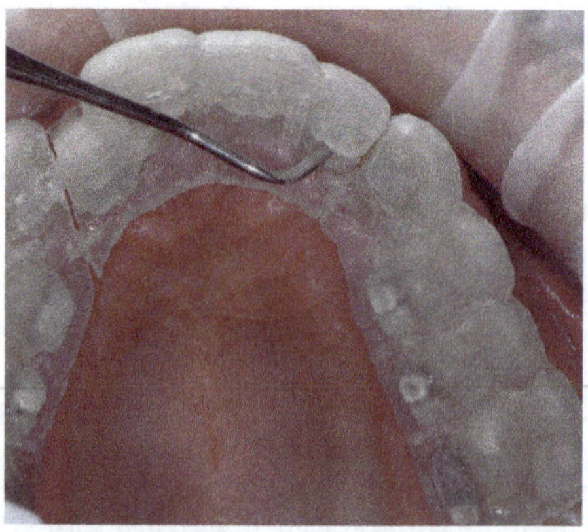

Figure 12: Transfer tray removal.

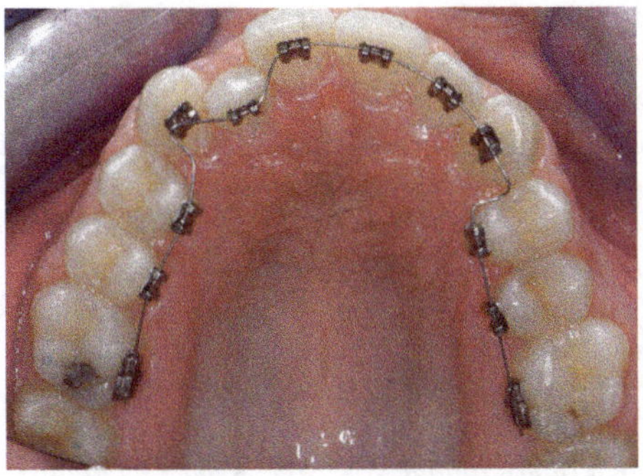

Figure 13: Wire placement.

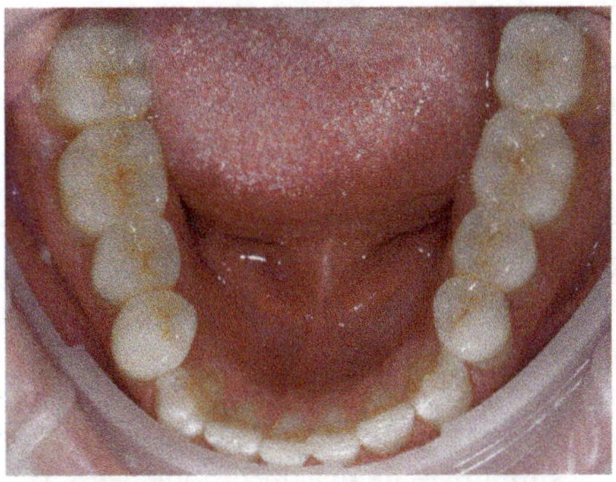

Figure 14: Setting of prototyped overlays.

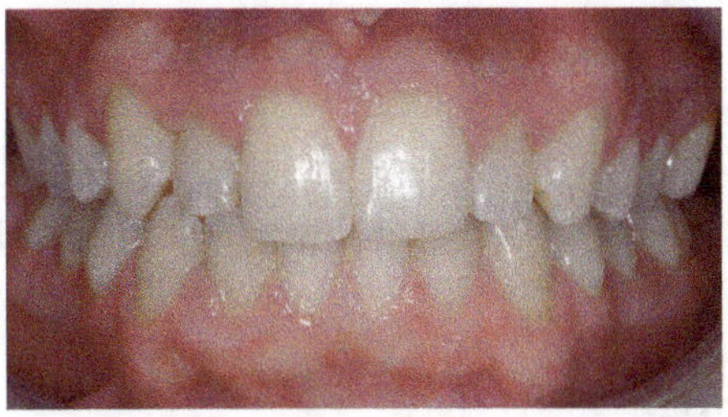

Figure 15: Front view of final occlusion.

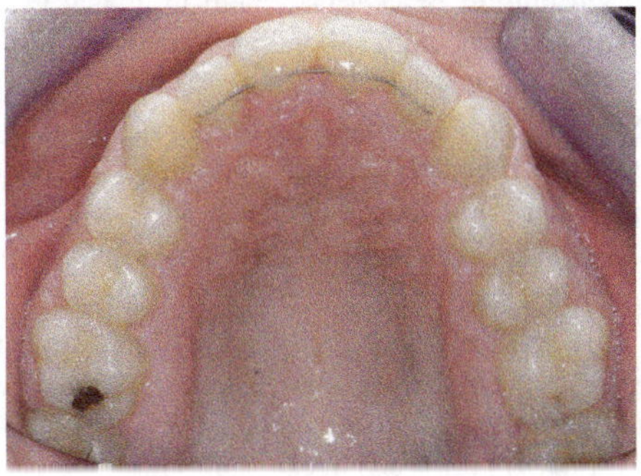

Figure 16: Occlusal view of final occlusion.

fracture line was created by the CAD software in order to be useful for an easy transfer tray removal.

On the lower jaw, prototyped overlay were set using an adhesive technique (Figure 14). Orthodontic treatment progress included 0.012 inch, 0.014 inch, and 0.016 inch nickel titanium archwires, followed by 0.16 stainless steel wire. The patient was checked each month, and wires were changed after 2 months each. Finally, brackets were removed, and teeth were polished (Figures 15 and 16). An upper splint and an upper Essix removable appliance were placed in order to guarantee posttreatment stabilization [23, 24].

3. Discussion

The virtual indirect bonding has been performed with lingual brackets with the treatment plan involving the upper teeth alone by resolution of the lateral incisor crossbite. The case has been planned with a digitalized workflow with CAD/-CAM digital impression taking presenting similar efficiency as traditional impression methods in orthodontics and being more comfortable for patients [25, 26]. The position of brackets on the patient teeth (Figure 13) corresponded to the position of the same brackets on the digital 3D models (Figure 4). This can be obtained as CAD/CAM technology shows a variety of possibilities in orthodontics from study design [25] to the construction of customized splints [15] and trays for vestibular appliances [27] or for maxillofacial surgery scopes [28]. To our knowledge in the literature, there are no studies that evaluated CAD/CAM preparation of transfer trays for standard lingual appliances realized by an independent dental technical laboratory. In fact, the CAD/-CAM transfer tray technique is performed only directly from the manufacturer for the use of customized lingual brackets [29], which present higher realization costs than standard lingual appliances using this technique [30].

Accurate surface imaging is required to digitally manufacture orthodontic appliances with 3D intraoral scanners reproducing precisely the image of the lingual dental surfaces [31]. Lingual surfaces vary more widely than labial surfaces [32]: for example, the bicuspid has a very slim and irregular lingual surface making bracket placement difficult. An advantage of the CAD design method is improved bonding of the lingual bracket base [33], which is important for adhesion performance [34]. The software can realize customized bracket bases which are useful in the case of bicuspids with very small lingual surfaces. Finally, the highest resolution of commercially available stereolithographic printers is about 0.3 mm, which is sufficient for providing both the bracket retention inside the prototyped transfer tray and the retention feature on the base of a stereolithographic prototype [35].

The computerized tool provides accuracy in bracket placement and significant reduction in chairside time. While software can provide precise reproducibility, orthodontists can incorporate alterations from the ideal placement to provide overcorrection of rotated teeth or accentuated tip to resist root motion in space closure [15]. Virtual indirect bonding can also be exported to other 3D CAD software, e.g., to realize customized occlusal bite raisers. Using the virtual articulation software, premature contacts on the brackets can also be eliminated.

Indirect bonding is currently used with 3D customized lingual brackets, and it is not used with the 2D lingual appliance, as the brackets can be placed directly. Moreover, 2D lingual brackets are a low cost option for mild cases where only the 1st- and 2nd-order corrections are required as there is no prescription in the bracket for torque correction (no 3rd-order modifications are possible). However, the present report evaluated indirect bonding for the 2D lingual system in order to reduce chair time of the bracket positioning appointment. Moreover, during direct bonding procedure on the lingual side of the tooth, often the clinician does not have a clear vision of the bonding area. Therefore, the advantage of a CAD/CAM indirect bonding is the possibility to zoom on details and provide a better position of the lingual bracket on the lingual surface. The implementation of a simplified lingual technique with CAD/CAM technology could offer orthodontic clinicians new interesting and feasible possibilities.

4. Conclusions

After an intraoral scan, a digital indirect bonding technique has been shown to be possible using the standard lingual brackets which is both repeatable and effective.

References

[1] N. Shpack, S. Geron, I. Floris, M. Davidovitch, T. Brosh, and A. D. Vardimon, "Bracket placement in lingual vs labial systems and direct vs indirect bonding," *The Angle Orthodontist*, vol. 77, no. 3, pp. 509–517, 2007.

[2] T. M. Hodge, A. A. Dhopatkar, W. P. Rock, and D. J. Spary, "The Burton approach to indirect bonding," *Journal of Orthodontics*, vol. 28, no. 4, pp. 267–270, 2001.

[3] A. Kotari, "Indirect bonding technique," *World Journal of Orthodontics*, vol. 7, no. 4, pp. 389–393, 2006.

[4] S. K. Carlson and E. Johnson, "Bracket positioning and resets: five steps to align crowns and roots consistently," *American Journal of Orthodontics and Dentofacial Orthopedics*, vol. 119, no. 1, pp. 76–80, 2001.

[5] T. M. Hodge, A. A. Dhopatkar, W. P. Rock, and D. J. Spary, "A randomized clinical trial comparing the accuracy of direct versus indirect bracket placement," *Journal of Orthodontics*, vol. 31, no. 2, pp. 132–137, 2004.

[6] D. A. Nichols, G. Gardner, and A. D. Carballeyra, "Reproducibility of bracket positioning in the indirect bonding technique," *American Journal of Orthodontics and Dentofacial Orthopedics*, vol. 144, no. 5, pp. 770–776, 2013.

[7] J. T. Kalange, "Indirect bonding: a comprehensive review of the advantages," *World Journal of Orthodontics*, vol. 5, no. 4, pp. 301–307, 2004.

[8] A. Menini, M. Cozzani, M. F. Sfondrini, A. Scribante, P. Cozzani, and P. Gandini, "A 15-month evaluation of bond failures of orthodontic brackets bonded with direct versus indirect bonding technique: a clinical trial," *Progress in Orthodontics*, vol. 15, no. 1, p. 70, 2014.

[9] B. C. Koo, C. H. Chung, and R. L. Vanarsdall, "Comparison of the accuracy of bracket placement between direct and indirect bonding techniques," *American Journal of Orthodontics and Dentofacial Orthopedics*, vol. 116, no. 3, pp. 346–351, 1999.

[10] Ö. P. Özsoy and H. Pamukçu, "Lingual treatment of an adult patient with a simplified extraction protocol," *Turkish Journal of Orthodontics*, vol. 31, no. 2, pp. 62–66, 2018.

[11] A. Scribante, M. F. Sfondrini, D. Fraticelli, M. Malfatto, and P. Gandini, "Adhesive systems for CAD-CAM customised lingual orthodontic brackets: which one is better?," *European Journal of Paediatric Dentistry*, vol. 18, no. 3, pp. 188–192, 2017.

[12] L. Binhuwaishel and T. Al-Jewair, "Lingual fixed orthodontic appliances may be associated with more adverse effects than buccal appliances," *The Journal of Evidence-Based Dental Practice*, vol. 18, no. 4, pp. 349–351, 2018.

[13] A. Scribante, M. F. Sfondrini, V. Collesano, G. Tovt, L. Bernardinelli, and P. Gandini, "Dental hygiene and orthodontics: effect of ultrasonic instrumentation on bonding efficacy of different lingual orthodontic brackets," *BioMed Research International*, vol. 2017, Article ID 3714651, 6 pages, 2017.

[14] M. F. Sfondrini, M. Debiaggi, F. Zara et al., "Influence of lingual bracket position on microbial and periodontal parameters in vivo," *Journal of Applied Oral Science*, vol. 20, no. 3, pp. 357–361, 2012.

[15] S. Y. Kwon, Y. Kim, H. W. Ahn, K. B. Kim, K. R. Chung, and S. H. Kim (Sunny), "Computer-aided designing and manufacturing of lingual fixed orthodontic appliance using 2D/3D registration software and rapid prototyping," *International Journal of Dentistry*, vol. 2014, Article ID 164164, 8 pages, 2014.

[16] M. J. Mayhew, "Computer-aided bracket placement for indirect bonding," *Journal of Clinical Orthodontics*, vol. 39, p. 653, 2005.

[17] F. Ciuffolo, E. Epifania, G. Duranti et al., "Rapid prototyping: a new method of preparing trays for indirect bonding," *American Journal of Orthodontics and Dentofacial Orthopedics*, vol. 129, no. 1, pp. 75–77, 2006.

[18] O. M. Tanaka, I. A. Fornazari, A. X. G. Parra, B. B. Castilhos, and A. Franco, "Complete maxillary crossbite correction with a rapid palatal expansion in mixed dentition followed by a corrective orthodontic treatment," *Case Reports in Dentistry*, vol. 2016, Article ID 8306397, 6 pages, 2016.

[19] M. F. Sfondrini, P. Gandini, T. Castroflorio et al., "Buccolingual inclination control of upper central incisors of aligners: a comparison with conventional and self-ligating brackets," *BioMed Research International*, vol. 2018, Article ID 9341821, 7 pages, 2018.

[20] J. A. Shaik and G. Guram, "A comparative evaluation of canine retraction using ceramic bracket and ceramic bracket with metal slot with conventional preadjusted edgewise appliance bracket systems: a clinical study," *Journal of International Society of Preventive and Community Dentistry*, vol. 8, no. 4, pp. 296–303, 2018.

[21] E. E. Hill, "Eye safety practices in U.S. dental school restorative clinics, 2006," *Journal of Dental Education*, vol. 70, no. 12, pp. 1294–1297, 2006.

[22] A. Scribante, R. Contreras-Bulnes, M. A. Montasser, and P. K. Vallittu, "Orthodontics: bracket materials, adhesives systems, and their bond strength," *BioMed Research International*, vol. 2016, Article ID 1329814, 3 pages, 2016.

[23] A. Scribante, M. F. Sfondrini, S. Broggini, M. D'Allocco, and P. Gandini, "Efficacy of esthetic retainers: clinical comparison between multistranded wires and direct-bond glass fiber-reinforced composite splints," *International Journal of Dentistry*, vol. 2011, Article ID 548356, 5 pages, 2011.

[24] A. Demir, H. Babacan, R. Nalcacı, and T. Topcuoglu, "Comparison of retention characteristics of Essix and Hawley retainers," *The Korean Journal of Orthodontics*, vol. 42, no. 5, pp. 255–262, 2012.

[25] M. F. Sfondrini, P. Gandini, M. Malfatto, F. Di Corato, F. Trovati, and A. Scribante, "Computerized casts for orthodontic purpose using powder-free intraoral scanners: accuracy, execution time, and patient feedback," *BioMed Research International*, vol. 2018, Article ID 4103232, 8 pages, 2018.

[26] L. Burhardt, C. Livas, W. Kerdijk, W. J. van der Meer, and Y. Ren, "Treatment comfort, time perception, and preference for conventional and digital impression techniques: a comparative study in young patients," *American Journal of Orthodontics and Dentofacial Orthopedics*, vol. 150, no. 2, pp. 261–267, 2016.

[27] R. Dewhurst, "Assessment of computer customized brackets and positioning jigs," *International journal of orthodontics*, vol. 23, no. 1, pp. 53–58, 2012.

[28] H. M. Kim, S. H. Baek, T. Y. Kim, and J. Y. Choi, "Evaluation of three-dimensional position change of the condylar head after orthognathic surgery using computer-aided design/computer-aided manufacturing-made condyle positioning jig," *The Journal of Craniofacial Surgery*, vol. 25, no. 6, pp. 2002–2007, 2014.

[29] C. Jacobs, M. Katzorke, D. Wiechmann, H. Wehrbein, and R. Schwestka-Polly, "Single tooth torque correction in the lower frontal area by a completely customized lingual appliance," *Head & Face Medicine*, vol. 13, no. 1, p. 18, 2017.

[30] G. E. Tynelius, "Orthodontic retention. Studies of retention capacity, cost-effectiveness and long-term stability," *Swedish Dental Journal Supplement*, vol. 236, no. 236, pp. 9–65, 2014.

[31] C. Zarauz, A. Valverde, F. Martinez-Rus, B. Hassan, and G. Pradies, "Clinical evaluation comparing the fit of all-ceramic crowns obtained from silicone and digital intraoral impressions," *Clinical Oral Investigations*, vol. 20, no. 4, pp. 799–806, 2016.

[32] T. Hiro and K. Takemoto, "Resin core indirect bonding system-improvement of lingual orthodontic treatment," *Journal-Japan Orthodontic Society*, vol. 57, pp. 83–91, 1998.

[33] K. S. Tamizharasi and D. S. Kumar, "Evolution of orthodontic brackets," *Journal of Indian Academy of Dental Specialist*, vol. 1, pp. 25–35, 2010.

[34] A. Scribante, M. F. Sfondrini, D. Fraticelli, P. Daina, A. Tamagnone, and P. Gandini, "The influence of no-primer adhesives and anchor pylons bracket bases on shear bond strength of orthodontic brackets," *BioMed Research International*, vol. 2013, Article ID 315023, 6 pages, 2013.

[35] B. Sager, D. W. Rosen, M. Shilling, and T. R. Kurfess, "Experimental studies in stereolithographic resolution," in *Proceedings of the Solid Freeform Fabrication Symposium*, pp. 70–81, Austin, Tex, USA, 2003.

12

Orthodontic Treatment of Bilateral Impacted Mandibular Canines and a Mupparapu Type 2 Transmigration

José Antonio Vera-Guerra,[1] José Rubén Herrera-Atoche,[2] and Gabriel Eduardo Colomé-Ruiz[2]

[1]*Department of Orthodontics, School of Dentistry, Universidad Autónoma de Nuevo León, Nuevo León, Mexico*
[2]*Department of Orthodontics, School of Dentistry, Universidad Autónoma de Yucatán, Yucatán, Mexico*

Correspondence should be addressed to José Rubén Herrera-Atoche; jose.herrera@correo.uady.mx

Academic Editor: Rui Amaral Mendes

Dental transmigration is a rare condition that mainly affects the mandibular canines. Since the tooth involved is usually impacted and its crown has crossed the midline towards the opposite side, the treatment options frequently are surgical removal or radiographic follow-up, and, in some cases, orthodontic traction is possible. In 2002, Mupparapu presented a classification for lower canines in transmigration according to their position within the mandible. This paper is aimed at describing the orthodontic treatment of a female patient with two impacted mandibular canines, one of them in a Mupparapu type 2 transmigration position (horizontal impaction position near the lower mandibular border and below the incisors' root apices). Additionally, the paper discusses the biomechanical orthodontic design and the alternative treatment options for these complex cases.

1. Introduction

Mandibular canine impaction is one of the most complex eruption dental anomalies to treat, and it occurs mainly when the crown of the affected tooth has crossed the midline and become a transmigration case [1]. According to the literature, the mandibular canines get impacted less frequently than the maxillary ones [2–5]; their prevalence is said to be between 0.92% and 5.1%, and they are usually accompanied by odontomas, cysts, and lateral incisor anomalies, which is the reason why those are associated with etiological factors [6]. Likewise, many studies in different populations report that bilateral impaction is less frequent than unilateral impaction [7–10].

Even though lower canine impaction is less common than upper canine impaction, the first type is much more affected by transmigration [5, 8] (approximately 40.4% of mandibular impacted canines) [11]. On the other hand, it is more frequent in women [1, 5, 7, 10, 12, 13].

According to Mupparapu in 2002, mandibular canines in transmigration might be classified into 5 different types: (1) in a mesioangular position across the lower midline, (2) when the affected canine is in a horizontal impaction position near the lower mandibular border and below the incisor's root apices, (3) when the canine erupts either mesial or distal to the canine of the opposite side, (4) in a horizontal impaction position near the mandibular lower border and below the molars or premolars' root apices of the opposite side, and (5) in a vertical position on the lower midline but with its long axis crossing it [1].

A 2017 systematic review regarding impacted canines found that the treatment options for this condition differ if the affected tooth is just impacted or if it is impacted and in a transmigration condition. For the first, surgical removal and orthodontic traction used to be the most common options; meanwhile, for the latter, surgical removal and a radiographic follow-up tended to be the most frequent [6].

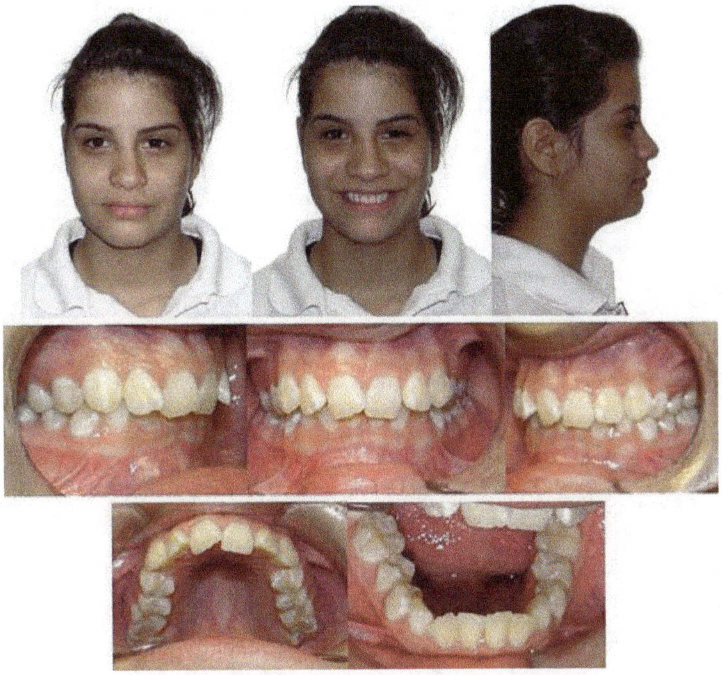

FIGURE 1: Pretreatment facial and intraoral photographs.

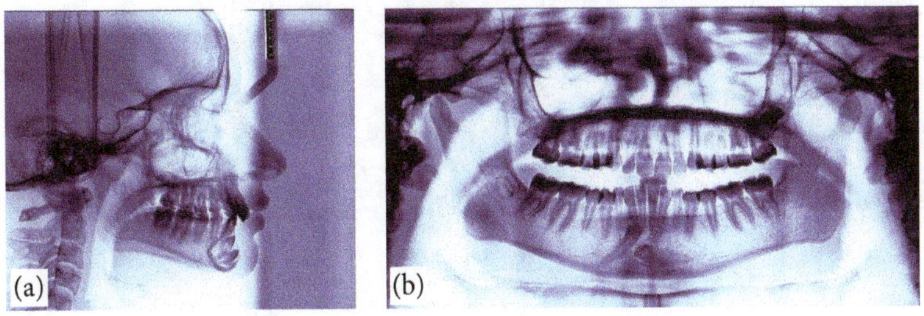

(a) (b)

FIGURE 2: (a) Pretreatment lateral cephalogram. (b) Pretreatment panoramic radiograph.

In any case, early diagnosis [11] and treatment [14] are recommended for eruption anomalies such as these, mainly due to the proven incidence of root resorption of the adjacent teeth [11].

This paper is aimed at describing the orthodontic treatment of a female patient with bilateral impaction of mandibular canines (one of them in Mupparapu type 2 transmigration) and at discussing the importance of the biomechanical design for successful treatment of these dental anomalies.

2. Case Report

2.1. Diagnosis and Etiology. A 14-year-old female patient was presented for orthodontic evaluation; her chief complaint was the absence of both lower canines. During the clinical assessment, it was noted that the deciduous lower canines were still present and a class I malocclusion with crowding, deep bite, and a straight profile was diagnosed (Figure 1). Dental casts, intraoral and extraoral photographs, and panoramic and lateral cephalogram X-rays were taken. On the panoramic X-ray, it was determined that both mandibular canines were impacted and the left one was in a Mupparapu type 2 transmigration position. Another critical issue was that the crown of the right canine was above the contralateral one. In the lateral cephalogram X-ray, it is possible to see that both canines were towards the vestibular side; however, the right one was closer to the incisors' roots (Figure 2). According to the Ricketts cephalometric analysis (Table 1), it was diagnosed that the lower incisors were retroclined, possibly because of the absence of the canines.

2.2. Treatment Objectives. The objectives of the treatment were (a) to open the space for the impacted and transmigrated canines, (b) to traction both canines to a functional position within the dental arch, (c) to improve the buccolingual inclination of the lower incisors, and (d) to correct the deep bite.

2.3. Treatment Alternatives. After the analysis of the studies, the patient was presented with the following treatment options: (a) surgical exposure of the canines and orthodontic traction and (b) surgical removal and an orthodontic opening of the spaces for future restoration. The orthodontist

Table 1: Ricketts cephalometric measurements.

	Initial	Final	Norm	Std dev
Dental relationships				
Molar relation (mm)	−0.1	−2.3	−3.0	1.0
Overjet (mm)	5.8	2.7	2.5	2.5
Overbite (mm)	4.8	−0.1	2.5	2.0
Mand incisor extrusion (mm)	2.4	−0.1	1.2	2.0
Interincisal angle (U1-L1) (°)	141.3	111.8	130.0	6.0
Skeletal/dental				
U-incisor protrusion (U1-APo) (mm)	3.3	6.3	3.5	2.3
L1 protrusion (L1-APo) (mm)	−2.0	3.6	1.0	2.3
U-incisor inclination (U1-APo) (°)	17.3	32.8	28.0	4.0
L1 to APo (°)	21.3	35.4	22.0	4.0
Occ plane to FH (°)	15.1	10.4	7.5	5.0
U6-PT vertical (mm)	9.5	16.5	17.0	3.0
Maxillo-mandibular relationships				
Convexity (A-NPo) (mm)	2.1	2.4	0.9	2.0
Mandibular arc (°)	36.7	43.8	29.7	4.0
Craniofacial relation				
FMA (MP-FH) (°)	30.2	20.4	24.2	4.5
Maxillary depth (FH-NA) (°)	87.0	97.1	90.0	3.0
Facial axis-Ricketts (NaBa-PtGn) (°)	92.4	92.0	90.0	3.5
Facial angle (FH-NPo) (°)	84.5	94.5	88.3	3.0
Facial taper (°)	65.3	65.1	68.0	3.5
Deep skeletal structure				
Porion location (mm)	−36.0	−37.6	−38.6	2.2
Cranial deflection (°)	19.6	29.8	27.3	3.0
Ramus position (°)	64.9	71.2	76.0	3.0
Lower face height (ANS-Xi-Pm) (°)	34.8	36.1	45.0	4.0
Esthetic				
Lower lip to *E*-plane (mm)	−1.7	−1.1	−2.0	2.0

explained to the patient's parents that the first option presented a risk of damaging the incisors roots, so the biomechanical design had to consider that. Also, the time of treatment could be longer than when choosing the second option. On the other hand, given her young age, the second option also had a disadvantage in that the patient would wear the restorations for a long time. Moreover, the increment in cost that the restorations would represent should be considered. In light of this information, the patient chose the first option of treatment.

2.4. Treatment Progress. Full fixed 0.018-inch metal Roth brackets were placed and bonded in both arches. The leveling and aligning phase was carried out in both arches using the next sequence of nickel-titanium wires: 0.012, 0.014, and 0.016. This phase lasted six months. Once the patient reached the 0.016 stainless steel (SS) wires, the canines were surgically exposed and two golden chains were cemented for traction. At the same time, to open the space for the canines, a couple of open coil springs were placed and the golden chain was ligated to the distal end of each one to initiate the traction with an up-and-distal vector (Figure 3).

Posteriorly, three wires were used, a 0.016 SS wire, which played an anchorage role, and two 0.014 nickel-titanium accessorial wires (one per side) to apply the traction force on the impacted teeth. As can be seen in Figure 4, the accessorial wires were tied around the SS wire and their mesial ends were introduced through the link closest to their respective chains (left and right). To prevent the mesial end of each accessorial wire from coming out, they were covered with a composite; meanwhile, their distal ends were bent to hold a power chain that would be tied to their respective first molar tube. With this system, the canines kept receiving a force with an up-and-distal vector. Given the caliber and the alloy of the accessorial wires, the forces were small and the moments were reduced. This scheme translated into having better control of the traction movement.

After seven months, the right canine made erupted and a bracket was fixed on it to be included in the arch. In addition, a new accessorial wire was made to move the crown of the left

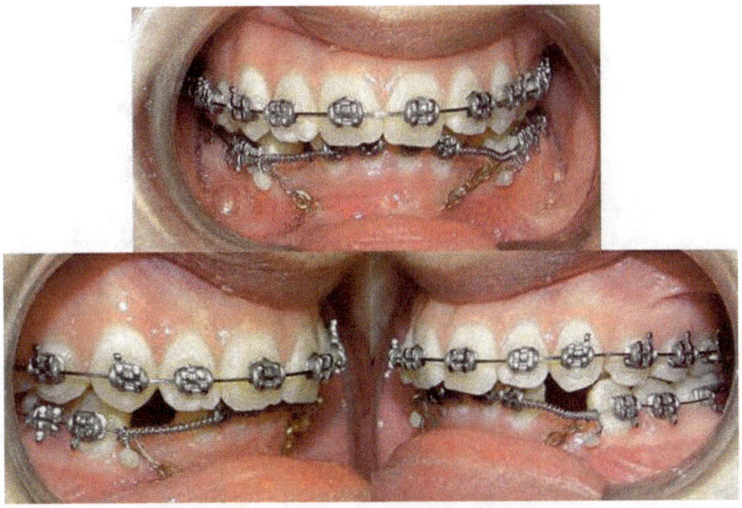

Figure 3: Intraoral photographs. Both golden chains are tied up to the distal end of their respective open coil to start the traction of the impacted canines.

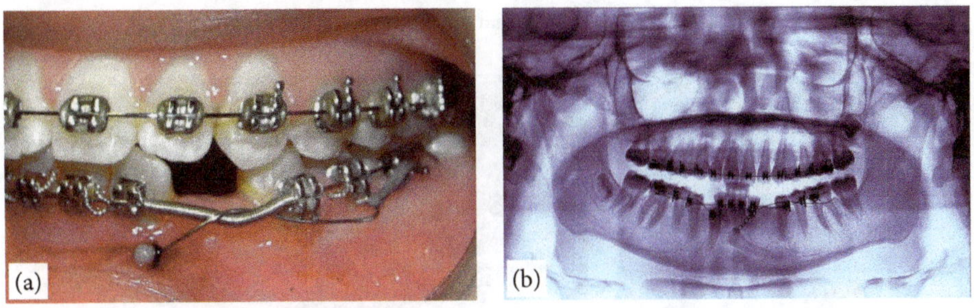

(a) (b)

Figure 4: (a) An intraoral photograph of the quadrant 3 accessorial wire tied up to the golden chain. (b) Progress panoramic radiograph.

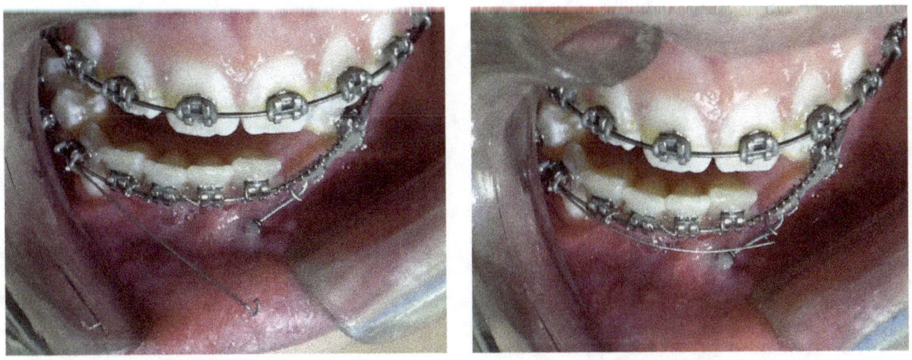

(a) (b)

Figure 5: Intraoral photographs showing the accessory wire used to move the crown of the left canine away from the incisors' roots: (a) in its passive manner; (b) once it has been activated.

canine away from the incisors' roots (0.018 nickel-titanium); this wire was tied at the right side (quadrant 4), and it would apply a force towards the vestibule. At the same time, the accessorial wire of quadrant 3 was changed to a 0.016 SS wire, and its mesial end was passed through the first link of the golden chain exposed in the mouth; to keep it from coming out, it was also covered with a composite. The distal end was bent to tie up a power chain that would exert a force with a distal vector (Figure 5). The new wire of quadrant 4 was tied up near the distal end of the sectional wire of quadrant 3; this way, the first would have the freedom to slide through the latter while tractioning the transmigrated canine towards the vestibular end.

Finally, after the eruption of the left canine, a bracket was fixed on it so it could be included in the dental arch. The next steps were to level the arch again, close the remaining spaces,

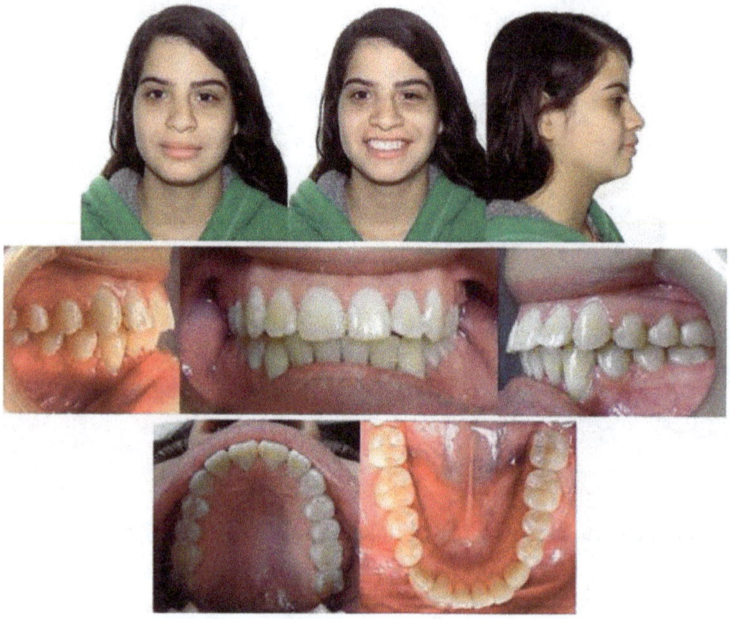

FIGURE 6: Posttreatment facial and intraoral photographs.

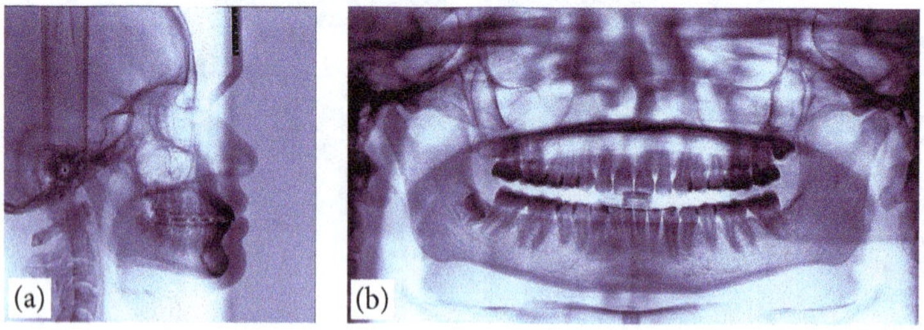

(a) (b)

FIGURE 7: (a) Final lateral cephalogram. (b) Final panoramic radiograph.

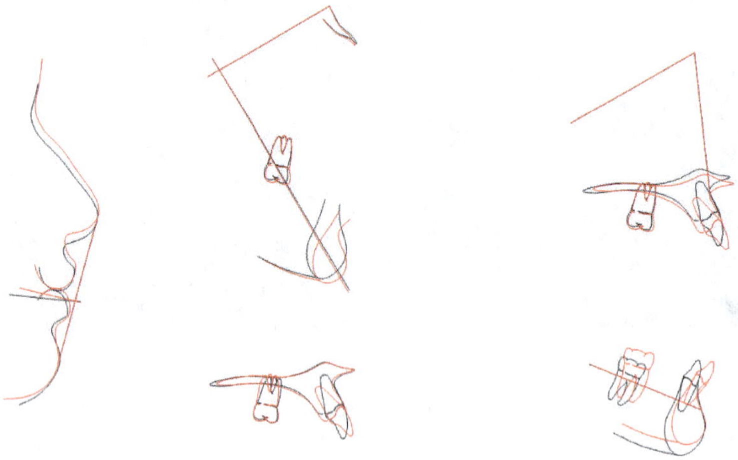

FIGURE 8: Ricketts superimpositions.

and do the final detailing. After three years of treatment, the brackets were removed and a fixed retainer was placed in the lower arch while a Hawley retainer was given for the upper section with the indication of full-time use. Figure 6 shows the case's final photographs.

3. Results

Both canines were successfully brought to a functional position within the dental arch and with a healthy periodontium. At the same time, the opening of the space for the canines helped to correct the buccolingual inclination of the lower incisors and the deep bite. The upper incisors suffered a slight proinclination; however, the patient's profile was kept inside the norm value (Table 1, Figures 7 and 8). Through orthodontic treatment, the crowding, irregularity, and rotations were resolved and, in the end, proper occlusion was achieved. Regarding the aesthetic aspect, a nice smile arc without buccal corridors or an excessive gingival display was obtained; in addition, the straight profile was maintained.

4. Discussion

The orthodontic treatment accomplished the goals of bringing both mandibular canines into the dental arch and correcting the crowding and the deep bite, thus achieving a proper occlusion. Moreover, the smile was improved, and at the same time, the treatment did not affect the original profile.

Scientific literature points out that the treatment of transmigrated mandibular canines usually involves a surgical extraction or a radiographic follow-up [6, 7, 11, 15]. Some authors indicate that the orthodontic traction treatment might be possible when the canine is in an angular position, which could be the reason why the Mupparapu type 1 cases are most commonly treated with this modality [16–19]. There are also reports of type 5 cases (vertical position on the lower midline but with its long axis crossing it) treated with orthodontic traction. In these cases, the canine is either tractioned or allowed to erupt, and then, it is shaped with restorative treatment to look like an incisor. Sometimes, this is done to replace some tooth that is missing or damaged by the transmigrated canine [20, 21].

The case described in this paper is the orthodontic traction of a Mupparapu type 2 transmigrated canine, which is unusual since those cases are frequently surgically removed [21, 22], left under radiographic follow-up [7, 18], or even surgically transplanted [23]. In the literature review, there was only one other report that found a Mupparapu type 2 canine that was orthodontically treated. In that case, the authors expressed their concern about damaging the lateral incisor's root during the treatment, so they instead chose to distalize it and then move the transmigrated canine towards its position. After this, both the lateral incisor and the canine were reshaped to resemble the teeth they were replacing [24]. Following other authors' recommendations in the case here described, the orthodontic traction was done with light force [14, 16] and with a biomechanical design that allowed for proper control of the vectors and the amount of force applied to the teeth involved [16]. In this regard, the use of the accessorial wires was critical to control the vectors in order to avoid damaging the adjacent structures.

As a further problem, the patient had the contralateral canine impacted, with its crown above the tooth in transmigration. Likewise, Kuftinec et al. in 1995 described a bilateral transmigration case where both canines were in a similar pattern to the case presented here; given its difficulty, the authors chose to extract both teeth [25]. On the other hand, as can be seen in the case discussed in this paper, it might be advantageous to traction the canine that is closest to the surface to liberate the path for the other.

Finally, in 1994, Wertz suggested that if the canine cusp has gone beyond the apex of the lateral incisor of the opposite side, it might be mechanically impossible to traction it [26]; it is interesting that, despite the fact that not all Mupparapu type 2 transmigrated canines reach this boundary determined by Wertz, most of them are surgically removed or left under radiographic follow-up, a fact that emphasizes the difficulty in treating these cases.

5. Conclusions

In conclusion, the traction of impacted mandibular canines is always a challenge for the orthodontist, especially when they are in a transmigrated position. The biomechanical design is critical for the success in these cases; it is recommended to use light forces for better control of vectors given that there is a high risk of damaging the adjacent tooth roots, even more so in Mupparapu type 2 cases.

References

[1] M. Mupparapu, "Patterns of intra-osseous transmigration and ectopic eruption of mandibular canines: review of literature and report of nine additional cases," *Dentomaxillofacial Radiology*, vol. 31, no. 6, pp. 355–360, 2002.

[2] U. Aydin, H. H. Yilmaz, and D. Yildirim, "Incidence of canine impaction and transmigration in a patient population," *Dentomaxillofacial Radiology*, vol. 33, no. 3, pp. 164–169, 2004.

[3] J. R. Herrera-Atoche, S. Diaz-Morales, G. Colome-Ruiz, M. Escoffie-Ramirez, and M. F. Orellana, "Prevalence of dental anomalies in a Mexican population," *Dentistry 3000*, vol. 2, no. 1, pp. 1–5, 2014.

[4] N. Watted and M. Abu-Hussein, "Prevalence of impacted canines in Arab population in Israel," *International Journal of Public Health Research*, vol. 6, no. 2, pp. 71–77, 2014.

[5] A. M. Aktan, S. Kara, F. Akgunlu, and S. Malkoc, "The incidence of canine transmigration and tooth impaction in a Turkish subpopulation," *European Journal of Orthodontics*, vol. 32, no. 5, pp. 575–581, 2010.

[6] D. Dalessandri, S. Parrini, R. Rubiano, D. Gallone, and M. Migliorati, "Impacted and transmigrant mandibular canines incidence, aetiology, and treatment: a systematic review," *European Journal of Orthodontics*, vol. 39, no. 2, pp. 161–169, 2017.

[7] R. M. Diaz-Sanchez, R. Castillo-de-Oyague, M. A. Serrera-Figallo, P. Hita-Iglesias, J. L. Gutierrez-Perez, and D. Torres-Lagares, "Transmigration of mandibular cuspids: review of published reports and description of nine new cases," *British Journal of Oral and Maxillofacial Surgery*, vol. 54, no. 3, pp. 241–247, 2016.

[8] G. Sharma and A. Nagpal, "A study of transmigrated canine in an Indian population," *International Scholarly Research Notices*, vol. 2014, Article ID 756516, 9 pages, 2014.

[9] M. Celikoglu, H. Kamak, and H. Oktay, "Investigation of transmigrated and impacted maxillary and mandibular canine teeth in an orthodontic patient population," *Journal of Oral and Maxillofacial Surgery*, vol. 68, no. 5, pp. 1001–1006, 2010.

[10] M. Isa-Kara, S. Ay, A. Murat-Aktan et al., "Analysis of different type of transmigrant mandibular teeth," *Medicina Oral, Patología Oral y Cirugía Bucal*, vol. 16, no. 3, pp. e335–e340, 2011.

[11] M. H. Bertl, C. Frey, K. Bertl, K. Giannis, A. Gahleitner, and G. D. Strbac, "Impacted and transmigrated mandibular canines: an analysis of 3D radiographic imaging data," *Clinical Oral Investigations*, vol. 22, no. 6, pp. 2389–2399, 2018.

[12] K. S. Al-Nimri and E. Bsoul, "Maxillary palatal canine impaction displacement in subjects with congenitally missing maxillary lateral incisors," *American Journal of Orthodontics and Dentofacial Orthopedics*, vol. 140, no. 1, pp. 81–86, 2011.

[13] M. R. Joshi, "Transmigrant mandibular canines: a record of 28 cases and a retrospective review of the literature," *The Angle Orthodontist*, vol. 71, no. 1, pp. 12–22, 2001.

[14] R. Cannavale, G. Matarese, G. Isola, V. Grassia, and L. Perillo, "Early treatment of an ectopic premolar to prevent molar-premolar transposition," *American Journal of Orthodontics and Dentofacial Orthopedics*, vol. 143, no. 4, pp. 559–569, 2013.

[15] K. Gündüz and P. Celenk, "The incidence of impacted transmigrant canines: a retrospective study," *Oral Radiology*, vol. 26, no. 2, pp. 77–81, 2010.

[16] S. Cavuoti, G. Matarese, G. Isola, J. Abdolreza, F. Femiano, and L. Perillo, "Combined orthodontic-surgical management of a transmigrated mandibular canine," *The Angle Orthodontist*, vol. 86, no. 4, pp. 681–691, 2016.

[17] S. Kumar, P. Jayaswal, K. C. Pentapati, A. Valiathan, and N. Kotak, "Investigation of the transmigrated canine in an orthodontic patient population," *Journal of Orthodontics*, vol. 39, no. 2, pp. 89–94, 2012.

[18] E. Mazinis, A. Zafeiriadis, A. Karathanasis, and T. Lambrianidis, "Transmigration of impacted canines: prevalence, management and implications on tooth structure and pulp vitality of adjacent teeth," *Clinical Oral Investigations*, vol. 16, no. 2, pp. 625–632, 2012.

[19] S. P. Plaza, "Orthodontic traction of a transmigrated mandibular canine using mini-implant: a case report and review," *Journal of Orthodontics*, vol. 43, no. 4, pp. 314–321, 2016.

[20] N. Umashree, A. Kumar, and T. Nagaraj, "Transmigration of mandibular canines," *Case Reports in Dentistry*, vol. 2013, Article ID 697671, 7 pages, 2013.

[21] M. K. Bhullar, I. Aggarwal, R. Verma, and A. S. Uppal, "Mandibular canine transmigration: report of three cases and literature review," *Journal of International Society of Preventive & Community Dentistry*, vol. 7, no. 1, pp. 8–14, 2017.

[22] R. Bahl, J. Singla, M. Gupta, and A. Malhotra, "Abberantly placed impacted mandibular canine," *Contemporary Clinical Dentistry*, vol. 4, no. 2, pp. 217–219, 2013.

[23] S. L. Verma, V. P. Sharma, and G. P. Singh, "Management of a transmigrated mandibular canine," *Journal of Orthodontic Science*, vol. 1, no. 1, pp. 23–28, 2012.

[24] L. Vaida, B. I. Todor, C. Corega, M. Baciut, and G. Baciut, "A rare case of canine anomaly – a possible algorithm for treating it," *Romanian Journal of Morphology & Embryology*, vol. 55, Supplement 3, pp. 1197–1202, 2014.

[25] M. M. Kuftinec, Y. Shapira, and O. Nahlieli, "A case report. Bilateral transmigration of impacted mandibular canines," *Journal of the American Dental Association (1939)*, vol. 126, no. 7, pp. 1022–1024, 1995.

[26] R. A. Wertz, "Treatment of transmigrated mandibular canines," *American Journal of Orthodontics and Dentofacial Orthopedics*, vol. 106, no. 4, pp. 419–427, 1994.

13

Orthodontic Treatment of Bilateral Transposition of Maxillary Canines and Lateral Incisors

Mandla Dominic Nyakale

Department of Orthodontics, Faculty of Dentistry, University of the Western Cape, Cape Town, South Africa

Correspondence should be addressed to Mandla Dominic Nyakale; mnyakale77@gmail.com

Academic Editor: John H. Campbell

Dental transposition is a severe disturbance of tooth position and its eruptive sequence. It may affect any tooth, and it may occur at any location within the dental arch, although some teeth may be more frequently affected than others. There are several types of dental transposition, and their classification depends on the type of teeth involved. The aetiology of transposition is not very clear and has always been the subject of controversies, and it is still not completely understood. The prevalence of dental transposition and the factors related to this dental anomaly have been well documented in the literature. When treating dental transposition, many factors which may affect the treatment results must be considered, such as aesthetics, occlusion, treatment duration, patient comfort, patient cooperation, and periodontal support. Various treatment options are currently available for the treatment of dental transposition. Successful treatment outcomes depend on the patient's age, concern about facial and dental aesthetics, motivation of the patient, functional requirements, type of malocclusion, and the position of the root apices. The present case report is aimed at outlining the orthodontic treatment of a young adult patient diagnosed with bilateral maxillary canine-lateral incisor transposition.

1. Introduction

Dental transposition was first described by Harris [1] as the positional interchange of two adjacent teeth within the same quadrant. Dental transposition may be considered to be complete when both the crowns and the roots of the involved teeth are completely interchanged and as incomplete when only the crowns of the involved teeth are interchanged, while their roots remain in their normal positions [2]. Dental transposition can adversely affect both the aesthetic and functional aspects of the dentition [3], and thus, it is important to understand the occurrence of this dental anomaly in order to manage it timeously and efficiently [4]. A multidisciplinary approach may be needed for the successful treatment of this dental anomaly in order to achieve long-term aesthetic and functional outcomes [3, 5–7]. The prevalence of dental transposition has been shown to vary in different populations. The highest prevalence of dental transposition has been reported in the Chinese population at 0.81% [8], followed by Africa estimated at 0.51% [9, 10], the United Kingdom estimated at 0.38% [11], and the European population with the least prevalence estimated at 0.26% [12]. Numerous studies have shown that dental transposition occurs more frequently in females than in males [3, 13–18] although other authors have reported a higher frequency in males [19–22]. The maxillary arch has been shown to be affected more frequently by dental transposition than the mandibular arch [22–24]. The tooth most frequently affected by dental transposition is the maxillary canine [14] with a prevalence of 0.14-0.51% [25, 26], and unilateral canine transpositions are more prevalent on the left than the right side [27]. Maxillary canine-first premolar transposition has been reported to be the most frequent, with a prevalence rate of approximately 0.13% [14, 28] in the general population [29]. Peck and Peck [16] classified dental transposition into five categories according to the type of teeth involved and also in the order of decreasing frequency as follows:

(1) *Class I*. Canine-first premolar transposition

(2) *Class II*. Canine-lateral incisor transposition

(3) *Class III*. Canine-first molar transposition

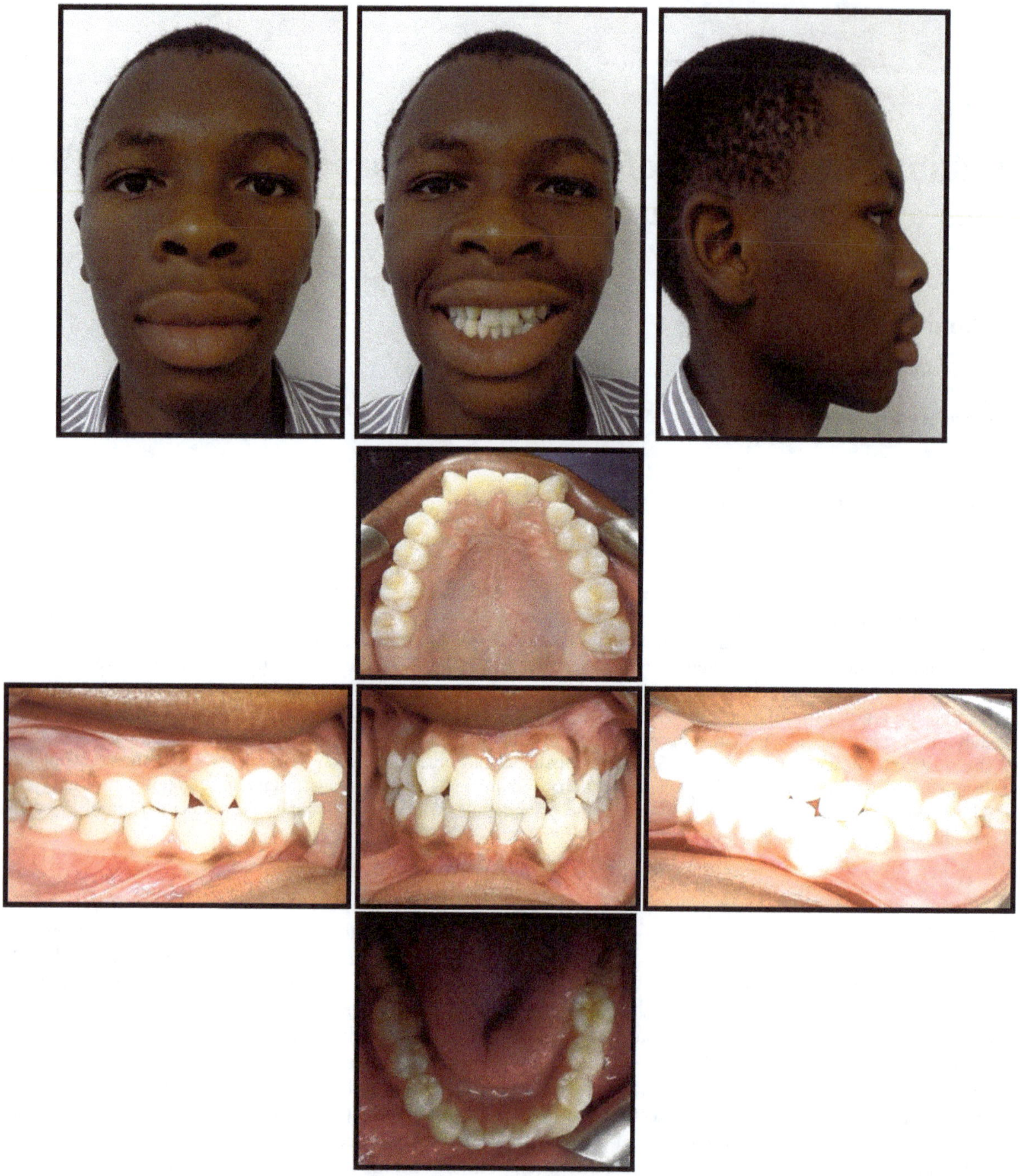

Figure 1: Pretreatment photograph.

(4) *Class IV*. Lateral incisor-central incisor transposition

(5) *Class V*. Canine-central incisor transposition

Several factors have been implicated in the aetiology of dental transposition, and these include genetic factors [2, 30], interchange in the position of the developing dental lamina during odontogenesis [14], trauma [13], mechanical interferences [16], and early loss of primary teeth [3, 15, 17, 18, 20, 21, 31]. Dental transposition may also occur with other dental anomalies such as tooth agenesis [15, 32], peg shaped lateral incisors [3], and retained primary teeth [33].

Diagnosis is usually made clinically; however, radiographs may be needed to confirm the severity of this dental anomaly. Early treatment is suggested for this condition [34]; however, this may require complex and lengthy treatment methods [35].

Presence of dental transposition can also be a very useful tool in the field of forensic odontology [36]. Over the years, dental transposition has been used successfully to identify unknown individuals, deceased victims, suspects of a crime, and also the victims of a mass disaster. Due to its extremely rare occurrence, dental transposition can be a very useful

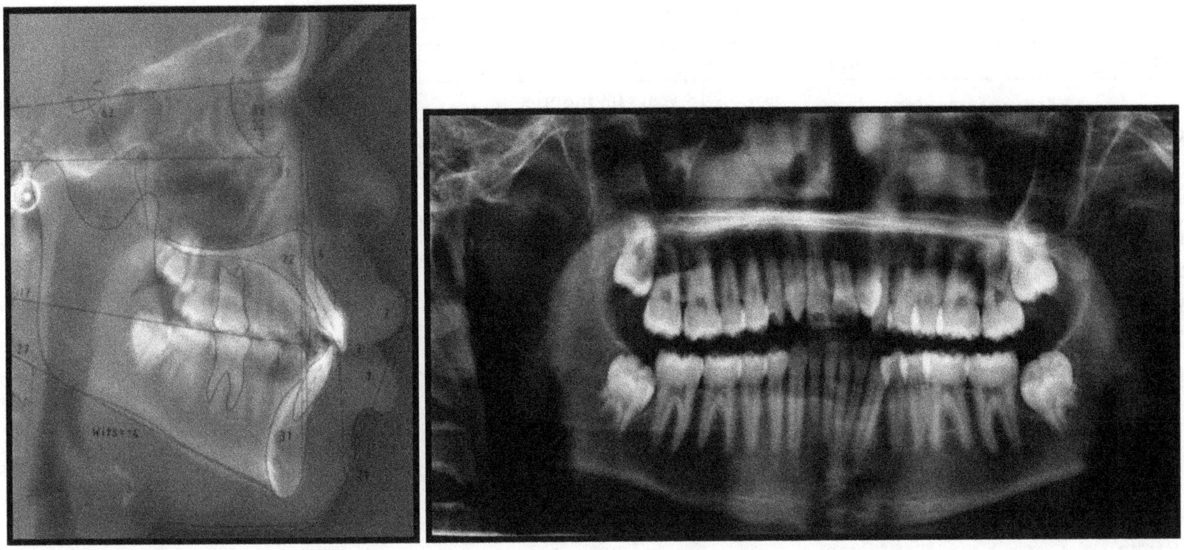

FIGURE 2: Pretreatment radiographs.

marker on the dental records which can be used to identify individuals, particularly when other comparative methods of identification are neither available nor adequate to establish the identity of the individual in question [36].

The objectives of treatment are to establish good static and functional occlusion and also to provide pleasing facial aesthetics while maintaining temporomandibular joint and periodontal health [37]. The treatment of dental transposition frequently requires a multidisciplinary approach in order to achieve long-term aesthetic and functional results [3, 4, 6, 7, 38]. When treating dental transposition, many factors that may affect the treatment results must be considered, such as the patient's age, dentofacial aesthetics, functional occlusal requirements, treatment duration, patient motivation and cooperation, periodontal support and type, and severity of malocclusion. Age is the single most important factor beyond all the other factors, which is directly correlated with the tissue regeneration. Available treatment options include alignment of the transposed teeth in their transposed positions [19, 39], extraction of one of the transposed teeth, or complete correction of the transposed teeth to their normal positions [40]. Many authors believe that the ideal treatment approach is to completely correct the transposed teeth to their normal positions; however, this may not be possible in many clinical situations. Risk to the teeth and adjacent tissues and treatment duration must be assessed and discussed with the patient prior to orthodontic treatment. The following case report is aimed at presenting the orthodontic treatment of a patient diagnosed with bilateral maxillary canine-lateral incisor transposition.

2. Case Presentation

An 18-year old male patient was referred to the orthodontic clinic at Pelonomi Tertiary hospital in Bloemfontein (Free State Province, South Africa) with the chief complaint of crowded anterior teeth and poor aesthetics. Ethical approval to publish this case report was obtained from the Health Sciences Research Ethics Committee of the University of the Free State (Ethics Reference number: UFS-HSD2019/0697/0110, Appendix A). The patient was in good general health, and the medical and dental history indicated no contraindications to orthodontic treatment. The patient had no history of trauma to the head and neck area. Extraoral examination revealed a normal face type, a convex facial profile with a symmetrical face. Intraoral examination showed the permanent dentition stage, good oral hygiene with no deleterious oral habits. The teeth were generally healthy with no carious lesions. The periodontal and gingival tissues were generally healthy with no evidence of bleeding or deep probing depths. Analysis of the occlusion revealed angle class I malocclusion with significant crowding of the maxillary and mandibular anterior teeth which were also protrusive. Bilateral transposition of maxillary canines and lateral incisors were also observed (Figure 1). Panoramic radiographic examination showed the teeth in a permanent dentition stage with bilateral complete transposition of maxillary canines and lateral incisors. The third molars were present in both jaws, and the mandibular third molars were developing in the ramus (Figure 2). No other pathologies were detected on the radiographs. Tracing and analysis of the lateral cephalogram showed a mild class III skeletal pattern with a horizontal growth pattern (Table 1).

3. Treatment Objectives

There were several potential treatment options available, ranging from extraction treatment, surgical repositioning of the transposed teeth, and alignment of the transposed teeth in their transposed positions. When planning to align the transposed maxillary canines and lateral incisors in their transposed positions, there are generally two problems to consider. The first problem is whether the lateral incisor will be able to function as a canine [7] and, the second is, whether we would be able to disguise the canine as a lateral incisor [41, 42]. This treatment option was not a preferred

TABLE 1: Lateral cephalometric readings.

Measurement	Norm	Before treatment	After treatment	14-month follow-up
Age		18 years 02 months	20 years 10 months	22 years 01 month
Skeletal pattern				
SNA (°)	87°	88°	87°	88°
SNB (°)	82°	85°	84°	84°
ANB (°)	5°	3°	3°	4°
Face plane angle	87°	89°	88°	90°
Convexity (NA-Apo) (mm)	4 mm	4 mm	3 mm	4 mm
Wits (mm)	-1-2 mm	-4 mm	-3 mm	-3 mm
Occipital plane to SN (°)	7°	7°	7°	7°
S.n. GoGn (°)	32-34°	27°	29°	28°
y-Axis (SGn.SN) (°)	66-68°	63°	65°	64°
Incisor relations				
U1-NA (°)	22°	22°	21°	23°
U1-NA (mm)	7 mm	7 mm	5 mm	6 mm
U1-NB (°)	38°	31°	29°	32°
L1-NB (mm)	10 mm	7 mm	6 mm	8 mm
APo (mm)	8 mm	7 mm	6 mm	8 mm
Soft tissues				
Holdaway angle (°)	20°	21°	20°	20°

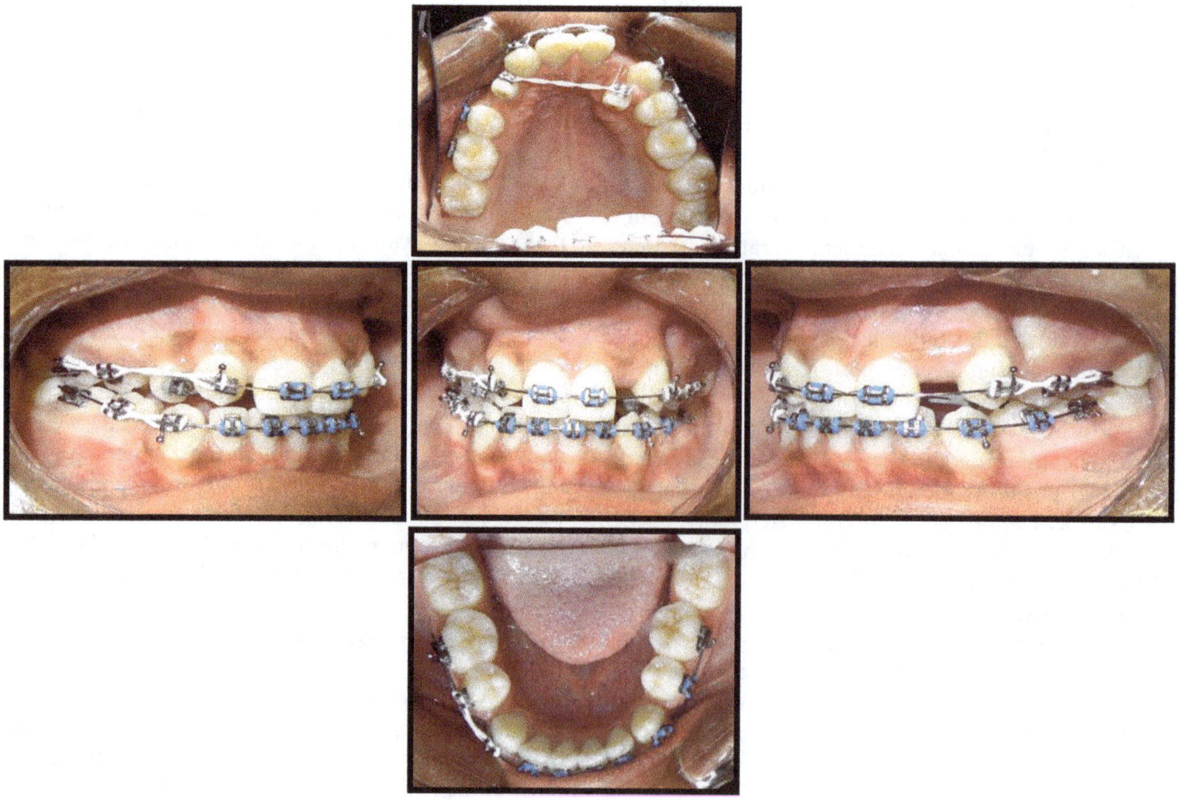

FIGURE 3: Intermediate intraoral photographs.

choice as our patient had significant crowding of the anterior teeth which required extraction of the first premolars to create space. The maxillary lateral incisors are also less favourable for canine guidance during functional occlusion because of their thin and short roots. Hence, conversion into group function may be beneficial for nonextraction cases

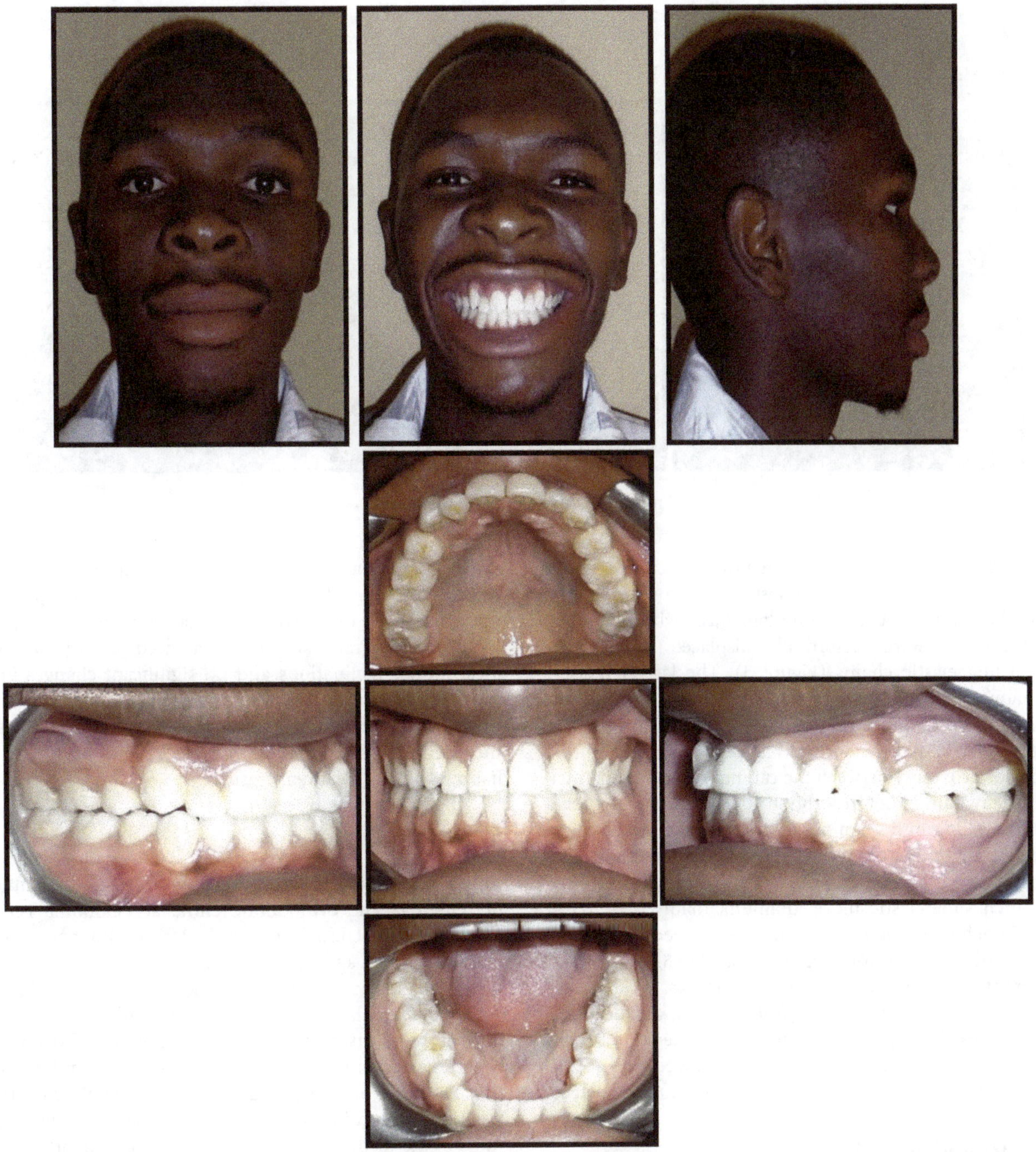

FIGURE 4: Posttreatment photographs.

[41, 42]. Similarly, camouflage of the maxillary canines will often require grinding of the tips, together with the addition of composite resin or porcelain veneers to improve the aesthetic appearance [41, 42]. The maxillary canine also has a broader and higher gingival contour when compared with the lateral incisor [7], and this option would have compromised the aesthetic appearance. It was mainly for these reasons that it was decided to correct the transposed teeth to their normal positions in the present case. The treatment objectives were to correct the transposed teeth to their normal positions, level and align the dental arches, and establish pleasing dentofacial aesthetics and good functional occlusion. The treatment plan included extraction of maxillary and mandibular first premolars in order to gain the space required to align and upright the crowded and protrusive anterior teeth.

4. Treatment Progress

Banding and bonding of the teeth were done with the standard preadjusted 0.018×0.025-inch slot Roth prescription edgewise appliances. Teeth were levelled and aligned with 0.012-inch, 0.014-inch, and 0.016-inch superelastic nickel titanium archwires, respectively. This was followed with

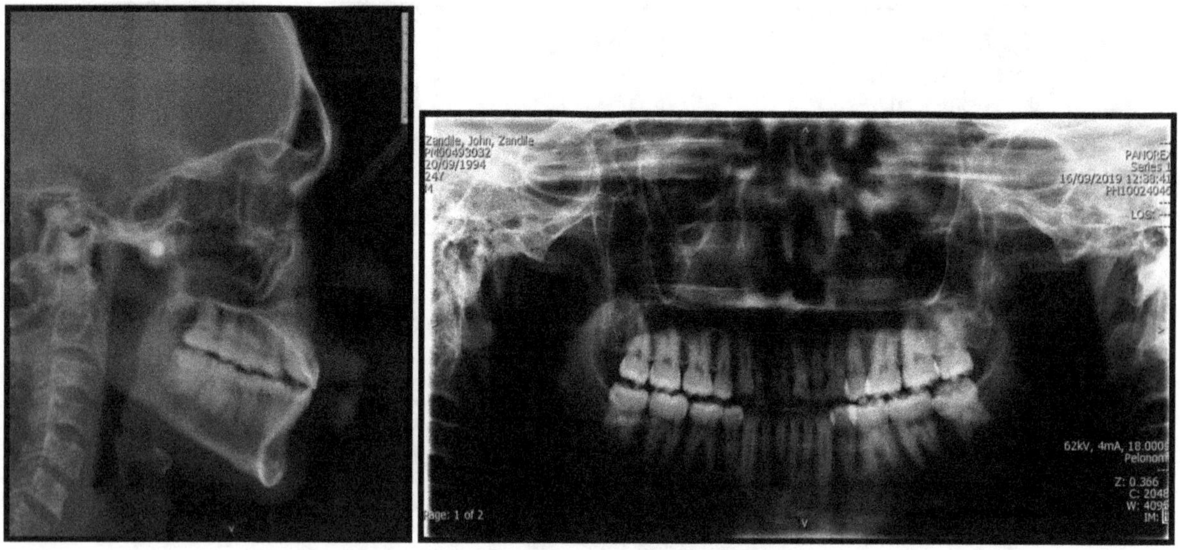

FIGURE 5: Posttreatment radiographs.

the retraction of maxillary and mandibular canines using elastic chains on 0.016-inch stainless steel archwires. Retraction of the canines was done simultaneously while maxillary lateral incisors were reciprocally displaced towards the palate using elastic chains (Figure 3). The lateral incisors were moved palatally in order to clear the way for the distal movement of the transposed canines. This was also done to prevent bony loss at the cortical plate of the canines and to avoid root proximity between the canine and the lateral incisor thus avoiding root resorption and periodontal breakdown. Levelling and aligning archwires were placed again to finalize alignment of all the teeth including the maxillary lateral incisors. Torque control was initiated with 0.016 × 0.022-inch superelastic nickel titanium, followed by 0.017 × 0.025-inch beta titanium archwires, respectively. Final detailing of the occlusion was done on 0.018 × 0.025-inch stainless steel archwires using finishing elastics. Final rectangular stainless steel wires were left in place for an additional 8 weeks to establish proper root torque. At the end of treatment, the orthodontic appliances were removed, and maxillary Hawley and mandibular fixed 3-3 retainers were placed.

5. Treatment Results

Treatment lasted for 24 months and at the end of orthodontic treatment, the teeth were well aligned, and canines and molars were in a class I relationship, with normal overjet and overbite. The maxillary and mandibular midlines were corresponding, and this improved the smile appearance. The gingival contour on the palatal aspect of the maxillary right lateral incisor was very high after orthodontic treatment (Figure 4). The patient was referred to the periodontist for the placement of a connective tissue graft to the affected area, but later he declined to have this treatment done. A posttreatment panoramic radiograph showed the optimal positioning of the maxillary and mandibular teeth with proper root parallelism with no signs of alveolar bone or root resorption (Figure 5). Periapical radiographs are more preferred to evaluate the presence of external apical root resorption [43], but unfortunately, these radiographs were not available in the hospital. A posttreatment lateral cephalometric radiograph showed a balanced facial profile with ideal incisor inclinations and no significant changes in the skeletal measurements (Figure 5/Table 1). No evidence of relapse or significant changes was observed 14 months after the retention period (Figure 6/Table 1), and the patient was happy with the treatment results.

6. Discussion

This is a case report of an 18-year old male patient who presented to the orthodontic clinic at Pelonomi Tertiary Hospital in Bloemfontein, South Africa. Our patient's age falls within the age range of the majority of patients who seek orthodontic treatment at Pelonomi Tertiary Hospital. Treatment results of this case will assist with treatment planning of future cases with a similar diagnosis. Although it has been reported in the literature that preventive and interceptive treatment of transposed teeth is best instituted early in the mixed dentition stage during the development of the roots of the teeth [3], the results of this case report will give us some insight into the management of transposition which may be diagnosed later in life. Dental transposition has also been reported to occur more frequently in female subjects than male subjects [3, 13–18]. Our patient was male, and this was in keeping with findings by other authors [19–22]. Our case was bilateral transposition of the maxillary canines and lateral incisors, and this has been reported as the second most frequent dental transposition to occur in the human dentition [16], with both dental and aesthetic complications [22]. As discussed earlier, dental transposition may be classified as complete or incomplete depending on the involvement of the crowns and roots [17]. Our case was a complete bilateral transposition of maxillary lateral incisors and canines. Since the maxillary canines are keystones in the dental arch, both for aesthetics and normal occlusal

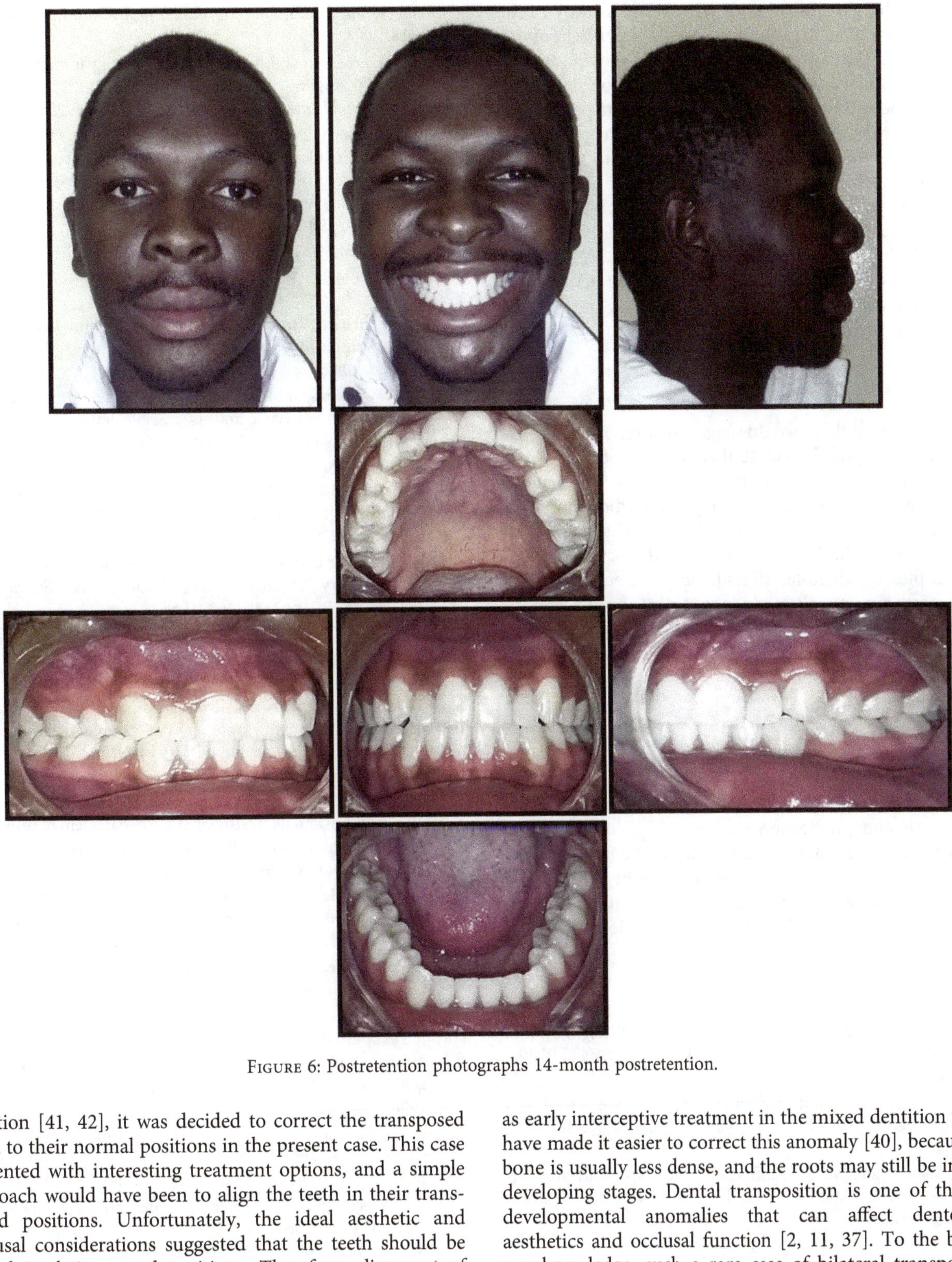

FIGURE 6: Postretention photographs 14-month postretention.

function [41, 42], it was decided to correct the transposed teeth to their normal positions in the present case. This case presented with interesting treatment options, and a simple approach would have been to align the teeth in their transposed positions. Unfortunately, the ideal aesthetic and occlusal considerations suggested that the teeth should be placed in their natural positions. Therefore, alignment of the transposed teeth to their natural positions in the dental arch was a preferred treatment option. It was then decided to extract the four first premolars to create the space needed to align the teeth and also to gain room to correct the transposed teeth. The treatment approach was planned in line with the patient's age, concern about dentofacial aesthetics, and also functional occlusal requirements. Preventive as well as early interceptive treatment in the mixed dentition would have made it easier to correct this anomaly [40], because the bone is usually less dense, and the roots may still be in their developing stages. Dental transposition is one of the rare developmental anomalies that can affect dentofacial aesthetics and occlusal function [2, 11, 37]. To the best of our knowledge, such a rare case of bilateral transposition of maxillary canines and lateral incisors has never been reported in the literature. The outcome of treatment of this case report will give us some insight with regards to the treatment options available to us regarding this dental anomaly. Complete dental transposition, although complicated, can be treated successfully by applying appropriate orthodontic mechanics [40]. The patient's needs should be assessed carefully as the anterior teeth relate directly to the psychological wellbeing of the patient [44]. Treatment of this case also presented with a few challenges, and the biggest challenge was poor buccal root torque control on the maxillary lateral incisors and also the recession on the palatal gingiva on the maxillary right lateral incisor. Proper torque control on the teeth requires a large moment to force ratio of at least 12 : 1 [45], and this can be achieved by placing a full thickness wire for a longer period of time, but unfortunately, the patient wanted to end the treatment as he was happy with the achieved results despite having been advised otherwise. The patient was also referred to the periodontist for the placement of a connective tissue graft, but he later declined to undertake this treatment.

7. Conclusion

Although many authors would suggest that repositioning the completely transposed teeth to their normal positions may be a complex and time-consuming process, it was decided in this case report to attempt to reposition the completely transposed maxillary canines and lateral incisors to their normal positions. In the present case, good functional occlusion and pleasing dentofacial aesthetics were achieved. This case report suggests that ideal treatment results can be obtained in difficult cases by meticulous treatment planning and proper mechanics in the shortest time and with the minimum tissue damage possible.

Consent

The patient has given consent for his images and other relevant clinical information to be published in this article solely for research and publication purposes (Appendix B). The patient understands that his name will not be revealed, and due efforts will be made to conceal his identity and ensure anonymity. A copy of the written informed consent is available for review by the Editor-in-Chief of this journal.

References

[1] C. A. Harris, *A Dictionary of Dental Sciences, Bibliography and Medical Terminology*, vol. 11, no. 36, 1849, Lindsay and Blakiston, Philadelphia, 1849.

[2] A. Chattopadhyay and K. Srinivas, "Transposition of teeth and genetic etiology," *Angle Orthodontist*, vol. 66, pp. 147–152, 1996.

[3] Y. Shapira and M. M. Kuftinec, "Maxillary tooth transpositions: characteristic features and accompanying dental anomalies," *American Journal of Orthodontics and Dentofacial Orthopedics*, vol. 119, no. 2, pp. 127–134, 2001.

[4] S. Chaushu, A. Becker, and M. Zalkind, "Prosthetic considerations in the restoration of orthodontically treated maxillary lateral incisors to replace missing central incisors: a clinical report," *Journal of Prosthetic Dentistry*, vol. 85, no. 4, pp. 335–341, 2001.

[5] R. Sabri, A. Zaher, and H. Kassem, "Tooth transposition: a review and clinical considerations for treatment," *Journal of the World Federation of Orthodontics*, vol. 9, no. 4, pp. 303–318, 2008.

[6] C. Beznos, "An alternative approach to replacement of a congenitally missing maxillary central incisor: a case report," *Quintessence International*, vol. 27, no. 11, pp. 759–762, 1996.

[7] V. G. Kokich, D. L. Nappen, and P. A. Shapiro, "Gingival contour and clinical crown length: their effect on the esthetic appearance of maxillary anterior teeth," *American Journal of Orthodontics and Dentofacial Orthopaedics*, vol. 86, no. 2, pp. 89–94, 1984.

[8] C. Shiu-yin, V. Chu, and Y. Ki, "A retrospective study on 69 cases of maxillary tooth transposition," *Journal of Oral Science*, vol. 54, no. 2, pp. 197–203, 2012.

[9] S. E. Burnett, "Prevalence of maxillary canine-first premolar transposition in a composite African sample," *Angle Orthodontist*, vol. 69, pp. 187–189, 1999.

[10] A. A. Umweni and M. A. Ojo, "The frequency of tooth transpositions in Nigerians, and its possible aetiologic factors and clinical implications," *Journal of the Dental Association of South Africa*, vol. 52, no. 9, pp. 551–554, 1997.

[11] A. Sandham and H. Harvie, "Ectopic eruption of the maxillary canine resulting in transposition with adjacent teeth," *Tandlaegebladet*, vol. 89, no. 1, pp. 9–11, 1985.

[12] B. Thilander and S. O. Jakobsson, "Local factors in impaction of maxillary canines," *Acta Odontologica Scandinavia*, vol. 26, no. 1-2, pp. 145–168, 1968.

[13] P. K. Dyal, K. H. Shodhan, and C. J. Dave, "Transposition of canine with traumatic etiology," *Journal of Indian Dental Association*, vol. 55, pp. 283–285, 1983.

[14] D. J. Plunket, P. S. Dysart, T. B. Kardos, and G. P. Herbison, "A study of transposed canines in a sample of orthodontic patients," *British Journal of Orthodontics*, vol. 25, no. 3, pp. 203–208, 1998.

[15] M. Budai, I. Ficzere, K. Gábris, and I. Tarjan, "Frequency of transposition and its treatment at the department of orthodontics of Semmelweis University in the last five years," *Fogorvosi Szemle Journal*, vol. 96, no. 1, pp. 21–24, 2003.

[16] S. Peck and L. Peck, "Classification of maxillary tooth transpositions," *American Journal of Orthodontics and Dentofacial Orthopaedics*, vol. 107, no. 5, pp. 505–517, 1995.

[17] L. Peck, S. Peck, and Y. Attia, "Maxillary canine-first premolar transposition associated dental anomalies and genetic basis," *Angle Orthodontist*, vol. 63, pp. 99–110, 1993.

[18] S. Peck, L. Peck, and M. Kataja, "Mandibular lateral incisor-canine transposition, concomitant dental anomalies, and genetic control," *Angle Orthodontist*, vol. 68, pp. 455–466, 1998.

[19] R. Ciarlantini and B. Melsen, "Maxillary tooth transposition: correct or accept?," *American Journal of Orthodontics and Dentofacial Orthopedics*, vol. 132, no. 3, pp. 385–394, 2007.

[20] E. C. Weeks and S. M. Power, "The presentations and management of transposed teeth," *British Dental Journal*, vol. 181, no. 11, pp. 421–424, 1996.

[21] C. Feichtinger, B. Rossiwall, and H. Wunderer, "Canine transposition as autosomal recessive trait in an inbred kindred," *Journal of Dental Restoration*, vol. 56, no. 12, pp. 1449–1452, 1977.

[22] M. A. Papadopoulos, M. Chatzoudi, and E. G. Kaklamanos, "Prevalence of tooth transposition," *Angle Orthodontist*, vol. 80, no. 2, pp. 275–285, 2010.

[23] K. Venkataraghavan, P. P. Anantharaj Athimuthu, and R. B.

Jagadeesh, "Transposition of mandibular lateral incisor – canine (Mn I2.C) associated with hypodontia: a review and rare clinical case," *Journal of Clinical and Diagnostic Research*, vol. 8, no. 4, pp. 4–6, 2014.

[24] C. R. Qamar and M. Riaz, "Transposition of teeth: a review of the literature," *Pakistan Orthodontic Journal*, vol. 2, no. 2, pp. 72–75, 2010.

[25] A. Demir, F. A. Basciftci, I. E. Gelgör, and A. I. Karaman, "Maxillary canine transposition," *Journal of Clinical Orthodontics*, vol. 36, no. 1, pp. 35–37, 2002.

[26] A. Ruprecht, S. Batniji, and E. El-Neweihi, "The incidence of transposition of teeth in dental patients," *Journal of Paedodontics*, vol. 9, pp. 244–249, 1985.

[27] M. R. Joshi and N. A. Bhatt, "Canine transposition," *Oral Surgery, Oral Medicine and Oral Pathology*, vol. 31, no. 1, pp. 49–54, 1971.

[28] C. Filho, M. A. Cardoso, T. L. An, and F. A. Bertoz, "Maxillary canine-first premolar transposition," *Angle Orthodontist*, vol. 77, no. 1, pp. 167–175, 2007.

[29] H. Tukkahraman, M. Sayın, and H. H. Yılmaz, "Maxillary canine transposition to incisor site: a rare condition," *Angle Orthodontist*, vol. 75, pp. 284–287, 2005.

[30] N. J. Ely, M. Sherriff, and M. T. Cobourne, "Dental transposition as a disorder of genetic origin," *European Journal of Orthodontics*, vol. 28, no. 2, pp. 145–151, 2006.

[31] Y. Shapira, "Transposition of canines," *Journal of American Dental Association*, vol. 100, no. 5, pp. 710–712, 1980.

[32] S. Camilleri, "Maxillary canine anomalies and tooth agenesis," *European Journal of Orthodontics*, vol. 27, no. 5, pp. 450–456, 2005.

[33] H. H. Yilmaz et al.et al, "Prevalence of tooth transpositions and associated dental anomalies in Turkish population," *Dentomaxillofacial Radiology*, vol. 34, no. 1, pp. 32–35, 2005.

[34] R. Cannavale, G. Matarese, G. Isola, V. Grassia, and L. Perillo, "Early treatment of an ectopic premolar transposition," *American Journal of Orthodontics and Dentofacial Orthopedics*, vol. 143, no. 4, pp. 559–569, 2013.

[35] L. J. Oesterle, R. J. Cronin Jr., and D. M. Ranly, "Maxillary implants and the growing patient," *International Journal of Maxillofacial Implantology*, vol. 8, pp. 377–387, 1993.

[36] S. Nambiar, S. Mogra, and S. Shetty, "Transposition of teeth: a forensic perspective," *Journal of Forensic Dental Sciences*, vol. 6, no. 3, pp. 151–153, 2014.

[37] Y. Shapira and M. M. Kuftinec, "Tooth transpositions- a review of the literature and treatment considerations," *Angle Orthodontist*, vol. 59, pp. 271–276, 1989.

[38] A. B. Rabie and R. W. Wong, "Bilateral transposition of maxillary canines to the incisor region," *Journal of Clinical Orthodontics*, vol. 33, no. 11, pp. 651–655, 1999.

[39] S. Kurodas and Y. Kurodab, "Nonextraction treatment of upper canine-premolar transposition in an adult patient," *Angle Orthodontist*, vol. 75, pp. 472–477, 2005.

[40] Y. Shapira and M. M. Kuftinec, "A unique treatment approach for maxillary canine-lateral incisor transposition," *American Journal of Orthodontics and Dentofacial Orthopedics*, vol. 119, no. 5, pp. 540–545, 2001.

[41] D. M. Sarver and M. B. Ackerman, "Dynamic smile visualization and quantification: part 1. Evolution of the concept and dynamic records for smile capture," *American Journal of Orthodontics and Dentofacial Orthopedics*, vol. 124, no. 1, pp. 4–12, 2003.

[42] D. M. Sarver and M. B. Ackerman, "Dynamic smile visualization and quantification: part 2. Smile analysis and treatment strategies," *American Journal of Orthodontics and Dentofacial Orthopedics*, vol. 124, no. 2, pp. 116–127, 2003.

[43] W. Luchessi and C. J. Nortjé, "Suitability of the panoramic radiograph for assessment of mesiodistal angulation of teeth in the buccal segments of the mandible," *American Journal of Orthodontics*, vol. 94, no. 4, pp. 303–310, 1988.

[44] D. P. Motloba, M. P. S. Sethusa, and O. A. Ayo-Yusuf, "The psychological impact of malocclusion on patients seeking orthodontic treatment at a South African oral health training centre," *South African Dental Journal*, vol. 71, pp. 200–205, 2002.

[45] R. Nanda, "Dr. Ravindra Nanda on his treatment philosophy part - I," *Journal of the Indian Orthodontic Society*, vol. 39, no. 2, pp. 68–78, 2005.

14

Physiologic Midtreatment Tooth Movement as a Correction Strategy for Iatrogenic Root Exposure

Adith Venugopal,[1] Paolo Manzano,[2] M. Srirengalakshmi,[3] Anand Marya,[1] Nikhilesh R. Vaid,[4] and S. Jay Bowman[5]

[1]*Department of Orthodontics, University of Puthisastra, Phnom Penh, Cambodia*
[2]*10:10 Dental Clinic, Manila, Philippines*
[3]*Department of Orthodontics, Saveetha Dental College, Tamil Nadu, India*
[4]*European University College, DHCC, Dubai, UAE*
[5]*Department of Orthodontics, University of Michigan, USA*

Correspondence should be addressed to Adith Venugopal; avenugopal@puthisastra.edu.kh

Academic Editor: Giuseppe Alessandro Scardina

In the case report showcased, we describe orthodontic treatment of a female patient with an excessive gingival display on smiling and severe dental crowding, with maxillary canines positioned excessively buccal (ectopic) to and in near transposition to the lateral incisors. The treatment involved extractions and initial use of unmitigated forces leading to excessive gingival thinning and buccal root positioning of the ectopic canines. Eventually, the root position was corrected and periodontal equilibrium was attained. On finishing the treatment, all objectives were achieved with a good esthetic outcome as well as excellent dental and occlusal relationships.

1. Introduction

Ectopic and buccally positioned canines are frequent occurrences in an orthodontic practice [1]. Various etiologies have been attributed to these ectopic and buccally erupting permanent canines. The most common of them is the lack of sufficient arch perimeter [2, 3], while others attribute this to the long and tortuous path of eruption that is usually buccal to the dental arch. Since they erupt after the laterals and first bicuspids, approximation of their roots may make it harder for the canines to erupt, in turn causing an ectopic eruption, most commonly manifested as an exaggeration in their buccal position [4, 5]. While treating ectopic canines, a biomechanical strategy is of extreme importance. Emphasis should be placed on avoiding unmitigated force systems to prevent iatrogenic complications.

In 1996, Behrents [6] defined iatrogenics as something unintentionally induced by treatment. Incorrect choice of dental procedures, poor treatment indications, adopting unaccounted treatment strategies, under estimation of treatment time, not changing a treatment plan when necessary, overambitious use of temporary anchorage devices as an anchorage strategy [7], and not establishing good communication with the patient are failures that may significantly affect outcomes, quality, and stability of correction. All these factors delay treatment efficiency [8].

Alveolar defects such as a fenestration or dehiscence are some common iatrogenic effects that may result as a consequence of improper force application to the dentition. Alveolar dehiscence is defined as a lack of the facial or lingual alveolar cortical plate, resulting in a denuded root surface [9]. These alveolar defects arise from different predisposing factors such as decreased thickness of the alveolar bone, labial placement of the tooth in the dental arch, contour of the roots, abnormal occlusal factors, orthodontic tooth movement, or periodontal and endodontic pathology. And more often than not, these conditions are commonly associated with the anterior region of the dental arch [10].

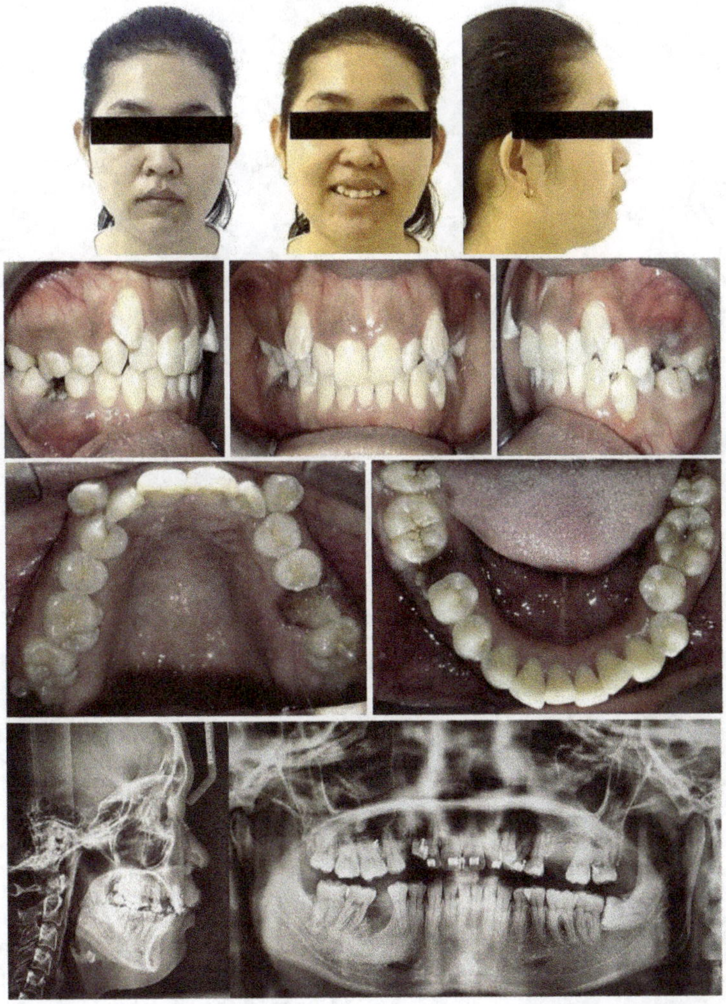

FIGURE 1: Pretreatment records with radiographs.

TABLE 1: Cephalometric analysis.

Values	Pretreatment	Posttreatment
Skeletal:		
SNA	78°	79°
SNB	70°	72°
ANB	8°	7°
SN-MP	41°	40°
FMA	34°	33°
ANS-GN	68 mm	66 mm
Dental:		
U1-NF	98°	105°
IMPA	97°	99°
Soft tissue:		
U lip-E line	-0.5 mm	1.2 mm
L lip-E line	1.4 mm	0.3 mm

2. Case History and Diagnosis

A 28-year-old female presented to the office, with the chief complaint of misaligned teeth. Her medical history reported her to be healthy. The clinical examination revealed a convex facial profile with a slightly increased lower third of the face, acute nasolabial angle, slight protrusion and incompetence of the lips, retruded and extruded maxillary incisors, high ectopic canines with a distal crown inclination, excessive display of the gingiva on smiling, and a lot of strain on the lower lip and chin soft tissue area (Figure 1). There was no deviation on mouth opening or mandibular closure. Also, no symptoms of any temporomandibular dysfunctions were reported.

Furthermore, the maxillary canines presented excessively buccal and the roots almost transposed over the laterals. The canines presented with mesial rotations and distal crown inclinations. The mandibular arch presented with moderate crowding and a curve of Spee measuring 3 mm. When in occlusion, the maxillary left lateral incisor showed a dental crossbite, in addition to an overbite of 2 mm and an overjet of 1 mm. The upper midline was coincident with the facial midline, but the lower midline was deviated to the left by

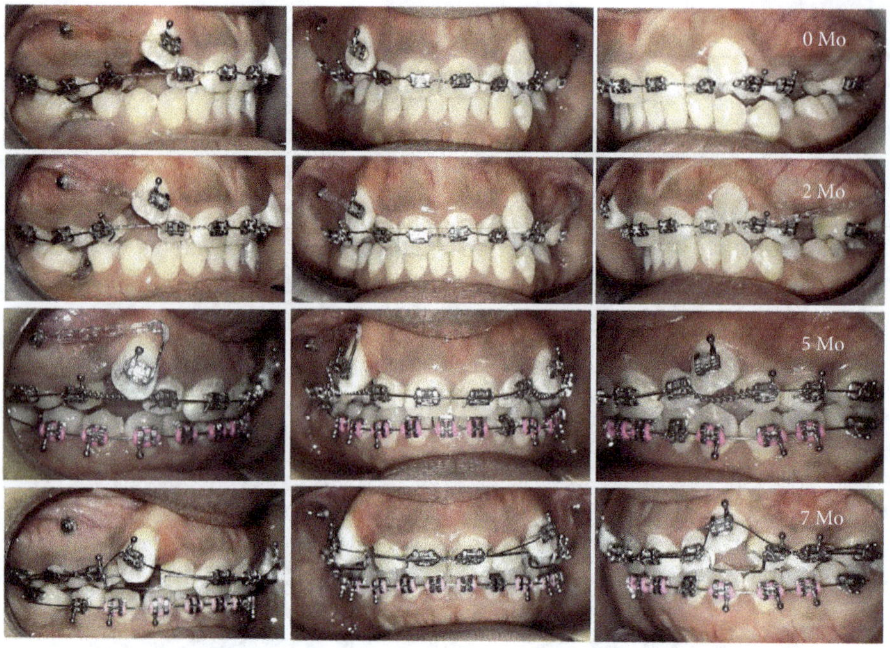

FIGURE 2: Usage of unmitigated forces causing distal crown tipping and buccalization of #13 root.

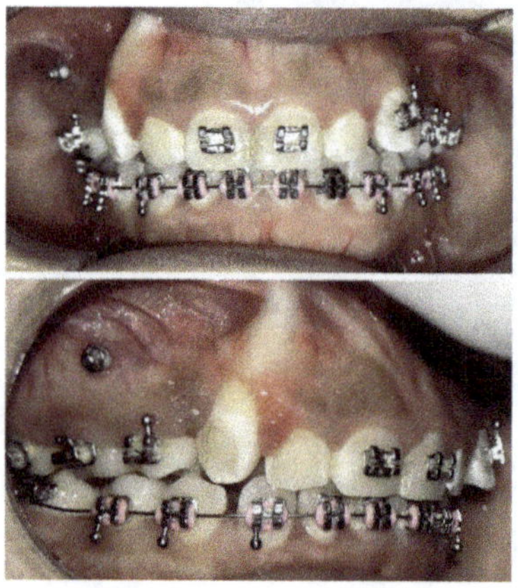

FIGURE 3: Extreme gingival thinning over the root of #13.

2 mm. The gingival contours of the maxillary anterior segment showed severe lack of leveling. The left mandibular canine and first premolar were almost in a crossbite (Figure 1).

The upper left first molar was freshly extracted because of a severe carious lesion on it. The lower right first molar was mutilated due to a previous carious infection, and the root stumps were referred for extractions prior to placing the brackets. Carious lesions on teeth #36, #37, #47, and #48 were referred for restorations.

Dental radiographic examination revealed the presence of all permanent teeth except #46 and #26. The lower left third molar was impacted and mesially angulated. No pathologic lesions were detected (Figure 1).

The cephalometric analysis (Table 1) showed a forward relationship of the maxilla to the mandible (ANB 8°), with retrusion of the maxilla (SNA 78°) and mandible (SNB 70°), and an increased vertical relationship (SN-MP 41°; FMA 34°). The maxillary incisors were projected palatally (U1-NF 98°), and the mandibular incisors were slightly proclined (IMPA 97°).

3. Treatment Objectives

The treatment objectives were to (1) improve the profile of the patient, (2) alleviate the crowding on the maxillary arch and make space for the traction of the ectopically placed canine, (3) establish class I canine relationship on both sides, (4) correct the left lateral incisor crossbite, (5) maintain ideal overjet and overbite, (6) eliminate excessive gingival display on smiling, (7) obtain good interdigitation, and (8) ensure stable results.

4. Treatment Alternatives

Due to the presence of localized crowding of the upper anteriors, the presence of maxillary canines with no space to align into the arch, a slightly convex facial profile with protruded upper lips, and an extraction space i.r.t. the already extracted upper left first molar, we proposed orthodontic treatment with extraction of either upper right first or second premolar and use of fixed appliances, followed by retraction and subsequent traction of the upper canines into occlusion with adequate anchorage control using TADs.

If the dental arches were to be leveled and aligned with a nonextraction approach or distalization of posterior teeth, the treatment may have resulted in further lip and bidental protrusions. Any approach involving distalization of teeth in the first quadrant to make space by different approaches (e.g., skeletal anchorage) might prove challenging and time-consuming and would inevitably require the extraction of the third molar.

Considering the patient's protruded lips, convex profile, severe crowding on the upper arch, and lack of space for

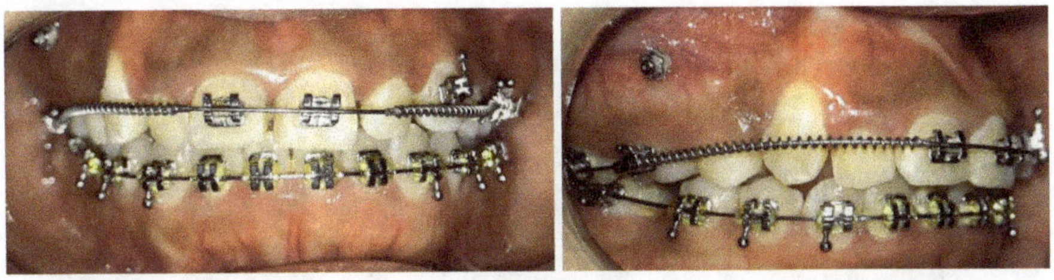

FIGURE 4: Three months of active space opening and spontaneously letting the canine root move into the alveolar bone.

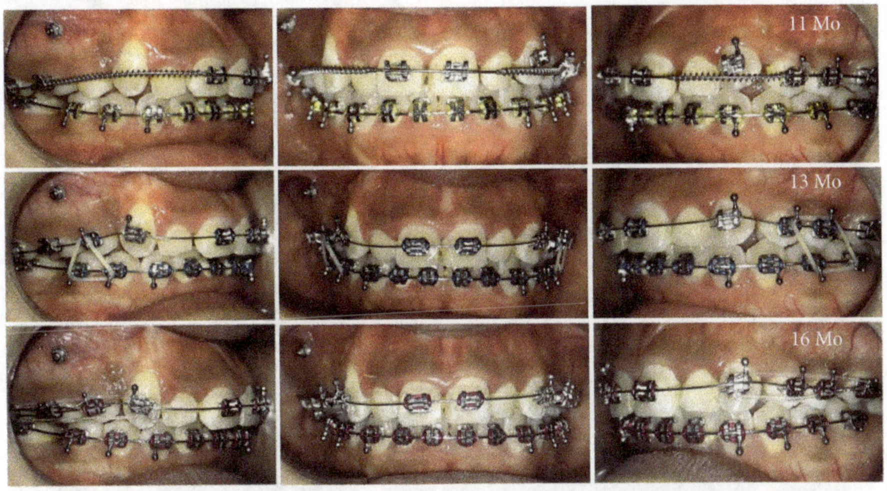

FIGURE 5: Light forces being used after spontaneous relapse of #13 into the bone in order to achieve intercuspation.

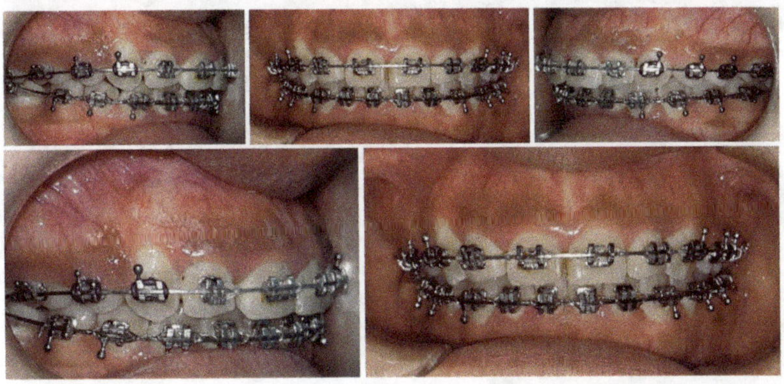

FIGURE 6: Finishing with coordinated $0.019'' \times 0.025''$ stainless steel archwires.

the ectopic maxillary canines to align, a nonextraction approach may have been unpredictable and lead to further complications.

After carefully considering all the options, it was decided to extract the upper right first premolar instead of the second as it was closer to the ectopic canine and would warrant quicker correction.

5. Treatment Progress

This case was treated using $0.022'' \times 0.028''$ slot preadjusted edgewise appliances with MBT prescription. Extraction of the upper right first premolar was performed, and interradicular TADs were placed, two of which were placed between the upper left first and second molars (#26-#27) and between the upper right first molar and second premolar (#16-#15).

A segment of the $0.016''$ NiTi wire was used from #17-#15 and #24-#25 to partially level the upper right and left posterior segments.

A light traction using a power chain measured using a Dontrix gauge to deliver 50 grams of force was applied to the bracket on the tooth #13 from the TAD on the right maxillary segment. A similar force was applied from the TAD on the left to #24 in order to distalize it in order to gain space for ectopic #23.

On subsequent review, the upper anterior teeth and the molars were included in the treatment using a light $0.014''$ NiTi wire. It was noticed that the crown of #13 was tipping

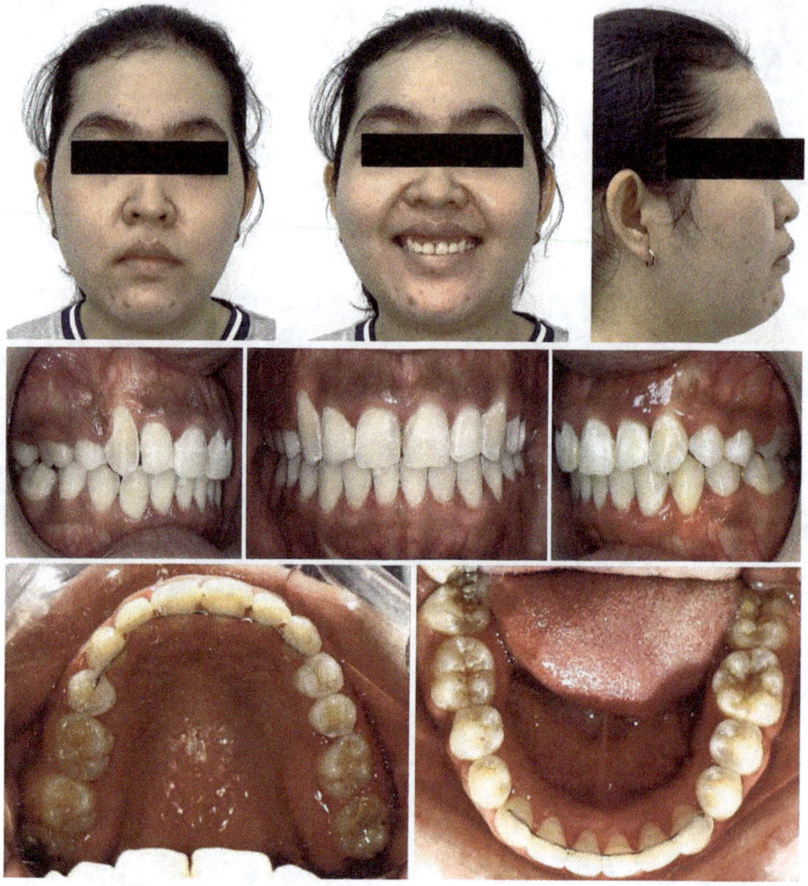

FIGURE 7: Posttreatment extraoral and intraoral pictures prior to gingivectomy.

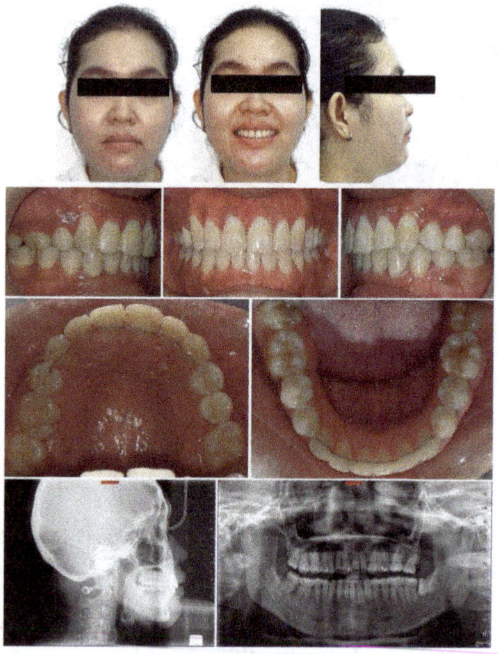

FIGURE 8: Posttreatment extraoral and intraoral pictures with radiographs after gingivectomy.

further distally, and so, it was decided to fabricate an attachment similar to a power arm, on #13 as shown in Figure 2, to approximate the forces closer to the CR of #13 in order to facilitate more bodily movement. To create more space for the left upper canine and to maintain space for the right canine, an open nickel titanium spring was compressed between #15-#12 and #22-#24.

Although efforts were made to reach closer to the CR of #13, further distal tipping along with increased root prominence was noticed. Once adequate space was achieved on both maxillary segments to get the canines into occlusion, the space was maintained using a rectangular stainless steel $0.016'' \times 0.022''$ bypass archwire and an overlay $0.012''$ NiTi wire was used for the further traction of canines into the arch (Figure 2).

After 7 months of active treatment, excessive gingival thinning over the root of #13 clearly indicated active dehiscence of the alveolar bone (Figure 3). It was then decided to remove all active forces from tooth #13. Brackets were removed from teeth #12, #13, #15, and #22, and nickel titanium open coil springs were placed between #16-#11 and #21-#24 to gain spaces and relieve the pressure on #13. Stops were placed distal to #11 and #21 in order to prevent excessive proclination as a side effect of the active open coil springs. Follow-up reviews over the next three months showed reduced root prominence over #13 indicating that the root moved physiologically into the alveolar housing (Figure 4).

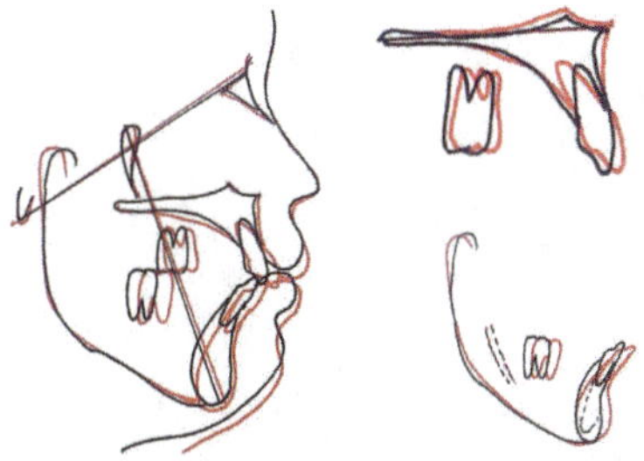

Figure 9: Superimpositions of pre- and posttreatment cephalograms.

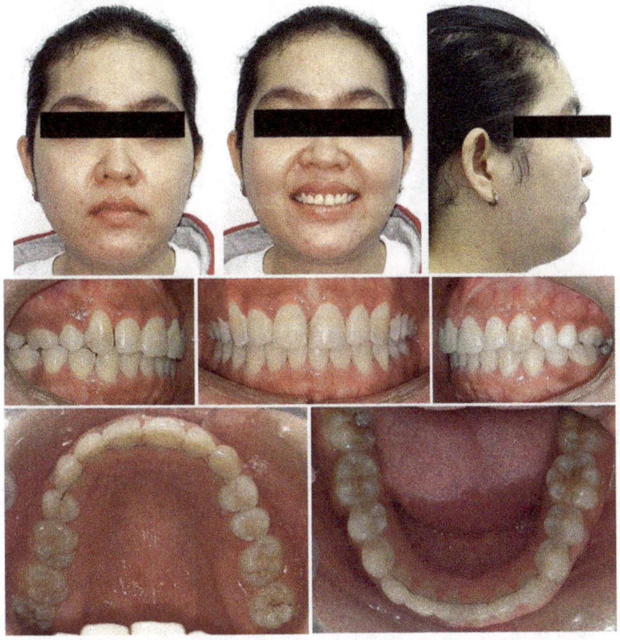

Figure 10: Treatment records at one-year follow-up review.

Brackets were now rebonded on #15 and #13, and a flexible continuous 0.014″ NiTi archwire was placed on the upper arch with light intermaxillary elastics for occlusal settling (Figure 5). Once #13 was brought vertically into occlusion, a stiff 0.021″ × 0.025″ NiTi archwire was inserted to correct all the third-order discrepancies. (Figure 6).

Symmetric and coordinated stiff archwires (0.019″ × 0.025″ stainless steel) were used for finishing stages, maintaining the original dental arch form. This phase required enhancing buccal root torque on the maxillary lateral incisors (Figure 6). Removable wraparound retainers were used on the upper and lower dentitions alongside fixed lingual bonded retainers to retain the orthodontic corrections.

Gingivectomy was performed on the upper dentition to even the gingival contours on all teeth and at the same time reduce the gingival display on smiling (Figures 7 and 8).

6. Treatment Results

Allowing physiologic midtreatment tooth movement of the upper right canine into the alveolar bone as a correction strategy for the iatrogenic root exposure enabled excellent gingival and periodontal harmony around the canine with stable results (Figures 7 and 8). There was no blanching or partial see through of the root contour through the gingiva over #13 at the end of treatment. Also, there was no tenderness or root prominence felt over #13 on palpation.

Satisfactory outcomes were achieved with an improved facial profile and smile harmony (Figure 8). Optimal occlusal contacts were obtained between all of the other teeth, especially the canines. Overjet and overbite were maintained, and the midlines were now coincident with each other and with the facial midline (Figures 7 and 8). A balanced gingival contour along with optimal gingival display on smiling was obtained, particularly by leveling the gingival margin of the upper dentition by performing a gingivectomy in the end (Figure 8).

Radiographic analysis (Figures 8 and 9; Table 1) revealed a good appearance of the alveolar ridges and bone, as well as appropriate root parallelism. The cephalometric analysis (Figure 8; Table 1) and superimposition of the tracings (Figure 9) indicate a forward relationship of the maxilla to the mandible with minimal changes in the chin position posttreatment (ANB 7, SNA 79, and SNB 72).

Improvement was noted in the facial profile and position of the lips with reduced mentalis muscle strain due to reduction in the lower facial height (pre-ANS-GN 68; post-ANS-GN 66). Superimposition showed a slight counterclockwise rotation of the mandible (pre-FMA 34; post-FMA 33). Upper incisors showed a good axial inclination compared to the pretreatment position (pre-U1-NF 98; post-U1-NF 105). Lower incisors showed a 2° proclination posttreatment. Furthermore, there was minimal loss of anchorage in the upper and substantial amount in the lower molars (Figure 9). Excellent gingival and periodontal harmony around the canine with stable occlusal contacts was documented even one year after removal of the fixed appliance (Figure 10).

7. Discussion

Incorrect estimations of the center of resistance of #13 with the use of unmitigated forces led to the alveolar dehiscence on #13 in this case. Bracket inversion, use of individual tooth torque on the wire, and placement of Warren springs or Goodman springs are alternatives suggested in the literature to correct the root angulations and place displaced teeth back into the alveolar housing [11, 12]. Unfortunately, the lack of adequate leveling and rotation on #13 made it impossible for a rectangular wire to be inserted into the slot to use the abovementioned torquing auxiliaries.

Removal of all active unmitigated orthodontic forces from the affected tooth has been known to improve the detrimental periodontal conditions [13]. Hence, it was best decided to remove all active forces from #13 in order to allow the root to physiologically move into the alveolar housing.

Excessive buccal or labial movement of the teeth into the labial cortical plate may cause thinning of the gingiva and a partial see through of the underlying root contour giving it a so called "washboard effect" and resultant bone loss or root resorption as teeth contact the cortical bone [14].

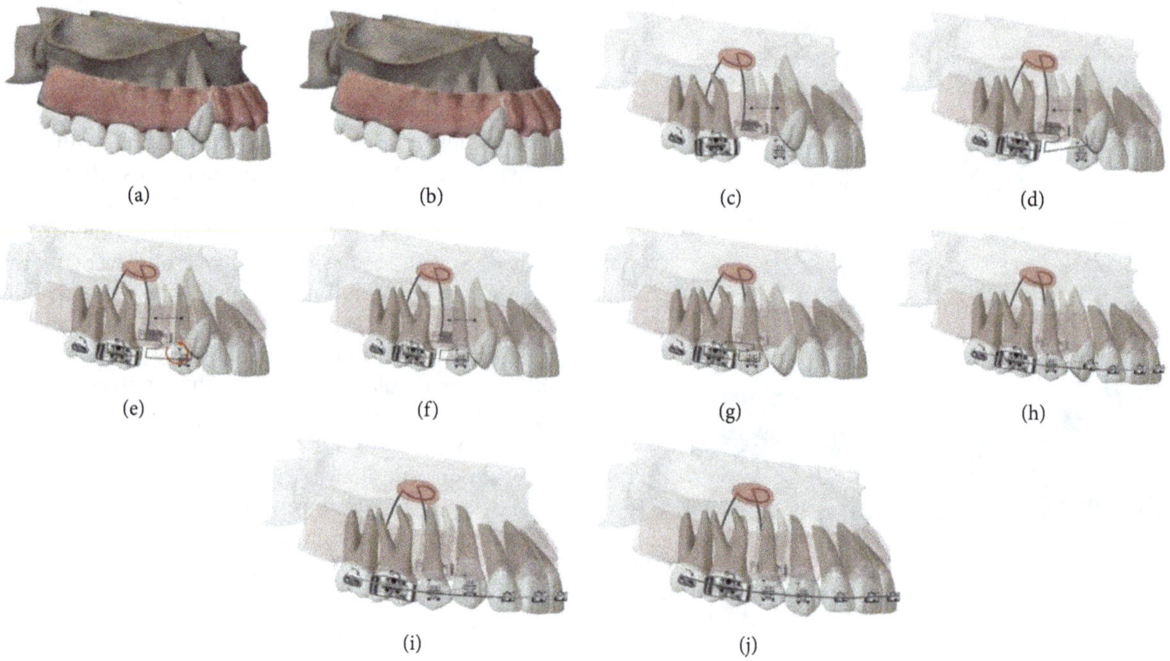

FIGURE 11: Illustration showing simulated movement of the ectopic canine into occlusion in a similar scenario following extraction of #15 (b). A segmented T loop being used for retraction of #14 into the extraction space and the transseptal fibers of #13 following #14 into occlusion (c–g). Overlay archwire to derotate and get #13 into alignment (h, i). Finishing on a 0.019″ × 0.025″ stainless steel archwire.

Wainwright [15], Karring et al. [16], and Thilander et al. [17] demonstrated the occurrence of dehiscence or fenestrations of the buccal alveolar plate on labial movement of teeth and subsequent healing and reforms when the tooth moved back into the alveolar housing. Only Engelking and Zachrisson [18] demonstrated no recovery of the recessed gingiva after the occurrence of dehiscence or fenestration, following movement back into the alveolar housing.

Cases like these suggest that the etiology of crowded permanent teeth is simply too much tooth structure for the available arch length. Teeth are forced to erupt out of the arch form when inadequate space is available, but they will spontaneously drift into a good arch form when adequate space is provided [19].

Although there were many challenges during the course of this case, it was finished well in less than 2 years, and furthermore, a one-year follow-up shows stable results and no gingival pathology w.r.t. #13.

On retrospective analysis, one of our treatment alternatives, in which we had planned the extraction of #15, could have possibly been a better option. The idea of retracting #14 using a segmented T loop with high alpha activation (to keep the root of #14 away from that of #13) for retraction would probably make more sense as it would cause simultaneous traction of #13 as well, due to the "pull" effect of the transseptal fibers [20]. As there would be no direct force application on #13, the chances of unwarranted forces causing excessive tipping and buccal root movements would be nullified, in turn simplifying the treatment. Once #14 was completely retracted, #13 should have been in a much better occlusal position to be involved with a simple overlay wire for vertical traction. This plan was initially not finalized upon because of the considerations of time. It was thought that extracting #14 may be a better option as it was closer to the ectopic canine and would warrant quicker correction.

8. Conclusion

This case demonstrates observations of such physiologic movements of the root into the alveolar bone when space was created. Extracting or making space to let the teeth out of the arch spontaneously align, depends on the fact that self-correction or self-separation occurs so rapidly. Orthodontists should be aware of possible complications and solution strategies whenever mechanics do not deliver desired outcomes. It is also prudent that clinicians analyze their completed cases on the basis of learning objectives for the future, after assessing both efficiency and efficacy of strategies employed.

Authors' Contributions

All coauthors have seen and agree with the contents of the manuscript.

References

[1] S. E. Bishara and D. Ortho, "Impacted maxillary canines: a review," *American Journal of Orthodontics and Dentofacial Orthopedics*, vol. 101, no. 2, pp. 159–171, 1992.

[2] S. Ericson and J. Kurol, "Early treatment of palatally erupting maxillary canines by extraction of the primary canines," *Euro-*

pean Journal of Orthodontics, vol. 10, no. 1, pp. 283–295, 1988.

[3] H. Jacoby, "The etiology of maxillary canine impactions," *American Journal of Orthodontics*, vol. 84, no. 2, pp. 125–132, 1983.

[4] A. Becker, *The Orthodontic Treatment of Impacted Teeth*, Taylor & Francis, 1997.

[5] J. B. Ferreira, G. S. Silveira, and J. N. Mucha, "A simple approach to correct ectopic eruption of maxillary canines," *American Journal of Orthodontics and Dentofacial Orthopedics*, vol. 155, no. 6, pp. 871–880, 2019.

[6] R. G. Behrents, "Iatrogenics in orthodontics," *American Journal of Orthodontics and Dentofacial Orthopedics*, vol. 110, no. 3, pp. 235–238, 1996.

[7] N. R. Vaid, "Temporary anchorage applications revisited!," *Seminars in Orthodontics*, vol. 24, no. 1, pp. 1-2, 2018.

[8] A. Venugopal, P. Manzano, and S. Rengalakshmi, "A novel temporary anchorage device aided sectional mechanics for simultaneous orthodontic retraction and intrusion," *Case Reports in Dentistry*, vol. 2020, Article ID 5213936, 8 pages, 2020.

[9] A. Edel, "Alveolar bone fenestrations and dehiscences in dry Bedouin jaws," *Journal of Clinical Periodontology*, vol. 8, no. 6, pp. 491–499, 1981.

[10] G. Chen, C. T. Fang, and C. Tong, "The management of mucosal fenestration: a report of two cases," *International Endodontic Journal*, vol. 42, no. 2, pp. 156–164, 2009.

[11] L. Bernstein, "Root torque with Warren springs," *Journal of Clinical Orthodontics*, vol. 5, no. 3, pp. 167–169, 1971.

[12] B. Mollenhauer, "An aligning auxiliary for ribbon arch brackets: rectangular boxes from ultrafine high tensile wires," *Australian Orthodontic Journal*, vol. 11, no. 4, pp. 219–226, 1990.

[13] L. Levin, S. Einy, H. Zigdon, D. Aizenbud, and E. E. Machtei, "Guidelines for periodontal care and follow-up during orthodontic treatment in adolescents and young adults," *Journal of Applied Oral Science*, vol. 20, no. 4, pp. 399–403, 2012.

[14] R. Blasi and R. Vanarsdall, *Periodontal–orthodontic interrelationships*, Chapter 22, Orthodontics: Current Principles and Techniques, Elsevier, St. Louis, 6th edition, 2017.

[15] W. M. Wainwright, "Faciolingual tooth movement: its influence on the root and cortical plate," *American Journal of Orthodontics*, vol. 64, no. 3, pp. 278–302, 1973.

[16] T. Karring, S. Nyman, B. Thilander, and I. Magnusson, "Bone regeneration in orthodontically produced alveolar bone dehiscences," *Journal of Periodontal Research*, vol. 17, no. 3, pp. 309–315, 1982.

[17] B. Thilander, S. Nyman, T. Karring, and I. Magnusson, "Bone regeneration in alveolar bone dehiscences related to orthodontic tooth movements," *European Journal of Orthodontics*, vol. 5, no. 2, pp. 105–114, 1983.

[18] G. Engelking and B. U. Zachrisson, "Effects of incisor repositioning on monkey periodontium after expansion through the cortical plate," *American Journal of Orthodontics*, vol. 82, no. 1, pp. 23–32, 1982.

[19] T. D. Creekmore, "Physiologic drift," *Journal of Clinical Orthodontics*, vol. 9, no. 12, pp. 749–773, 1975.

[20] W. R. Proffit, H. W. Fields Jr., and D. M. Sarver, *Contemporary Orthodontics*, Mosby, St. Louis, 4th edition, 2007.

15

Distalization in Orthodontics: A Review and Case Series

Yahya A. Alogaibi,[1,2] Ahmad A. Al-Fraidi,[2] Manar K. Alhajrasi,[3] Saleh S. Alkhathami,[2] Abdulkarim Hatrom,[4] and Ahmed R. Afify[5,6]

[1]*Bisha Dental Center, Ministry of Health, P.O. Box 418, Bisha 61922, Saudi Arabia*
[2]*Department of Orthodontic, King Fahad Hospital, Specialized Dental Center, Madina, Saudi Arabia*
[3]*Department of Orthodontic, North Jeddah Specialty Dental Center, MOH, Jeddah, Saudi Arabia*
[4]*Department of Orthodontic, Ministry of Health, P.O. Box 4137, Makkah, Saudi Arabia*
[5]*Orthodontic Department, Faculty of Dentistry, King Abdulaziz University, P.O. Box 80209, Jeddah 21589, Saudi Arabia*
[6]*Orthodontic Department, Faculty of Dentistry, Mansoura University, Mansoura, Egypt*

Correspondence should be addressed to Yahya A. Alogaibi; y1010@hotmail.com

Academic Editor: Maria Beatriz Duarte Gavião

Distalization is a conservative method that is utilized in orthodontics to gain space by moving posterior teeth distally. It may be combined with other space gaining strategies, such as expansion, or can be used alone. Many methods have been used for distalization. These methods differ significantly in their place, whether to be extraoral or intraoral, site of action in upper and/or lower arch, and cooperation needed by the patient if it is removable or fixed. This review illustrates some of the most commonly used methods for distalization with a brief presentation of three cases that incorporated successful distalization techniques.

1. Introduction

Molar distalization is a term that is commonly used now for referring to the procedure of increasing the length of the dental arch by the rearward movement of the buccal segment teeth [1, 2]. For more than 100 years, maxillary molar distalization has been successfully used in orthodontics to treat many cases, most notably are cases with class II malocclusion. This technique is usually utilized to gain space to relieve crowding and to reduce the increased overjet [3]. A primary advantage in this technique is the ability to gain space in a conservative way without the need for extraction [4–6].

Other treatment options to gain space are expansion (which is commonly used in combination with distalization), proclination of anterior teeth, interproximal stripping, extraction, and orthognathic surgery. All these methods are available for orthodontic treatment but not all of them are suitable for every case. The severity of malocclusion and the facial profile usually govern these choices [7].

Class II malocclusion is one of the most frequent problems in orthodontics, and distalization is considered one of the conservative ways to treat such cases [1, 8]. Nonextraction treatment of class II malocclusion has become very popular in the last decade [9].

One of the common methods to achieve distalization is the incorporation of extraoral appliances such as headgears. These appliances are commonly utilized either for anchorage to support maxillary molars or for distalization of molars to correct the molar relation and to increase the arch length. These methods were found to be both efficient and reliable when used correctly [10, 11].

However, these appliances depend mainly on patient compliance and have a problem of bad esthetics, which led to the preference of intraoral distalizing appliances by some patients.

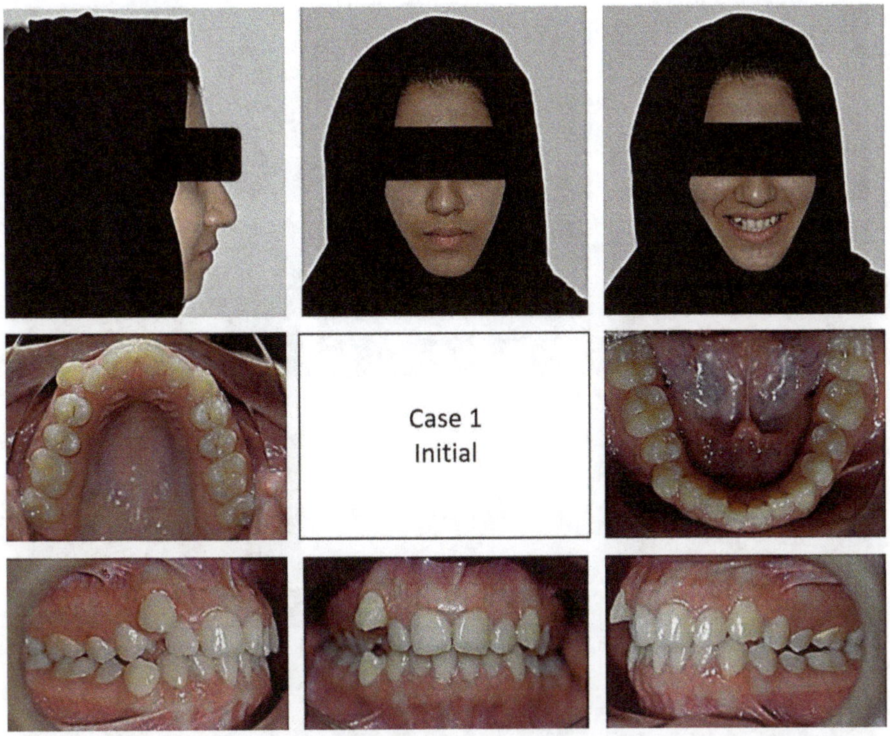

FIGURE 1: Pretreatment extraoral and intraoral photographs of the patient.

Intraoral appliances are more accepted by the patient and allow more control for the orthodontist on teeth [12].

2. Search Strategy

A search was done on PubMed to find all the available literature on distalization and orthodontics. This search showed total articles of 556, which showed only 95 articles were related to this topic. The Endnote software (version X7) was utilized to file the articles and to remove duplicates.

2.1. Indications for Molar Distalization

(i) To mesially position the maxillary first molar

(ii) Preferred in patients with low mandibular plane angle (brachy-cephalic type) or normal (meso-cephalic type)

(iii) Mild to moderate class II molar relationship, which are not indicated for extraction

(iv) To correct the second molar position

(v) To achieve ideal overbite and overjet

(vi) To early correct class II pattern

(vii) To regain the lost space (space regainer)

2.2. Contraindications for Molar Distalization

(i) Patients with high mandibular plane angle and excessive lower anterior facial height

(ii) Patients with skeletal or dental open bite

(iii) Severe class II skeletal pattern with an orthognathic maxilla and retrognathic mandible

(iv) Excessive overjet and proclination of anterior teeth

(v) Crowding in the posterior segment

(vi) Patients with temporomandibular joint problems

2.3. Various Modalities to Distalize Molars

2.3.1. Extraoral Appliances. In 1892, Norman Kingsley described for the first time a device called headgear, which can achieve maxillary molar distalization. This was the beginning of the universal use of headgears [13]. The force utilized for molar distalization by headgears should be constant and steady to allow for effective teeth movements and should be relatively light as it is mainly concentrated on the first molars. The amount of the recommended force is about 100 grams, which allows for a rate of tooth movement of 1 mm per month. This duration of wear should be as long as possible as the more the patient will wear the appliance, the better and faster the expected results. However, the minimum recommended time for headgear is 14 to 16 hours daily [14, 15]. Orthopedic force, on the other hand, which is a force aiming to modify craniofacial bones, should be much higher than the orthodontic force required for tooth movement. These forces should be ranging from 150 to 300 gams [16].

Headgear type is usually determined according to the type of vertical problem. In cases of deep bite, cervical headgear is usually recommended to extrude the molars during distalization and thus correct the deep bite anteriorly. On

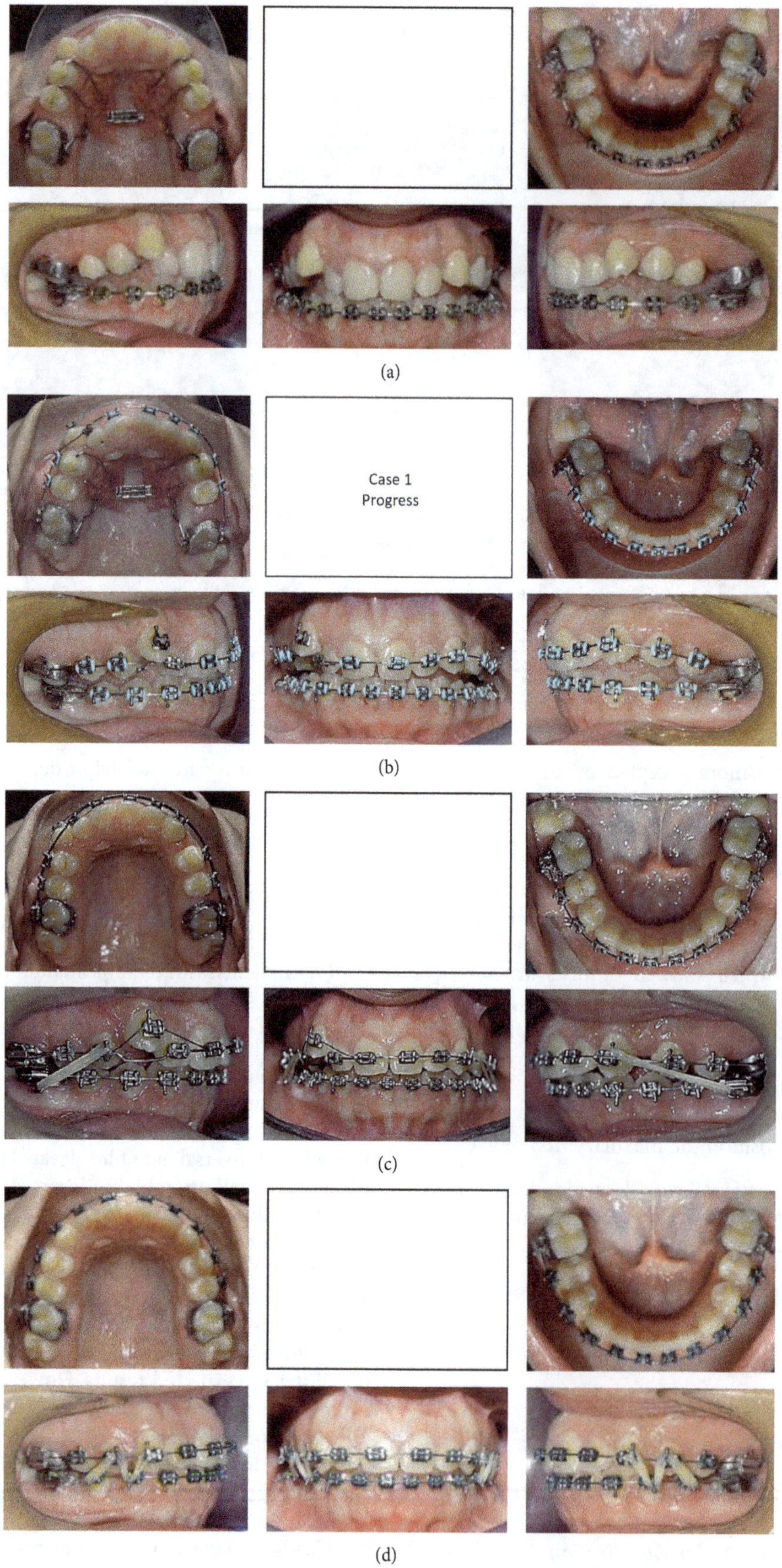

FIGURE 2: (a) Progress treatment intraoral photographs of the patient. (b) Progress treatment intraoral photographs of the patient. (c) Progress treatment intraoral photographs of the patient. (d) Progress treatment intraoral photographs of the patient.

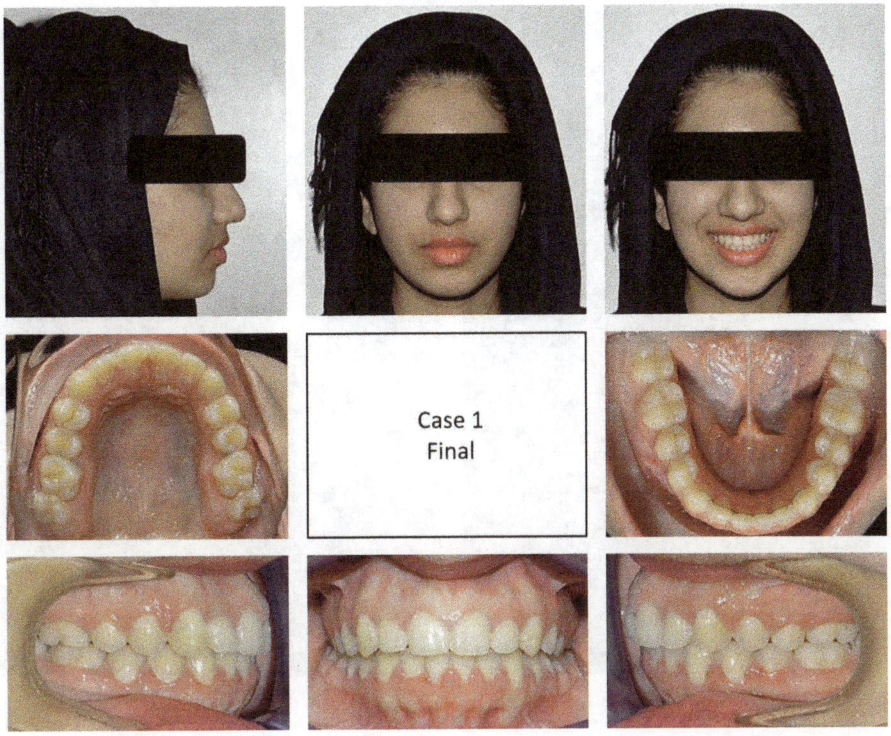

FIGURE 3: Posttreatment extraoral and intraoral photographs of the patient.

the other hand, a case with open bite a high pull headgear is usually indicated as it leads to both intrusion and distalization of molars. Straight headgear can be utilized in cases where no vertical problems exist [17–19].

2.3.2. Intraoral Appliances. There are many examples of intraoral distalizing appliances including but not limited to the following: Pend-X appliance, Lip Bumper, Forsus appliance, Herbst Appliance, Twin block, modified Nance holding arch, Japanese NiTi coils, molar distalizing system using magnets, Distal Jet, Pendulum appliance, Ghoshgarian TPA, Carriere appliance with class II elastics, and Sliding Jig with miniscrews combined with closed coil. However, not all of these appliances are commonly used among orthodontists. Only some of them were found to be more preferred to be used [3, 20].

(1) Distalizing the Upper Arch (Class II Correctors). In 1992, an appliance called pendulum was described by Hilgers, which was found to be an efficient method for distalization the upper molars. This appliance consisted of palatal button similar to Nance holding arch, which is retained by wires bonded to the occlusal surface of premolars and two coil springs distal to the palatal button that are attached to the palatal sheaths of molar bands. These coils act as the active component for distalizing the molars. Soon after the introduction of this appliance, it was updated by adding an expansion screw inside the palatal button, which was named "Pend-X." The Pend-X appliance was found to be a reliable method for distalization as it prevents the tendency of crossbite in molars during distalization by slight expansion of the arch. Also, it can be utilized in cases that need both arch expansion and distalization [21].

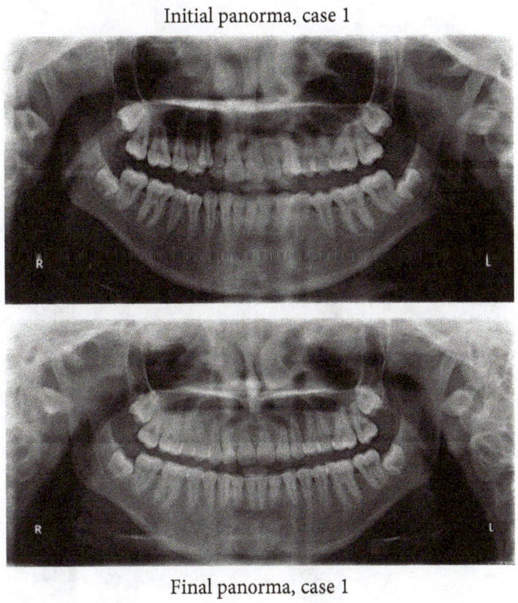

FIGURE 4: Initial and final panoramic radiographs.

Forsus class II appliance is a newer version of functional appliance that has the ability for upper molar distalization. It is composed of a specially designed telescopic spring, which does not bend on the cheek, and its spring is comfortable and easily brushed and cleaned [22, 23].

Herbst appliance is a fixed functional device designed by Emil Herbst in 1909, and Pancharz popularized it in 1979. It is composed of bilateral telescopic device that can protrude the mandible causing a reactive force on maxillary molars leading to its distalization. This device

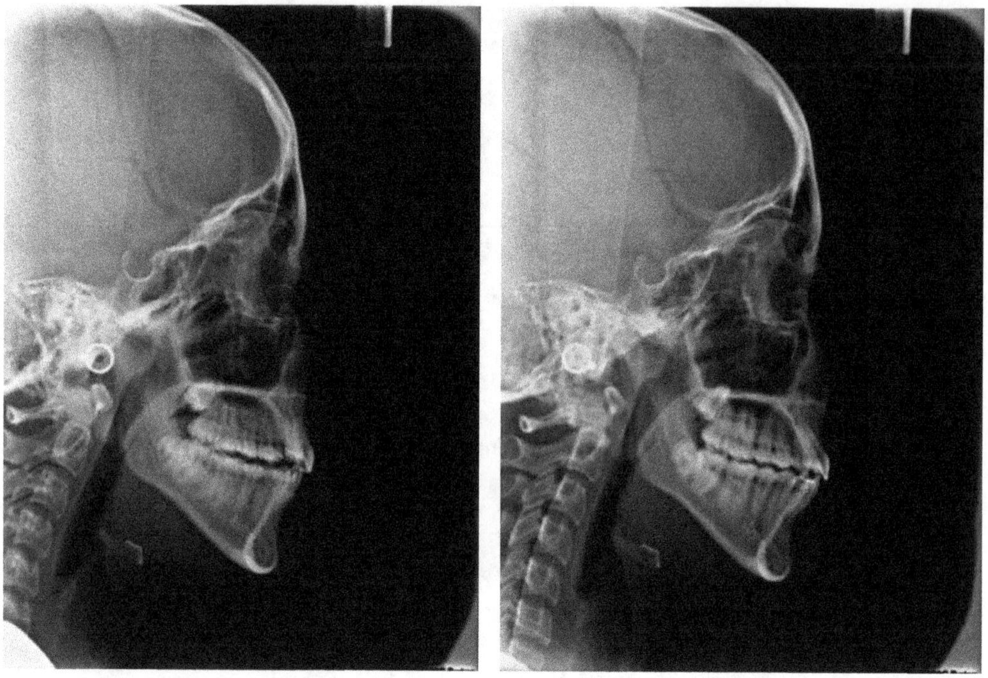

Initial cephalometric, case 1 Final cephalometric, case 1

FIGURE 5: Initial and final cephalometric radiographs.

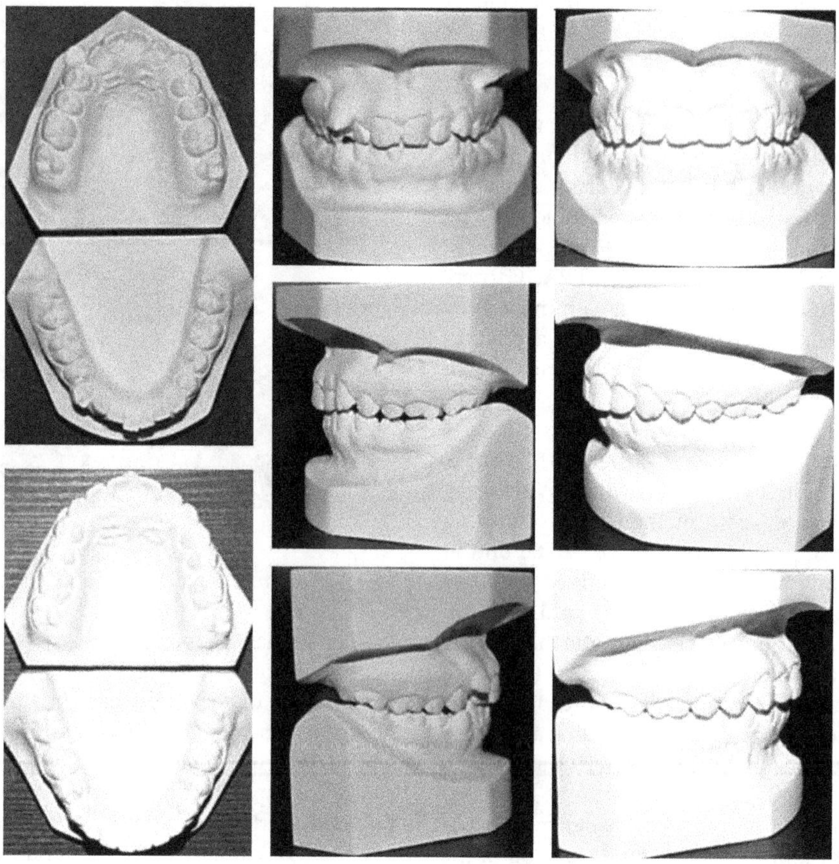

FIGURE 6: Initial and final study cast.

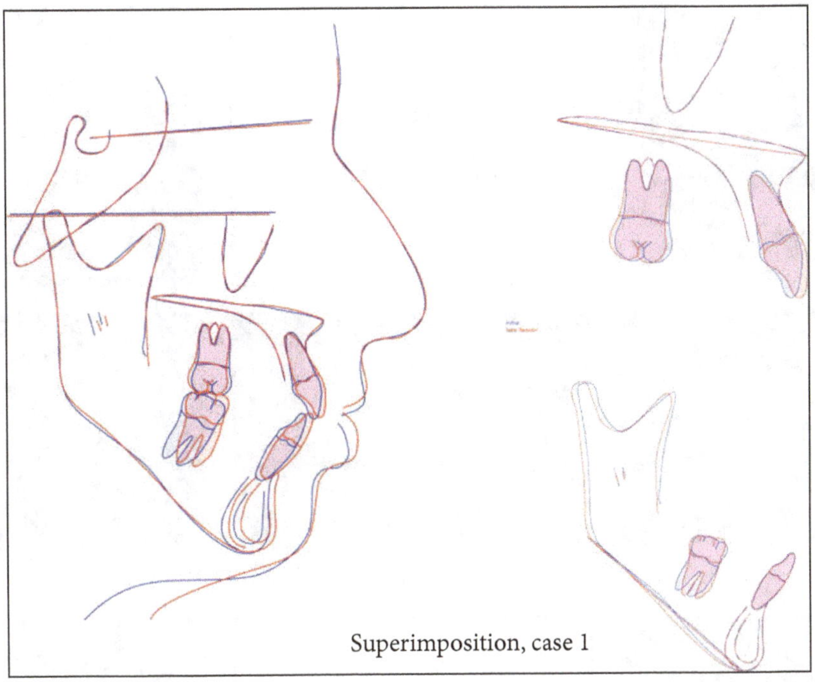

FIGURE 7: Superimposition.

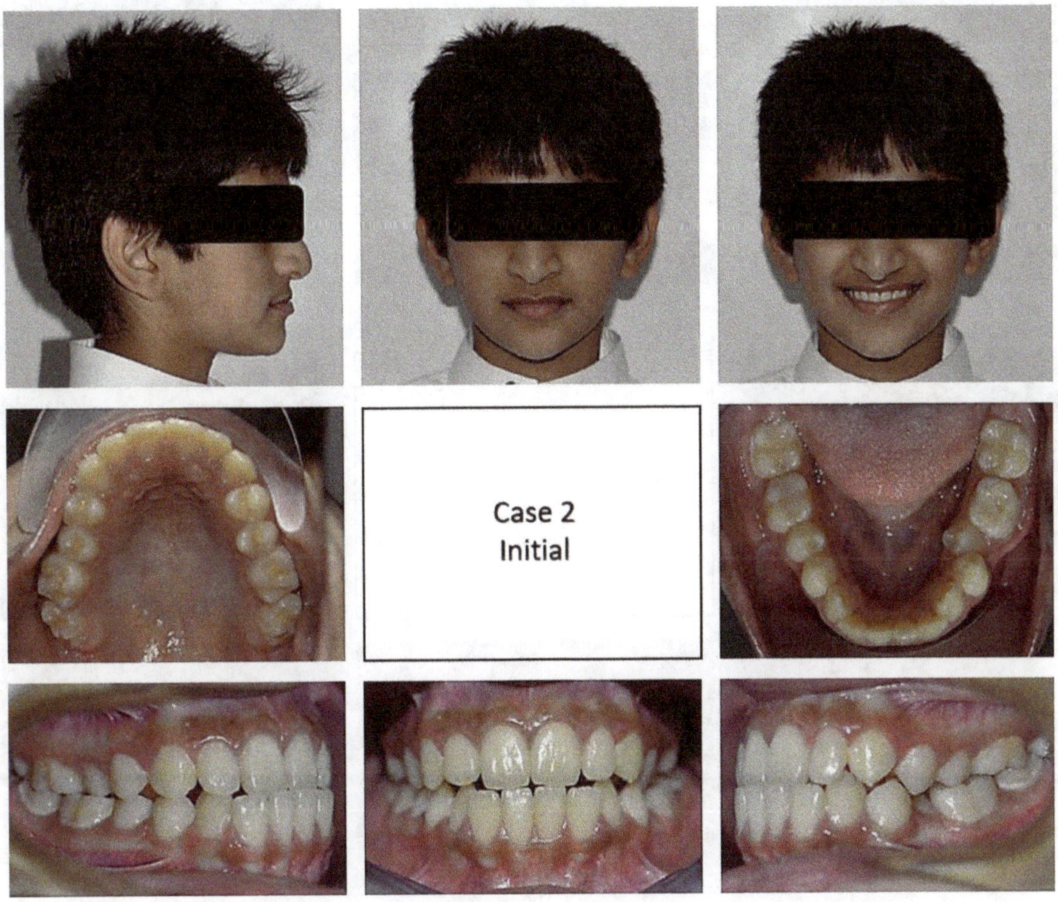

FIGURE 8: Pretreatment extraoral and intraoral photographs of the patient.

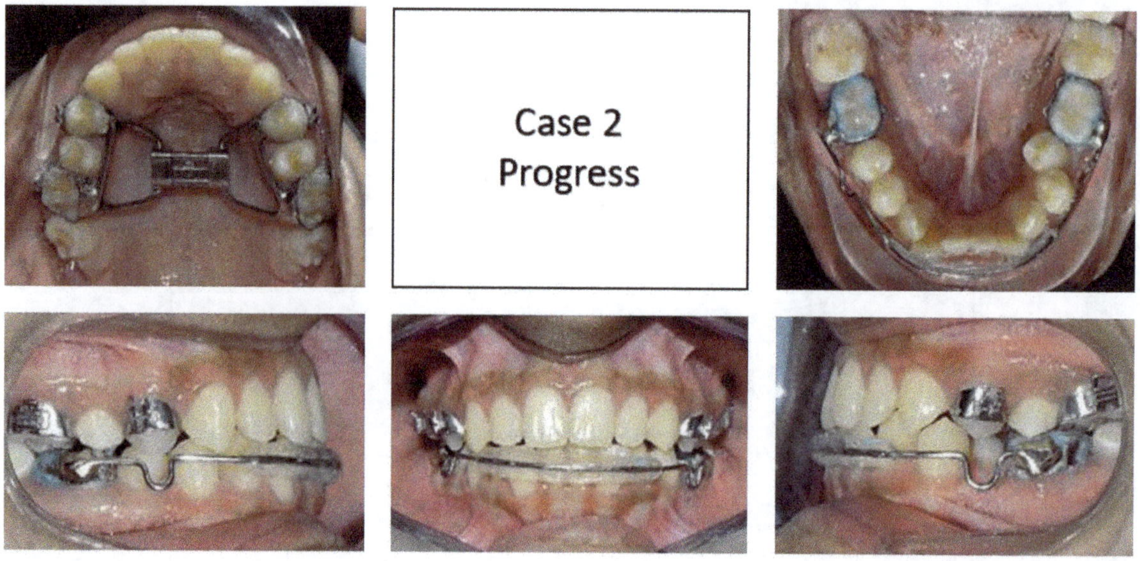

(a)

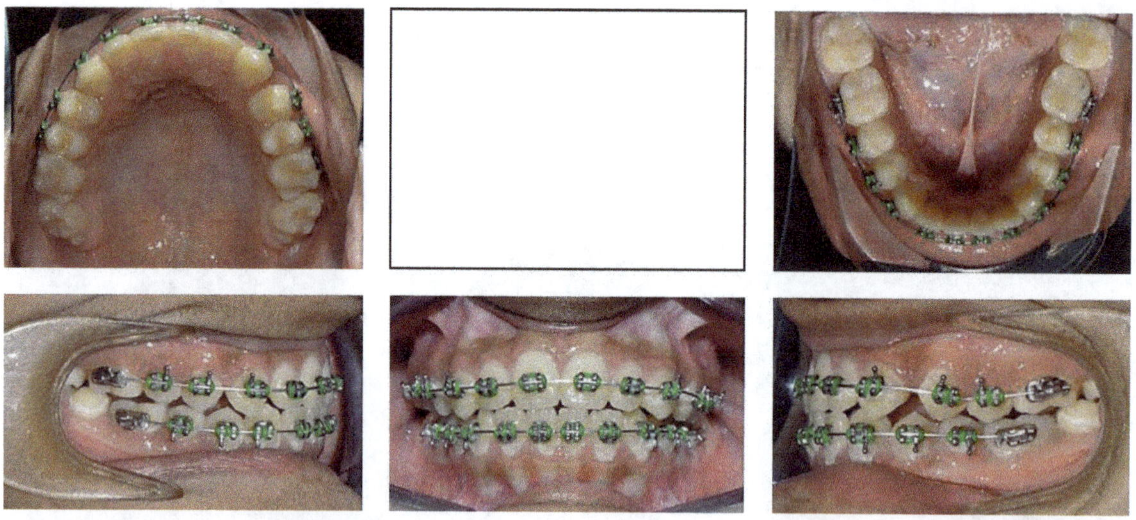

(b)

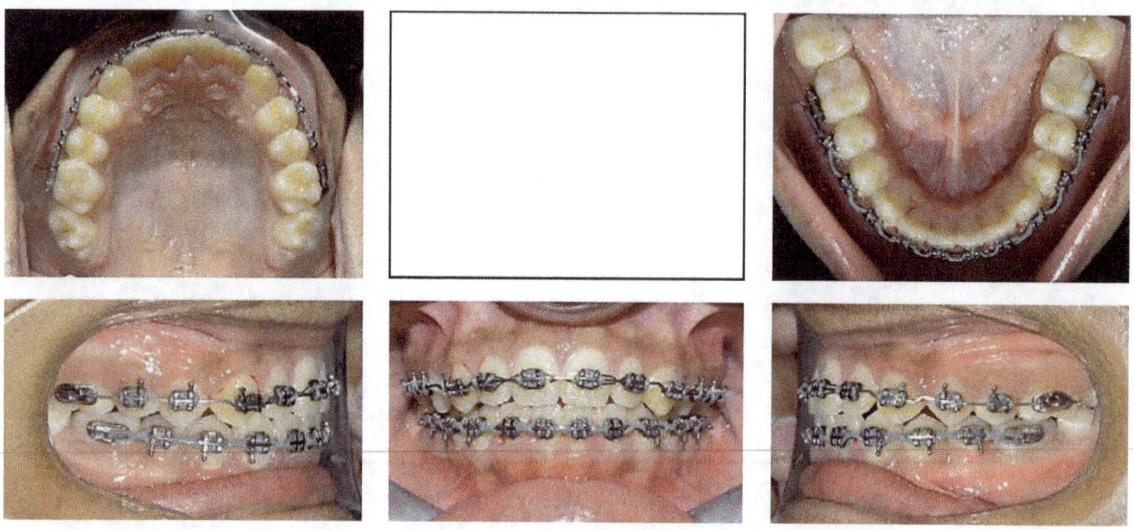

(c)

FIGURE 9: (a–c) Progress treatment intraoral photographs of the patient.

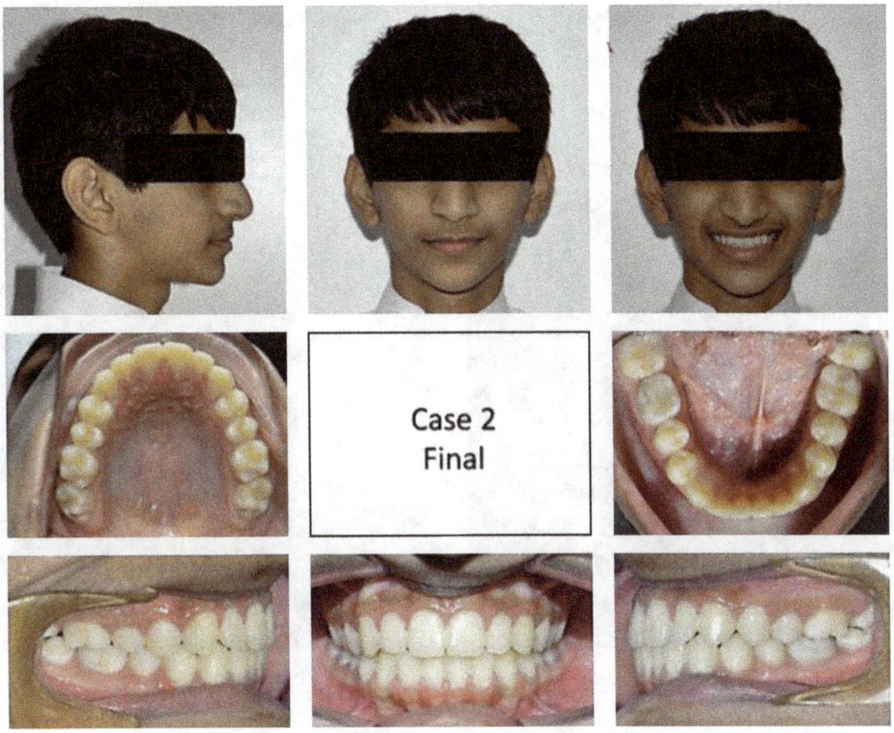

FIGURE 10: Posttreatment extraoral and intraoral photographs of the patient.

can produce both skeletal and dental changes in growing patients [24].

Twin blocks are those appliances having upper and lower bite blocks that incorporate inclined planes on the occlusal surfaces. These inclined planes with a 70-degree angle exert a distal force on the upper posterior teeth that may lead to distalization. Twin block is well tolerated by patients and relatively smaller than many other functional appliances. It also has an advantage of having minimal interference with speech [25, 26].

(2) Distalizing the Lower Arch. Lip bumper is another functional distalizing appliance that is composed of a stainless steel wire covered labially by acrylic to avoid ulceration of the lower lip. This appliance is inserted in the tubes of the lower molars and extends anteriorly to contact the lower lip. The labial portion is positioned 2-5 mm from the lower incisors causing distal forces from the lower lip to the molars. It has also an effect on incisor proclination as it alters the equilibrium between the lower lip and the tongue [27, 28].

Active lingual arch is another effective method for molar distalization in the lower arch. It has many modifications that enable the operator to distalize the molars unilaterally or bilaterally. However, this may come on the expense of the lower anteriors as it may lead to a reactive incisor proclination. So this appliance is usually recommended when lower incisors are retroclined and molars are in need of distalization [29, 30].

Franzulum is another appliance, which was introduced by Buyoff et al., in the year 2000. It was composed of a button made of acrylic that is situated inferior and lingual to the lower canine on each side. Additionally, there are two rests situated on the first premolar and the canine. The appliance utilizes a nickel titanium coil spring as an active component to produce the forces of distalization [31].

Initial panorama, case 2

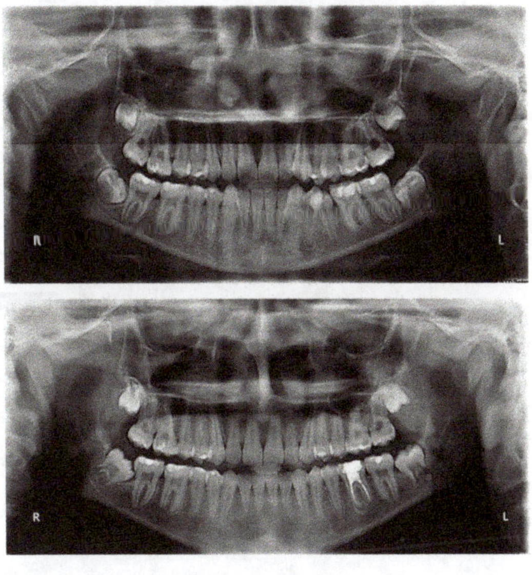

Final panorama, case 2

FIGURE 11: Initial and final panoramic radiographs.

(3) Universal Distalizing Methods for Upper and/or Lower Arches. Miniscrews have been reliably used as a method

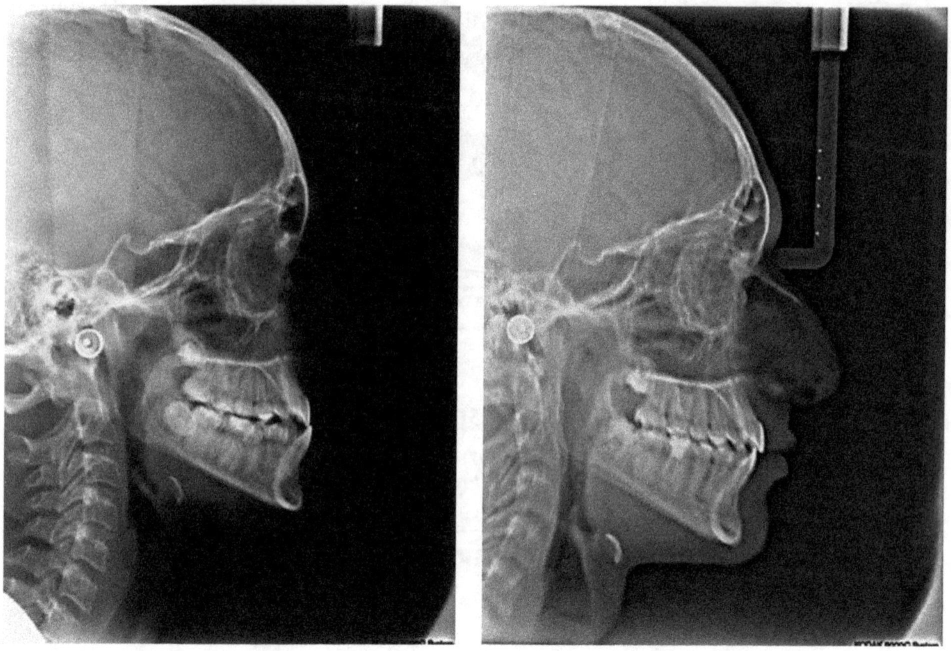

Initial cephalometric, case 2

Final cephalometric, case 2

FIGURE 12: Initial and final cephalometric radiographs.

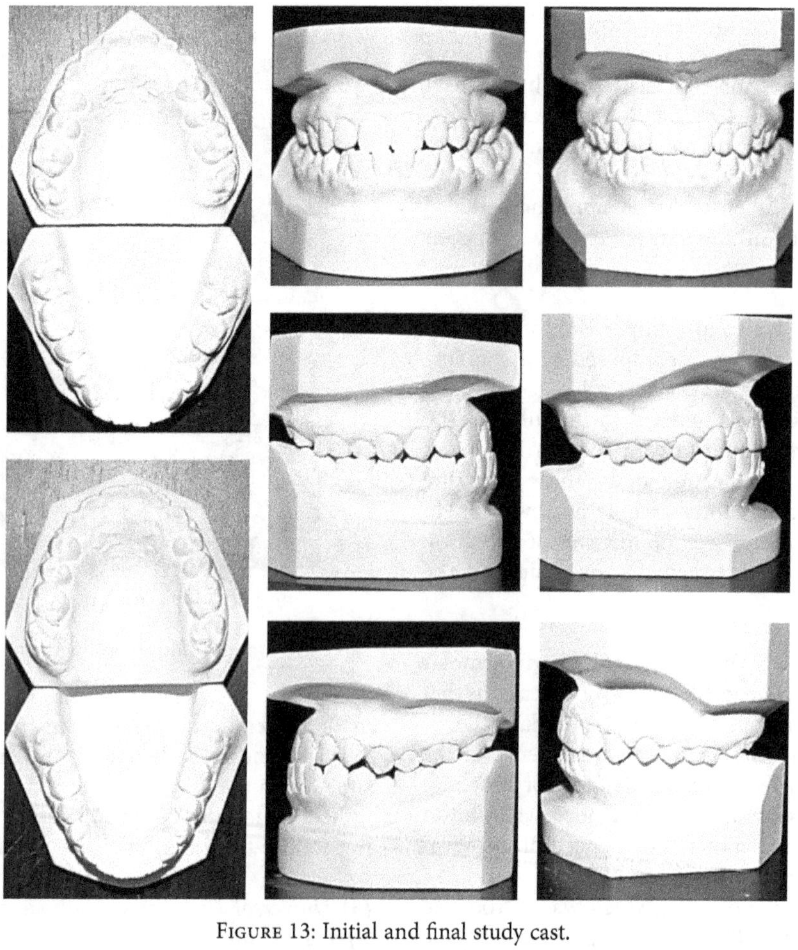

FIGURE 13: Initial and final study cast.

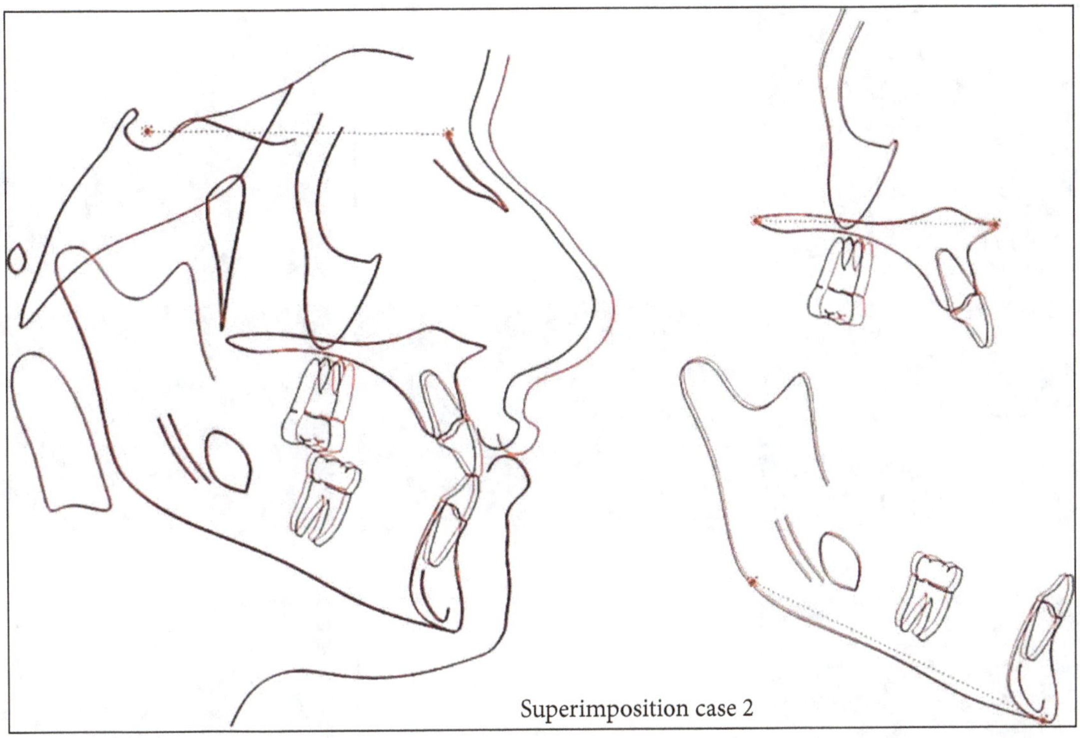

FIGURE 14: Superimposition.

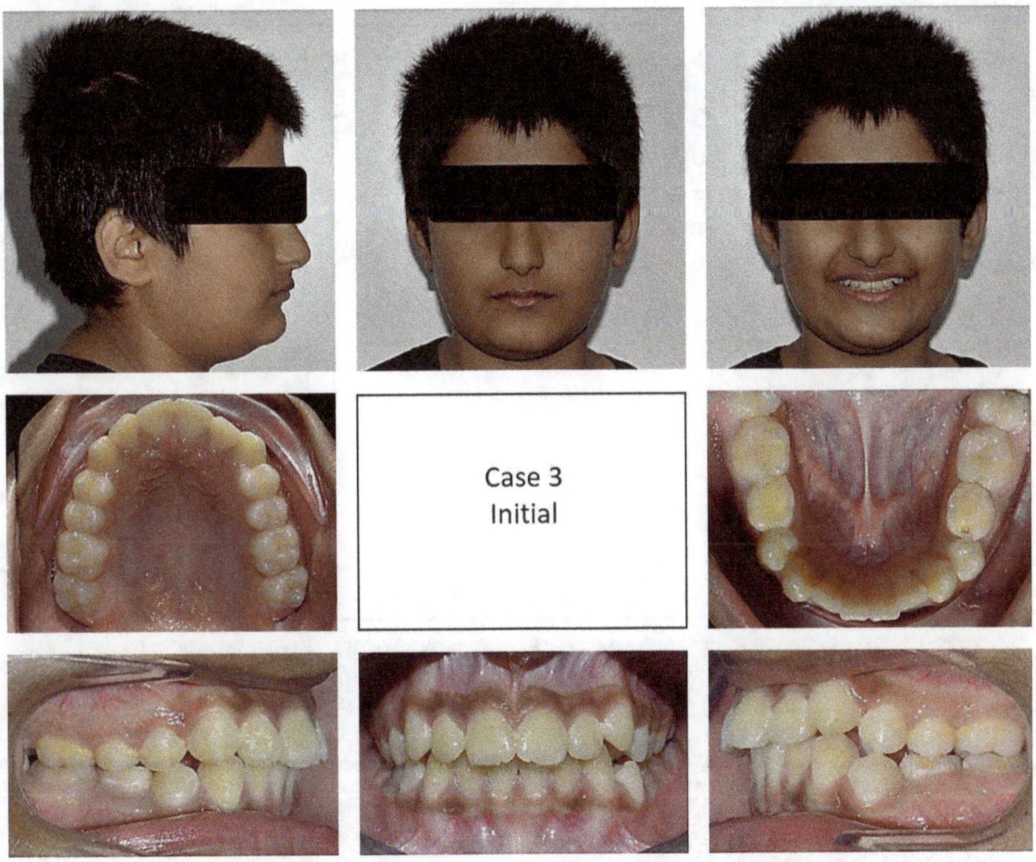

FIGURE 15: Pretreatment extraoral and intraoral photographs of the patient.

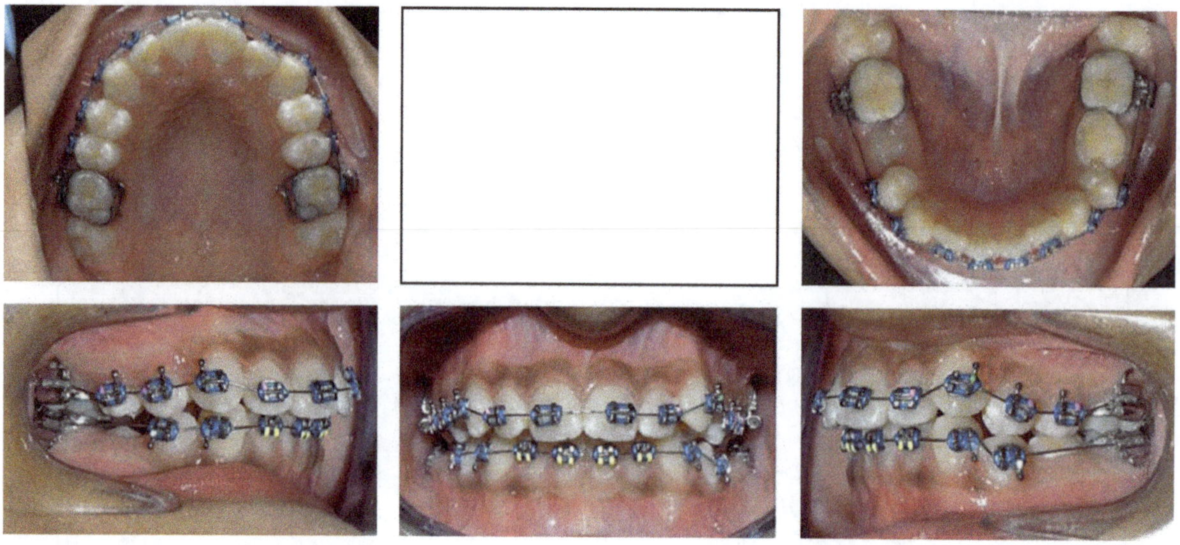

(a)

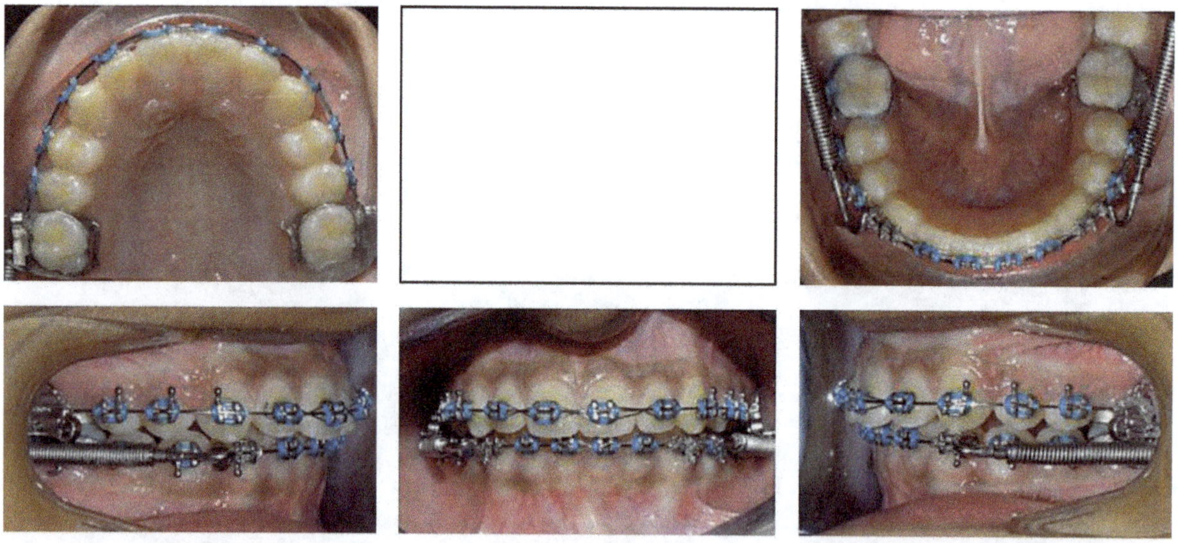

(b)

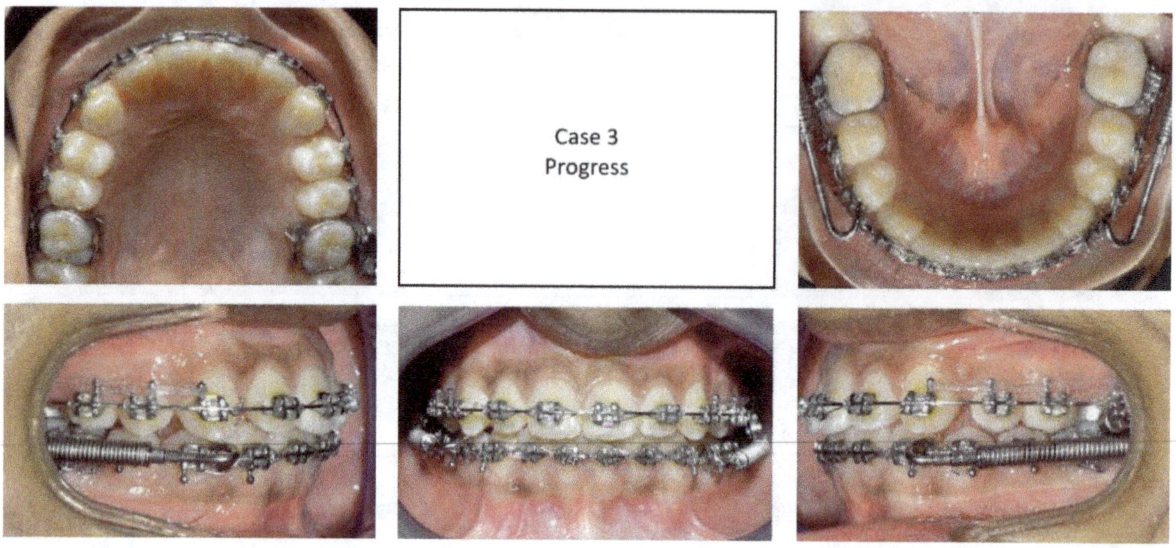

(c)

Figure 16: (a–c) Progress treatment intraoral photographs of the patient.

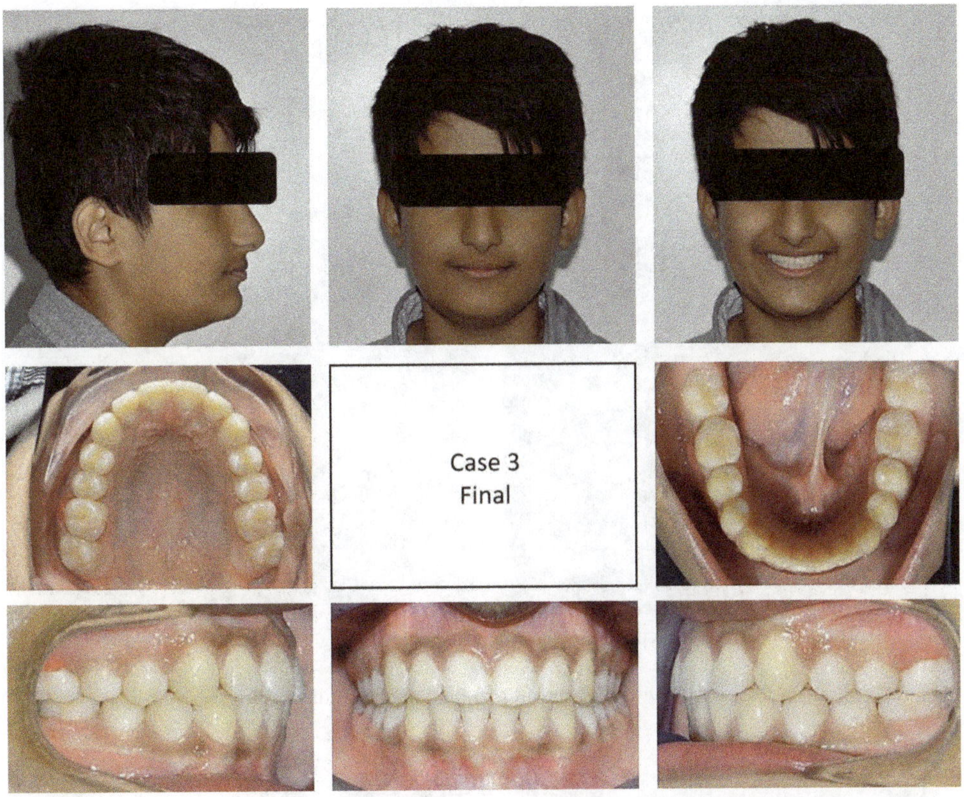

Figure 17: Posttreatment extraoral and intraoral photographs of the patient.

to gain absolute anchorage by either direct or indirect methods. Direct method of anchorage means that the active component causing the movement is directly attached to the miniscrew(s) while indirect attachment means that a tooth or teeth are attached to the miniscrew(s), and then, this tooth or teeth are utilized for anchorage. However, indirect anchorage was reported to be less reliable than direct anchorage as it may show some degree of anchorage loss. Nevertheless, miniscrews in general were able to efficiently distalize both molars and premolars without affecting the position of anterior teeth and minimal distal tipping [32, 33].

2.3.3. First Case. A 17-year-old female presented with class I incisors relationship on class II skeletal base with average vertical proportions. Her chief complaint was from crooked teeth and high canine. The molar relationship was 1/2 unit class II at left side and 1/3 unit class II at right side. The upper midline was shifted to the right by 2 mm. The crowding in the upper arch was moderate and in the lower was mild. Treatment initially was held using Pend-X appliance for distalization. This was followed by fixed appliance (0.018″ slot size) Roth prescription, on nonextraction basis. Pend-X appliance was able to correct the molar relationship into class I relation and to gain a space to relief the incisor crowding and the ectopically erupted right canine by both expansion and distalization (Figures 1–7).

Initial panorama, case 3

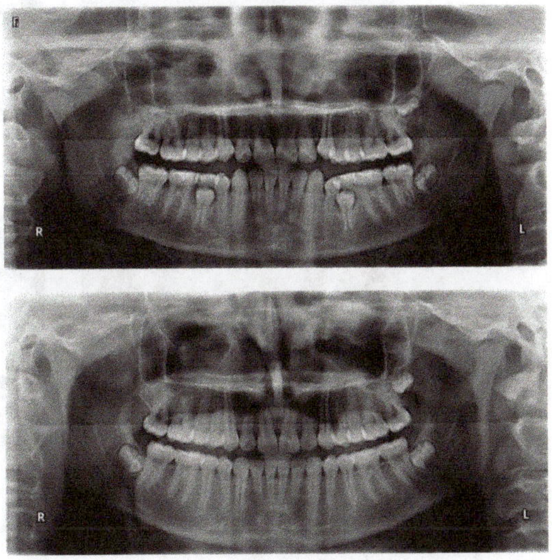

Final panorama, case 3

Figure 18: Initial and final panoramic radiographs.

2.3.4. Second Case. A 13-year-old male came to the clinic with a chief complaint of unpleasant teeth. Upon examination, the patient revealed class III incisor relation with anterior crossbite, minimal overbite, and skeletal class III base with horizontal growth pattern. The patient had class III molar relation on both sides. The canine relation was class III on the right side and class I on the left side. The lower left second

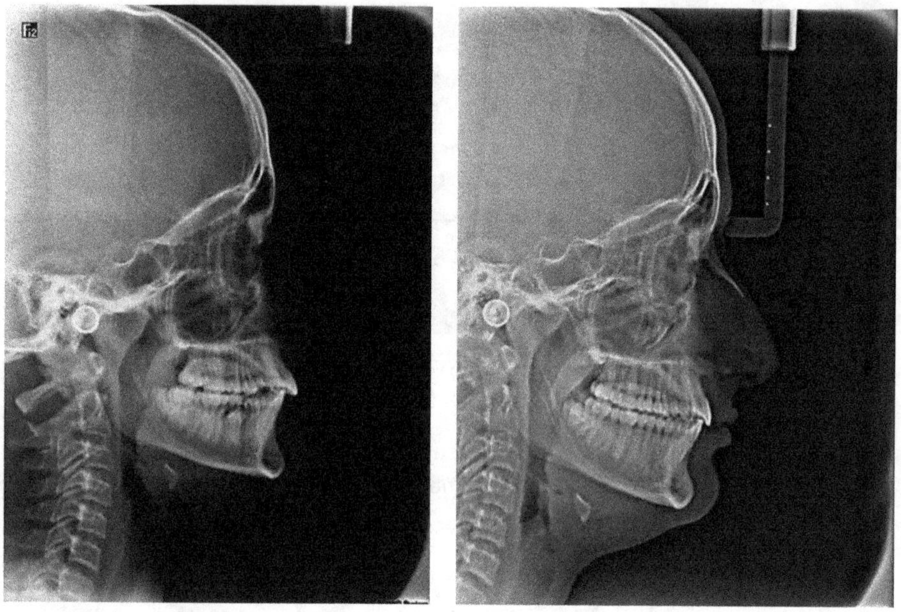

Initial cephalometric, case 3 Final cephalometric, case 3

FIGURE 19: Initial and final cephalometric radiographs.

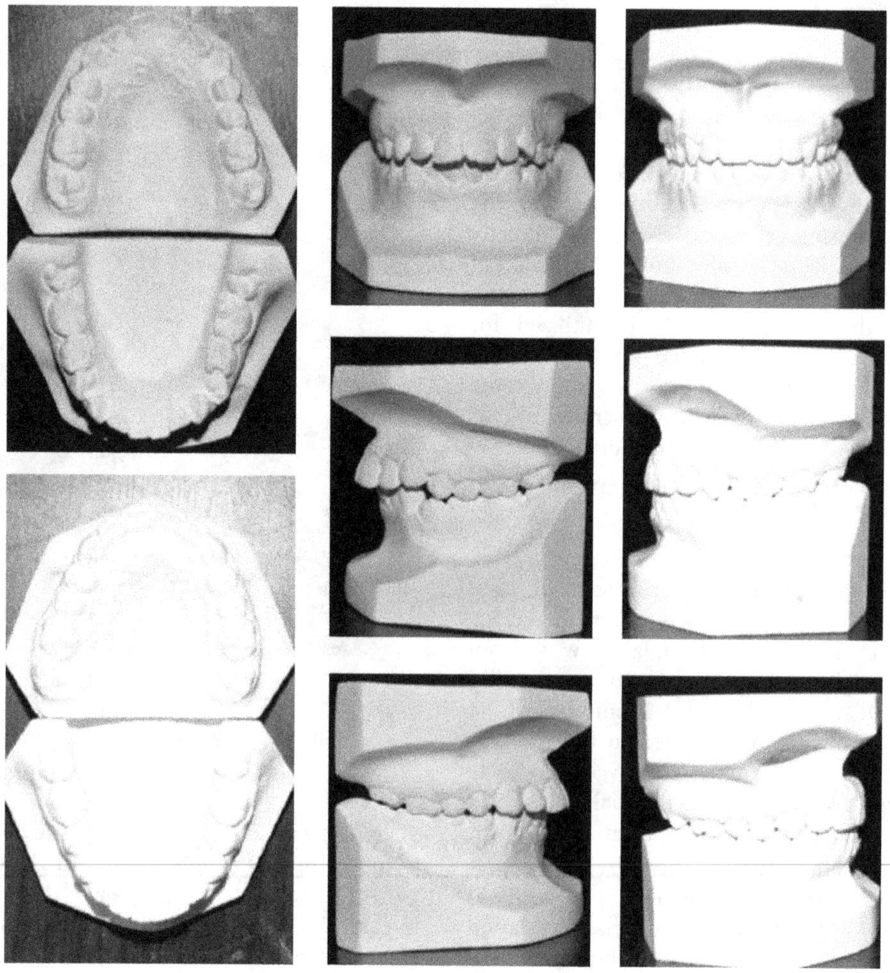

FIGURE 20: Initial and final study cast.

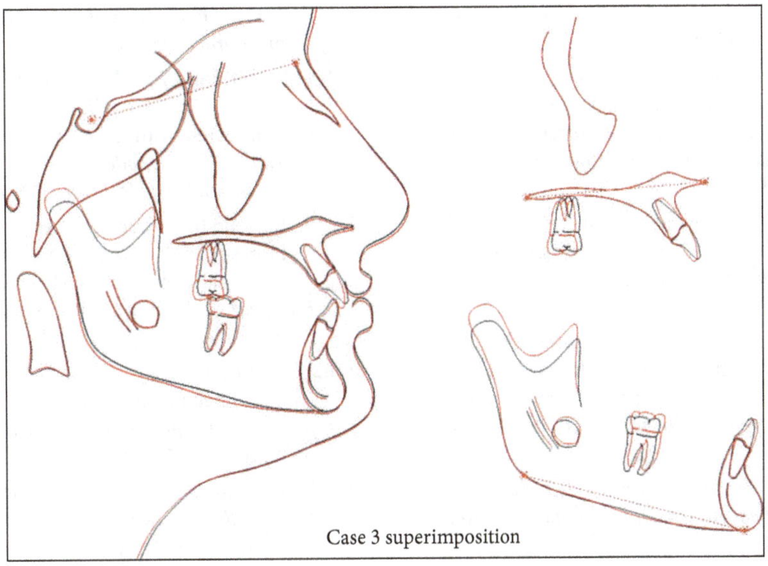

FIGURE 21: Superimposition.

premolar was ectopically erupted to the lingual side. Treatment plane was aimed at protracting the maxilla forward and at distalizing the lower molars to correct the class III molar relation and to give a space for alignment of the lower left second premolar. Maxillary protraction was achieved by utilizing facemask combined with rapid maxillary expansion using hyrax to disarticulate the maxilla from its sutures. Lip bumper was utilized to distalize the lower molars and was able to successfully correct the class III molar relation and to gain a space for the lower left second premolar (Figures 8–14).

2.3.5. Third Case. A 13-year-old male patient was presented with a class II division 1 incisor relationship on mild class II skeletal base and decreased vertical proportions. This was complicated with mild crowding in the upper and lower arches and 6 mm over jet. Molar and canine relations were class II on both sides. Because the patient was still growing, treatment plan was aimed at achieving skeletal and dental correction using nonextraction protocol. Functional appliances were the method to achieve these corrections. Forsus fixed functional appliance was chosen as it requires minimal patient cooperation and can increase the lower anterior facial height and achieve proper proclination of the retruded lower incisors. Positive response for treatment was found, and both skeletal and dental problems were corrected by in increasing the lower anterior facial height, reducing overjet, and correction of class II molar and canine relation (Figures 15–21).

3. Conclusion

Molar distalization is one of the fundamental approaches for nonextraction therapy, especially in class II malocclusion cases. Many methods have been utilized to achieve molar distalization, including extraoral app and intraoral appliances, either removable or fixed. Innovative devices continue to evolve as the trend changing from headgears to intraoral appliances that attempt to favorably distalize teeth without requiring much patient compliance. To ensure good results, a comprehensive clinical assessment of the case must be done to understand which method will mostly be suitable for this case in terms of cost, cooperation, treatment time, and stability of the results.

References

[1] M. Sfondrini, V. Cacciafesta, and G. Sfondrini, "Upper molar distalization: a critical analysis," *Orthodontics & craniofacial research*, vol. 5, no. 2, pp. 114–126, 2002.

[2] A. O. Cambiano, G. Janson, A. Fuziy, D. G. Garib, and D. C. Lorenzoni, "Changes consequent to maxillary molar distalization with the bone-anchored pendulum appliance," *Journal of Orthodontic Science*, vol. 6, no. 4, pp. 141–146, 2017.

[3] M. Almuzian, F. Alharbi, J. White, and G. McIntyre, "Distalizing maxillary molars–how do you do it?," *Orthodontic Update*, vol. 9, no. 2, pp. 42–50, 2016.

[4] N. Patil, V. Kerudi, H. A. Patil, P. D. Tekale, P. Bonde, and S. Dolas, "Molar distalization by miniplates-a review," *Journal Of Applied Dental and Medical Sciences*, vol. 2, 2016.

[5] S. Y. Jo, M. Bayome, J. Park, H. J. Lim, Y.-A. Kook, and S. H. Han, "Comparison of treatment effects between four premolar extraction and total arch distalization using the modified C-palatal plate," *The korean journal of orthodontics*, vol. 48, no. 4, pp. 224-235, 2018.

[6] K. Anasart, A. Pattarahirun, E. Y. Suzuki, B. Suzuki, and C. Sukjamsri, "Comparison of molar distalization devices in a treatment of malocclusion class II: finite element analysis," in *Paper presented at: Proceedings of the 2019 9th International Conference on Biomedical Engineering and Technology*, Tokyo, Japan, 2019.

[7] J. Pindoria, P. Fleming, and P. Sharma, "Inter-proximal enamel reduction in contemporary orthodontics," *British dental journal*, vol. 221, no. 12, pp. 757–763, 2016.

[8] G. S. Antonarakis and S. Kiliaridis, "Maxillary molar distalization with noncompliance intramaxillary appliances in class II

malocclusion: a systematic review," *The angle orthodontist*, vol. 78, no. 6, pp. 1133–1140, 2008.

[9] S. A. Bellini-Pereira, D. C. Pupulim, A. A.-D. Castillo, J. F. C. Henriques, and G. Janson, "Time of maxillary molar distalization with non-compliance intraoral distalizing appliances: a meta-analysis," *European journal of orthodontics*, vol. 41, no. 6, pp. 652–660, 2019.

[10] S. Haydar and O. Üner, "Comparison of Jones jig molar distalization appliance with extraoral traction," *American Journal of Orthodontics and Dentofacial Orthopedics*, vol. 117, no. 1, pp. 49–53, 2000.

[11] J.-M. Kang, J. H. Park, M. Bayome et al., "A three-dimensional finite element analysis of molar distalization with a palatal plate, pendulum, and headgear according to molar eruption stage," *The Korean Journal of Orthodontics*, vol. 46, no. 5, pp. 290–300, 2016.

[12] N. Jeckel and T. Rakosi, "Molar distalization by intra-oral force application," *The European Journal of Orthodontics*, vol. 13, no. 1, pp. 43–46, 1991.

[13] A. Geramy, N. Kizilova, and L. Terekhov, "Finite element method (FEM) analysis of the force systems produced by asymmetric inner headgear bows," *Australian orthodontic journal*, vol. 27, no. 2, pp. 125–131, 2011.

[14] J. Julku, K. Pirilä-Parkkinen, M. Tolvanen, and P. Pirttiniemi, "Comparison of effects of cervical headgear treatment on skeletal facial changes when the treatment time is altered: a randomized controlled trial," *European journal of orthodontics*, vol. 41, no. 6, pp. 631–640, 2019.

[15] T. Talvitie, M. Helminen, S. Karsila, R. Varho, L. Signorelli, and T. Peltomäki, "Adherence to instructions and fluctuation of force magnitude in cervical headgear therapy," *The Angle Orthodontist*, vol. 89, no. 2, pp. 268–274, 2018.

[16] J. J. Mao, X. Wang, and R. A. Kopher, "Biomechanics of craniofacial sutures: orthopedic implications," *The Angle Orthodontist*, vol. 73, no. 2, pp. 128–135, 2003.

[17] C. O. Park, N. L. Sa'aed, M. Bayome et al., "Comparison of treatment effects between the modified C-palatal plate and cervical pull headgear for total arch distalization in adults," *The korean journal of orthodontics*, vol. 47, no. 6, pp. 375–383, 2017.

[18] C. A. Brierley, A. DiBiase, and P. Sandler, "Early class II treatment," *Australian dental journal*, vol. 62, pp. 4–10, 2017.

[19] E. E. Bilbo, S. D. Marshall, K. A. Southard et al., "Long-term skeletal effects of high-pull headgear followed by fixed appliances for the treatment of Class II malocclusions," *The Angle Orthodontist*, vol. 88, no. 5, pp. 530–537, 2018.

[20] P. Chandra, S. Agarwal, D. Singh, and S. Agarwal, "Intra oral molar distalization-a review," *Journal of Dentofacial Sciences*, vol. 1, no. 1, pp. 15–18, 2012.

[21] J. Hilgers, "The pendulum appliance: an update," *Clin Impressions*, vol. 2, pp. 15–17, 1993.

[22] D. Amarnath, K. Patil, and M. R. Manohar, *A cephalometric evaluation of skeletal class II patients treated with premolar extraction and fixed functional appliance (Forsus)*, International Journal of Applied Dental Sciences, 2017.

[23] R. Varshan, K. Selvarasu, and S. Pandian, "A review on Forsus appliance on skeletal Class II management," *Drug Invention Today*, vol. 12, no. 3, 2019.

[24] J. Hourfar, J. A. Lisson, U. Gross, L. Frye, and G. S. M. Kinzinger, "Soft tissue profile changes after Functional Mandibular Advancer or Herbst appliance treatment in class II patients," *Clinical oral investigations*, vol. 22, no. 2, pp. 971–980, 2018.

[25] L. R. Toth and J. A. McNamara, "Treatment effects produced by the Twin-block appliance and the FR-2 appliance of Frankel compared with an untreated Class II sample," *American Journal of Orthodontics and Dentofacial Orthopedics*, vol. 116, no. 6, pp. 597–609, 1999.

[26] S. Ehsani, B. Nebbe, D. Normando, M. O. Lagravere, and C. Flores-Mir, "Short-term treatment effects produced by the Twin-block appliance: a systematic review and meta-analysis," *European Journal of Orthodontics*, vol. 37, no. 2, pp. 170–176, 2015.

[27] W. S. Osborn, R. S. Nanda, and G. F. Currier, "Mandibular arch perimeter changes with lip bumper treatment," *American Journal of Orthodontics and Dentofacial Orthopedics*, vol. 99, no. 6, pp. 527–532, 1991.

[28] D. Jamshir and A. Castaldo, *Effectiveness of Mandibular Lip Bumper therapy in mixed dentition patients-A review of literature*, WebmedCentral Journal, 2019.

[29] G. Kinzinger, U. Fritz, and P. Diedrich, "Combined therapy with pendulum and lingual arch appliances in the early mixed dentition," *Journal of orofacial orthopedics = Fortschritte der Kieferorthopadie : Organ/official journal Deutsche Gesellschaft fur Kieferorthopadie*, vol. 64, no. 3, pp. 201–213, 2003.

[30] M. M. Brennan and A. A. Gianelly, "The use of the lingual arch in the mixed dentition to resolve incisor crowding," *American journal of orthodontics and dentofacial orthopedics*, vol. 117, no. 1, pp. 81–85, 2000.

[31] F. Byloff, M. A. Darendeliler, and F. Stoff, "Mandibular molar distalization with the Franzulum Appliance," *Journal of clinical orthodontics: JCO*, vol. 34, no. 9, pp. 518–523, 2000.

[32] M. Cozzani, M. Fontana, G. Maino, G. Maino, L. Palpacelli, and A. Caprioglio, "Comparison between direct vs indirect anchorage in two miniscrew-supported distalizing devices," *The Angle Orthodontist*, vol. 86, no. 3, pp. 399–406, 2016.

[33] T. E. Bechtold, Y.-C. Park, K.-H. Kim, H. Jung, J.-Y. Kang, and Y. J. Choi, "Long-term stability of miniscrew anchored maxillary molar distalization in Class II treatment," *The Angle Orthodontist*, vol. 90, no. 3, pp. 362–368, 2020.

Management of the Vertical Dimension in the Camouflage Treatment of an Adult Skeletal Class III Malocclusion

Manuel Gustavo Chávez Sevillano,[1] Gina Judith Flores Diaz,[1] Luciane Macedo de Menezes,[2] Livia Kelly Ferraz Nunes,[3] José Augusto Mendes Miguel,[3] and Cátia Cardoso Abdo Quintão[3]

[1]*Department of Orthodontics, National University of San Marcos, Lima, Perú. Av. GermánAmézaga 375, Cercado de Lima-Lima, Peru*
[2]*Orthodontics Professor of the School of Health and Life Science-Pontifícia Universidade Católica do Rio Grande do Sul (PUCRS), Brazil. Ipiranga Avenue, 6681 Partenon-Porto Alegre RS, Brazil*
[3]*Department of Orthodontics, Rio de Janeiro State University, Rio de Janeiro, RJ, Brazil. Boulevard 28 de Setembro, 157; Vila Isabel – Rio de Janeiro, RJ, Brazil*

Correspondence should be addressed to Manuel Gustavo Chávez Sevillano; mchavezs@unmsm.edu.pe

Academic Editor: Mariano A. Polack

Treating skeletal class III malocclusions is one of the biggest challenges in Orthodontics. Given the complexity of these cases, orthognathic surgery is often the best treatment option. However, many patients refuse this treatment due to its risks, morbidity, and costs involved. Alternatively, dental compensation can be planned for some of these skeletal problems. This case report presents a dentoalveolar compensation in the orthodontic treatment of a 20-year-old female patient with class III malocclusion, concave profile, anterior crossbite, mandibular prognathism, maxillary retrusion, and a vertical deficiency in the posterior region. Treatment planning involved a multiloop edgewise archwire (MEAW) associated with intermaxillary elastics with counterclockwise rotation of the occlusal plane in the posterior region of the maxilla aiming at obtaining an increased posterior vertical dimension. After 24 months of treatment, the severe anterior crossbite was corrected, and the skeletal class III relationship was camouflaged. At the end of the orthodontic treatment, it was possible to observe an improved facial profile, a nice smile, and a functional occlusion. The results remained stable at a three-year follow-up. The MEAW, associated with the use of elastics, seems to be an effective treatment option for class III camouflage with reduced posterior vertical dimension with no need for additional anchoring devices but requiring adequate bending of wires and patient compliance.

1. Introduction

The diagnosis, treatment, and prognosis of class III malocclusion are often a challenge for orthodontists [1]. The main features of skeletal class III anatomy include mandibular prognathism, maxillary atresia, anterior crossbite, and a reduced skull base angle [2]. However, there are different types of class III malocclusions depending on the predominance of the facial growth (vertical or horizontal) and the mandibular plane angle (open or closed) [3].

Class III malocclusion with a closed mandibular plane angle is characterized by poor vertical growth of the maxillary posterior segment, and, as a consequence, there is a deficiency in the posterior vertical dimension. In such cases, the occlusal plane, in the posterior region, presents a clockwise rotation, with a lack of proportion of the vertical maxillary growth and the mandibular ramus, with an excessive counterclockwise rotation of the mandible. As a consequence, there can be an anterior crossbite with negative overbite [2, 4, 5].

The vertical dimension is believed to be significantly different in skeletal malocclusions, playing an important role in establishing the various sagittal bone relationship morphologies [6]. The primary objective in treating class III malocclusion, with a predominance of horizontal growth, is to restore

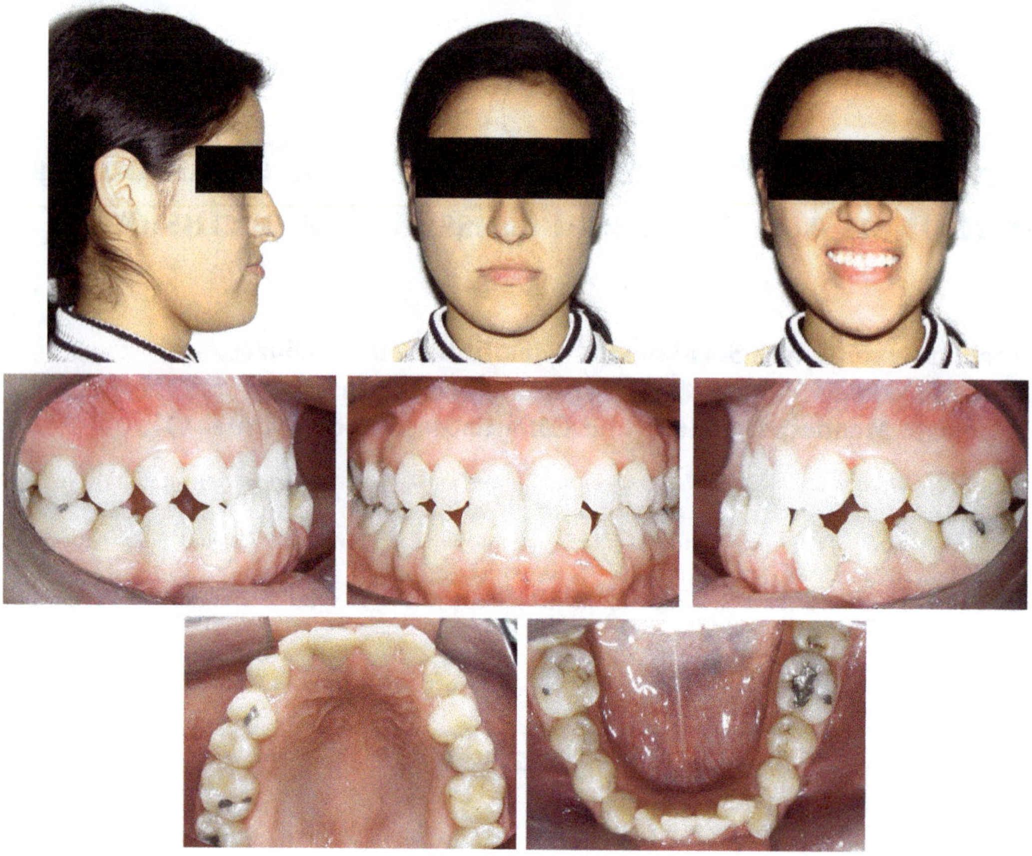

Figure 1: Pretreatment facial and intraoral photographs.

the skeleton harmony by controlling the occlusal plane and obtaining an appropriate posterior vertical dimension, thus improving the balance between the mandibular ramus height and the posterior maxillary vertical dimension [3, 7].

Multiloop Edgewise Archwire Wires (MEAW), which were introduced by Kim [8, 9], are effective in treating class III malocclusion basically with vertical occlusal plane alteration and distal mass movement of the lower arch. The distal movements of the posterior lower teeth occur through the boot loops and second-order bends (tip-back), along with class III intermaxillary elastics, promoting counterclockwise rotation of the occlusal planes. This improves both the sagittal bone and teeth relationship, allowing a good intercuspal relationship in a short period of time [3].

In the present case, due to the rejection of the patient's surgical treatment and to the lack of vertical harmony between the jaws with a moderate facial aesthetic compromise, counterclockwise rotation of the occlusal plane and a clockwise rotation of the mandible were promoted through orthodontic mechanics and no surgical intervention and without any type of skeletal anchorage. Verticalization and extrusion of the upper and lower molars as well as vestibular proclination of the upper incisors were part of the compensatory treatment of this adult skeletal class III malocclusion with the MEAW technique. The profile and the smile were significantly improved and maintained after a three-year posttreatment follow-up.

2. Case Presentation

2.1. Diagnosis and Etiology. A 20-year-old female was referred to the Orthodontics Department of the School of Dentistry, National University of San Marcos. Her chief complaint was the anterior crossbite, crowded teeth, and a large jaw. She presented a good general state of health and no history of systemic disease. The extraoral frontal examination revealed a mesofacial aspect, a lower prognathic third, and a symmetrical face. The smile showed adequate gingival exposure with upper dental crowding. In the lateral view, a total and concave lower third profile was observed, an apparent lack of development in the sub nasal region, and a protruding lower lip. Intraorally, she had a class III molar and canine relationship, with a negative overjet and overbite of −1 mm and −3 mm, respectively. The space deficiency of the upper arch was -3 mm and -6 mm in the lower arch. The lower midline was 0.5 mm shifted to the left. In the lower arch, the incisors showed a severe lingual inclination and the premolars and molars showed an increased mesial inclination (Figures 1 and 2). No symptoms of temporomandibular joint dysfunction were detected during jaw function and palpation.

The panoramic X-ray (Figure 3) revealed the presence of the four third molars, and endodontic treatment on the upper right central incisor (11) and the left upper premolar (25), with no presence of caries. It was identified the

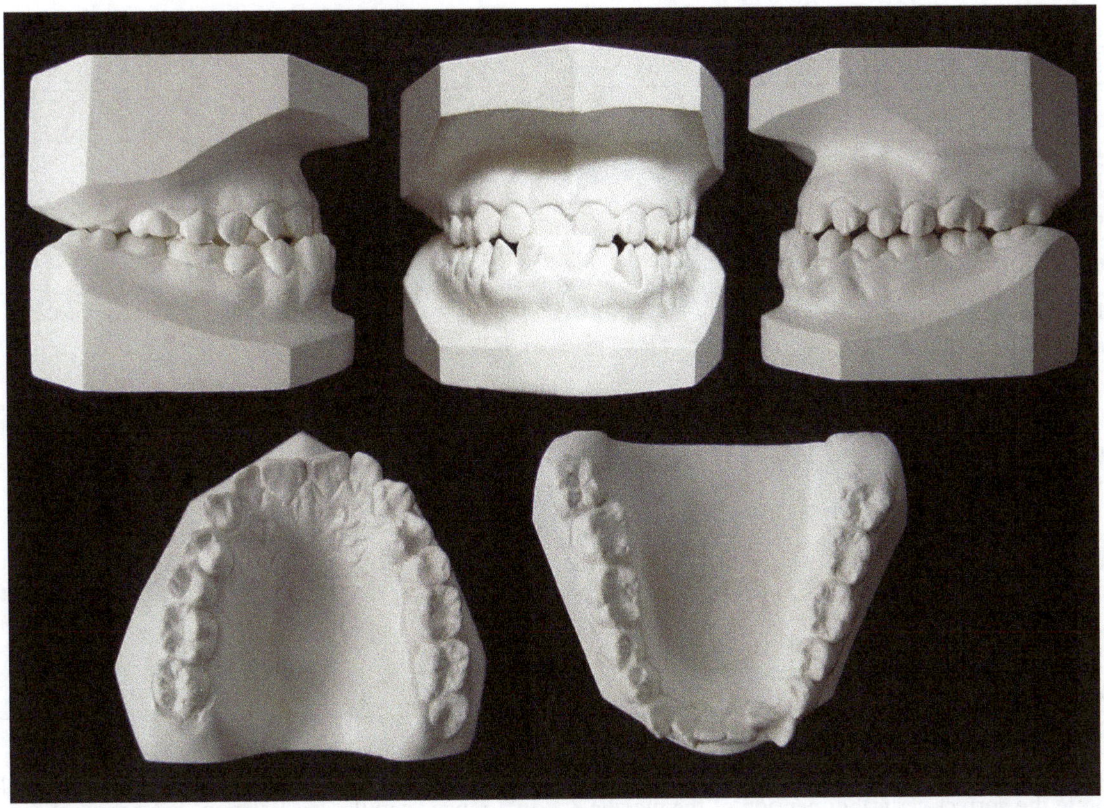

Figure 2: Pretreatment dental casts.

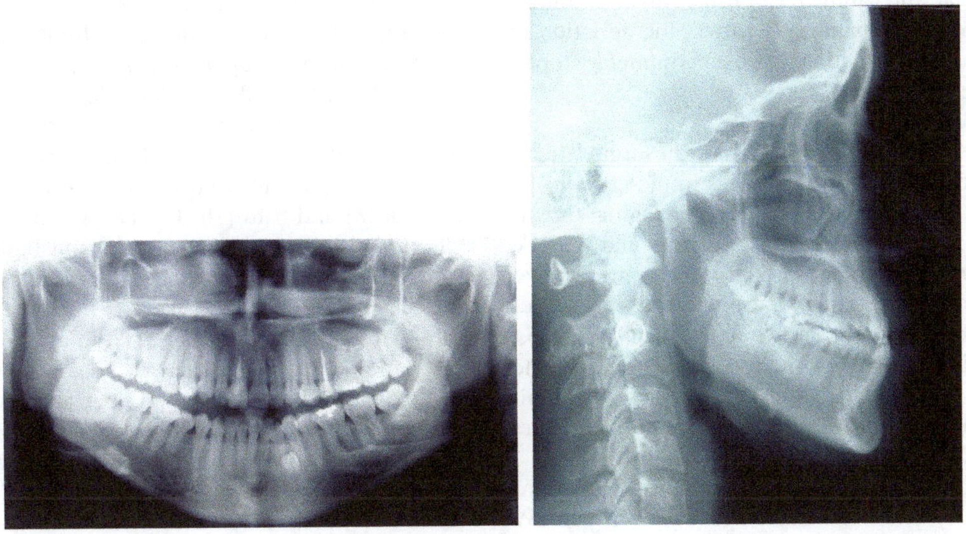

Figure 3: Pretreatment radiographs.

presence of a supernumerary tooth between the left lower canine and the first premolar (33 and 34). The condyles were morphologically asymmetrical. The cephalometric analysis revealed a slight maxillary retrusion (SNA: 79°) and mandible protrusion (SNB: 82°), resulting in a skeletal class III (ANB: −3°; Wits: -11 mm). Facial growth was hypodivergent (FMA: 20.5^0) and the occlusal plane showed clockwise rotation (Occlusal-SN plane: 22.5°) indicating a deficiency in maxillary posterior vertical dimension.

Cephalometric radiography also showed an increased distal angulation of the maxillary molars and upper and lower incisors retroinclined (1-NA: 15° and 1-NB: 17°) (Figure 3, Table 1).

2.2. Treatment Objectives. The overall goals of the treatment plan were to achieve a good skeletal relationship, improve the profile, and establish a stable occlusion. The specific objectives were (1) to correct the sagittal skeletal relationship,

Table 1: Pretreatment and posttreatment cephalometric values.

Measurement	Norm	Pretreatment	Posttreatment
SNA (°)	82	79	81.5
SNB (°)	80	82	80.5
ANB (°)	2	-3	1
Wits	-1	-11	-5
Convexity (°)	0	-4.5	1
y-axis (°)	59.9	50.5	51.5
Facial angle (FH-NPo) (°)	87.8	102	100
Mandibular plane to SN (SN-GoGn) (°)	32	38.5	38
FMA (°)	25	20.5	23
IMPA (°)	90	75.5	83
Occlusal plane to SN (OP-SN) (°)	14	22.5	14
Maxillary incisor-NA (U1-NA) (°)	22	15	34
Maxillary incisor-NA (U1-NA) (mm)	4	11	22
Mandibular incisor-NB (L1-NB) (°)	25	17	23
Mandibular incisor-NB (L1-NB) (mm)	4	11.5	20
1–1 (°)	130	150	121
LS-S (mm)	0	-11	-5
LI-S (mm)	0	4	4

(2) promote a counterclockwise rotation of the occlusal plane to incorporate the correct vertical dimension of the maxilla, (3) achieve a clockwise rotation of the jaw to improve facial profile, (4) establish a correct overbite and overjet, (5) establish a class I molar and canine relationship, (6) to eliminate the negative tooth discrepancy, (7) correct the deviation of the lower midline, (8) extraction of the supernumerary tooth, and (9) improve the smile.

2.3. Treatment Alternatives. Initially, an orthosurgical treatment was presented for the patient. This would consist of a maxillary Lefort I advancement and a ramus sagittal osteotomy to achieve mandibular clockwise rotation and setback. Due to economic constrains and fear, the surgery was rejected. Therefore, an orthodontic camouflage was considered as an alternative, based on five biomechanics options: (1) teeth extractions (lower first premolars and upper second premolars); (2) intermaxillary Class III elastics; (3) miniplates; (4) extraalveolar miniscrews; and (5) Multiloop Edgewise Archwire (MEAW) technique.

The patient has not accepted extractions apart from third molars nor the use of skeletal anchorage. Thus, the MEAW technique was the chosen option as the occlusal plane could be rigorous controlled. The patient was aware of the need for collaboration regarding the use of intermaxillary elastics and of the need of third molars extractions.

2.4. Treatment Progress. Treatment began with third molar extractions to facilitate distal movements of the upper and lower second and first molars. A cone-beam computed tomography (CBCT) scan was performed to assess the area of the supranumerary tooth; an initial segmentation of the compromised teeth was performed and showed no contact or damages to the adjacent teeth (Figures 4 and 5). The distances between the teeth measured in the tomography were in a range from 0.55 to 1.30 mm. Extraction of the supernumerary tooth was requested but the patient refused the proposal due to unsuccessful previous extraction attempting procedure. Therefore, it was decided to keep the supernumerary tooth as long as annual controlling exams were performed. Full-fixed appliance was placed in both dental arches (0.022×0.028-inch slot, 3 M Unitek). First and second molars were banded with prescription tubes MBT 0.022×0.028-inch slot (3 M Unitek). Treatment with MEAW arches was divided into five phases, as proposed by Kim [8] and Sato [10, 11]: (1) Alignment and Leveling, where the 0.016-inch, 0.018-inch, and $0.016" \times 0.022$-inch slot Nickel-Titanium (NiTi) (Unitek-3 M) arches were installed. Short intermaxillary 3/16 in elastic, 2.5 oz of upper canine to lower canine was placed to avoid excessive buccal inclination of the lower incisors. The objectives were to correct rotations, coordinate the upper and lower arches, and facilitate the insertion of the MEAW arch (Figure 6(a)); (2) Elimination of Interferences, which was initially performed by installing an upper MOAW (Modified Offset Arch Wire) arch, made with 0.016×0.0022-inch blue elgiloy (RMO) wire. It was used to produce intrusion and buccal inclination of the upper incisors facilitating the crossbite correction (Figure 6(b)). To eliminate dental interference from the posterior segments, upper and lower MEAW arches with 0.016×0.022-inch blue elgiloy (RMO) wires were installed. Step-up bends for the upper and lower molars associated with tip-back bends for molar and lower premolar verticalization and class III (3/16-in, 6.5 oz) intermaxillary elastics were incorporated. (Figure 6(c)); (3) Mandibular displacement, with downward and backward rotation, helped achieving an adequate molar and canine Class I relationship, as well as correcting the overbite and

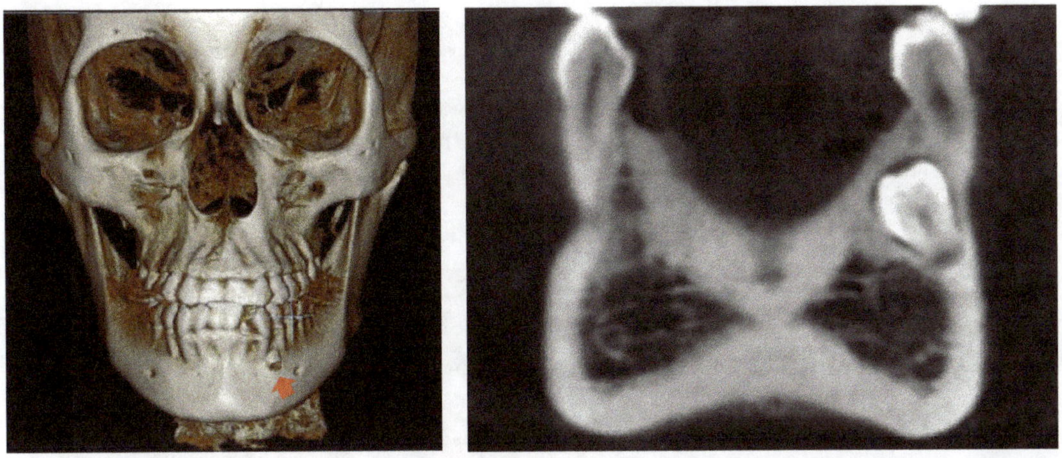

(a) (b)

FIGURE 4: (a) 3D frontal view of the CBCT where the supernumerary tooth is visualized (red arrow) and (b) Coronal section of the supernumerary tooth showing no evidence of contact with the first lower premolar.

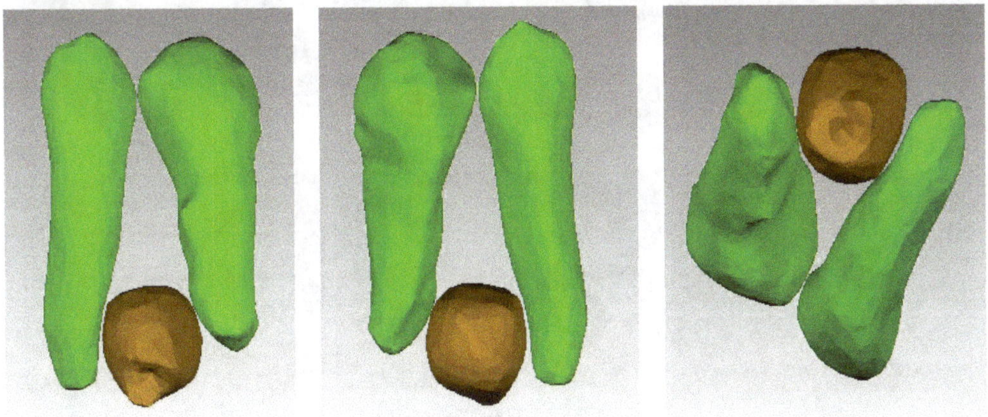

(a) (b) (c)

FIGURE 5: 3D reconstruction of supernumerary, cuspid, and premolar teeth: (a) vestibular view of segmented tooth, (b) lingual view, and (c) Inferior view.

overjet (Figure 6(c)); (4) Reconstruction of the Occlusal Plane, modification of the posterior occlusal plane by incorporating a step down of the upper molars and a tip-back of the lower molars. In this phase, the occlusal plane was rotated (counterclockwise) increasing the vertical dimension of the maxilla (Figure 6(d) and 7(b)); and (5) Obtaining a Physiological Occlusion, with the use of a 0.020-inch stainless steel (SS) continuous arch and class III intermaxillary elastics, to achieve a good intercuspation (Figure 6(e)).

After 15 months of MEAW mechanics, the treatment continued with a 0.020-inch and 0.018×0.025-inch rectangular stainless steel arches and Class III elastics (3/16 in, 4.5 oz) to extrude the upper molars and continue increasing the posterior occlusal dimension. Treatment was completed within 24 months. A Hawley removable appliance associated to bonded canine to canine lower lingual wire were used as retainers (0.7 mm SS), supervised from 3 to 3 months.

2.5. Treatment Results. The final registries showed that the majority of treatment targets were accomplished. Extraoral photographs indicated significant improvement of the facial profile and lip position. The lack of development in the subnasal region, and the protrusion of the lower lip were camouflaged. The smile became more aesthetic, and the patient reported great satisfaction with the results. Intraorally, the anterior crossbite was corrected, a Class I Canine and a Class III molar functional relationship was achieved, with adequate overjet and overbite. The dental arches were aligned and leveled and the upper and lower dental midlines were coincident (Figure 8). Panoramic X-ray showed a verticalization of the upper and lower molars and premolars, with acceptable parallelism and no signs of significant bone or root resorption (Figure 9). In order to reevaluate the position of the remaining, a CBCT was required and the area segmented using ITK-SNAP 3.8 (USA) (Figure 10). There was no contact nor damages between the extra tooth and neighbouring teeth. Final Cephalometric radiography—taken immediately before appliance removal—(Figure 9, Table 1) revealed an improved skeletal relationship (ANB: 1°, SNA: 81.5°, SNB: 80.5°, Wits: -5 mm). Regarding the dentoalveolar changes, it

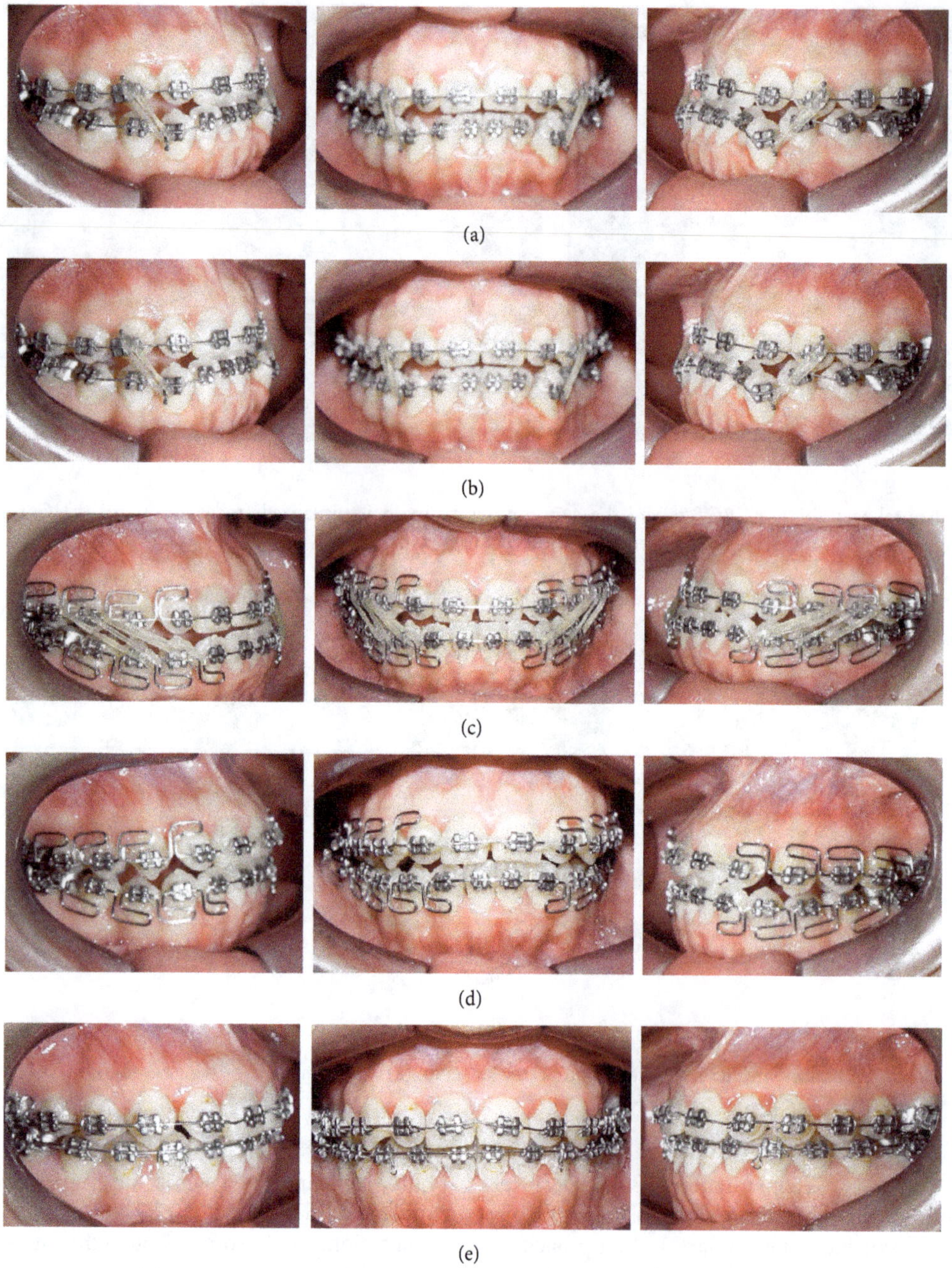

Figure 6: (a) Alignment and leveling with wires 0.014-inch NiTi, (b) MEAW arches with blue elgiloy 0.016 × 0.022-inch, (c) MEAW arches with blue elgiloy 0.016 × 0.022-inch and elastic 3/16 in, 4.5 oz elastic with Class III component, (d) MEAW arches and canine Class I, (e) 0.020-inch Stainless Steel continuous arches with the use of 3/16-in Class III elastics 4.5 oz.

is possible to observe the protrusion of the upper and lower incisors (1-NA: 34°, 1-NB: 23° and IMPA: 83°) and a decrease in the inclination of the occlusal plane (Occ. Plane-SN: 14°), which reflected an increase in the vertical dimension of the maxilla (Figure 7). Cephalometric superposition revealed the improvement of the facial profile with a slight increase in facial height (as shown in Table 1: FMA: 23°).

The upper and lower molars were uprighted and the upper extruded as well resulting in an anticlockwise rotation of the occlusal plane (OccPlane-SN: 14°). The vestibuloversion of the upper and lowers incisors can be observed (Figure 11). Three-dimensional (3D) superposition of the jaws was performed using Geomagic Qualify 2013 (USA), highlighting the extrusion of the upper molars and the vestibuloversion of the upper incisors (Figure 12). In the 3D superposition of the mandible, no extrusion of the lower molars and mild vestibuloversion of the lower incisors was observed (Figure 13).

After three years of posttreatment, the position of the lips was maintained and profile remained straight. The patient underwent nasal plastic surgery, with a significant improvement of the facial profile. Functional molar Class III and canine Class I were maintained, although the patient lost the lower retention after24 months of control. A slight

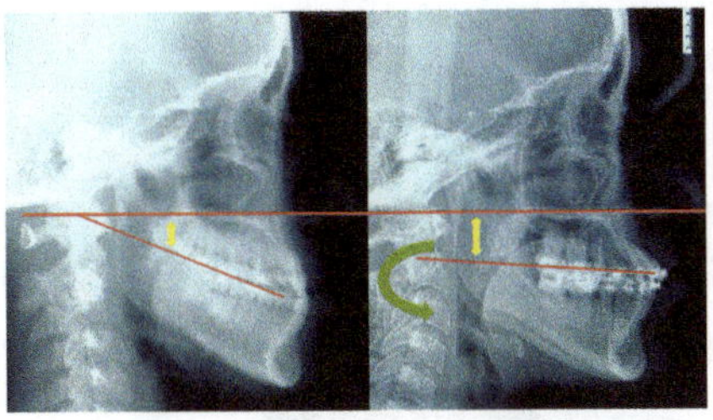

(a) (b)

FIGURE 7: Occlusal plane evaluation, before (a) and at the end (b) of treatment. (a) Deficiency of vertical dimension (short yellow arrow), (b) increase of the vertical dimension (long yellow arrow) with counterclockwise rotation of the occlusal plane (green arrow).

relapse was observed in the lower incisors; however, an occlusion with acceptable stability was observed (Figure 14).

3. Discussion

For correct diagnosis and orthodontic treatment plan, it is important to evaluate the morphological characteristics of the different vertical and sagittal skeletal alterations types, observed in Class III malocclusion, dolichofacial, mesofacial, or brachyfacial, each one with its own characteristics [2–4]. A close relationship has also been identified between the vertical behavior of the occlusal plane and the establishment of a certain sagittal skeletal alteration [6]. Thus, there are certain types of Class III malocclusions with an imbalance between the vertical growth of the mandibular ramus and the vertical growth of the maxilla in the posterior region, which is hypodeveloped causing a deficiency of vertical descent of the occlusal plane. As a consequence, the lower jaw loses the adequate vertical occlusal support and moves forward [3]. This morphological feature is present in our patient. The deficiency of the occlusal support and in the vertical dimension can be identified in the facial and dentoalveolar analysis and mainly, in radiographic evaluation (Figure 7 and Table 1). The patient reported that she had already consulted other specialists, and that all had proposed orthognathic surgery as the only treatment option for her case. Traditionally, this type of treatment has been the most effective way to correct skeletal discrepancies. The first treatment choice for this patient was orthognatic surgery. However, the patient refused the surgical inter-vention. Therefore, a compensatory orthodontic treatment was considered and the options were the use of class III intermaxillary elastics, treatment with miniplates [12] or extraalveolar mini implants [13, 14], treatment with premolar extractions [10], and the adoption of the MEAW [7, 8] technique.

Since the patient had an FMA of 20.50°, a treatment with premolars extractions could reduce even more the occlusal support in the posterior region. The maintenance or increase of the occlusal support is fundamental to prevent the clockwise mandibular rotation and also to improve the facial profile. The use of Class III intermaxillary elastics alone would cause a counterclockwise rotation of the occlusal plane by increasing the posterior vertical dimension, but would not be sufficient to upright the lower molars and premolars as well as to perform a thorough control of the occlusal plane. The use of miniplates would involve minor surgical procedures, also rejected by the patient. The use of extraalveolar mini implants may provide adequate anchorage for the verticalization of the premolars and lower molars, along with a counterclockwise rotation of the occlusal plane, but with minimal extrusion and verticalization of the upper molars, which is required to increase the vertical dimension. In addition, this technique seems to be effective for Dolichofacial Class III patients [13]. Seeking to obtain counterclockwise rotation of the occlusal plane and a clockwise rotation of the mandibular plane, we opted for the MEAW technique to correct the vertical imbalance between the mandibular and the maxillary arches [3]. This treatment modality was developed by Kim [15–18] and is considered effective for class III corrections, severe open bite, lateral deviation of the mandible, and TMJ problems. The technique does not require skeletal anchoring devices; however, the loops require manual operator skills, and patient collaboration is of utmost importance.

The tip-back, step-up, and/or step-down bends incorporated into the arches, associated to intermaxillary elastics, generate significant vertical dental displacement, allowing the occlusal planes to be reconstructed effectively through moving the posterior teeth vertically [19–22]. The presence of the loops provides versatility and flexibility to the MEAW technique; therefore, the forces produced are more physiological than the ones generated by the continuous arches [9]. This alveolar compensation process takes place in a relatively short period of time due to the simultaneous movement that occurs in all teeth.

The treatment performed consists of several phases, beginning with the alignment of the dental arches with light and continuous wires seeking to prepare it for a more passive insertion of the MEAW arch (Alignment and leveling phase). Then, the anterior crossbite was corrected with the MOAW (modified offset archwire) arch and all types of occlusal contact of the molars and second premolars were eliminated, with posterior intrusion. This gave the mandible more freedom for a sagittal movement (Interference elimination phase). Once the occlusal interference was eliminated, the jaw was relocated in the posterior direction (clockwise rotation) and the adequate vertical dimension is obtained, with occlusal contacts just at the level of the first premolars. At this point, a class I canine relationship and a functional class III molar relationship were achieved. The facial profile was favorably modified (mandibular replacement phase). The relocated mandible was stabilized so that intercuspidation of all molars and second premolars was sought, now with extrusive movements, mainly of the upper molars (Occlusal plane reconstruction phase). Thus, the stability of the jaw was achieved and an acceptable canine and molar relationship were sought to increase occlusion throughout the arch (phase of obtaining a physiological occlusion) [5]. All phases required the use of 3/16 in, 6.5 oz elastics, which were installed from the second upper loop to the first lower loop. When using double elastics per side, the elastic force should be reduced (4.5 oz) (Figure 6(c)).

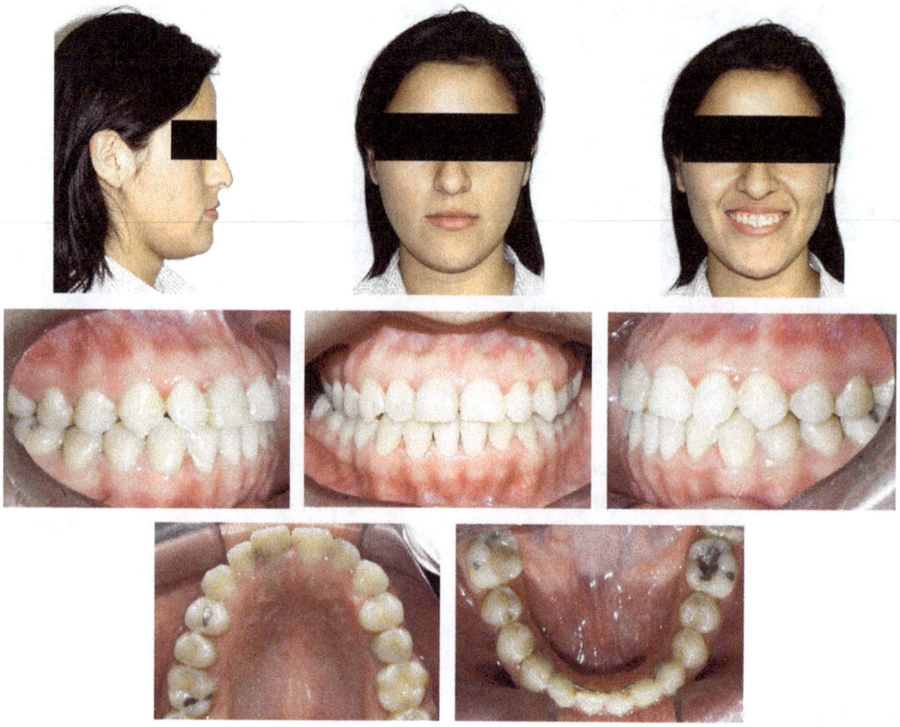

FIGURE 8: Posttreatment extraoral and intraoral photographs.

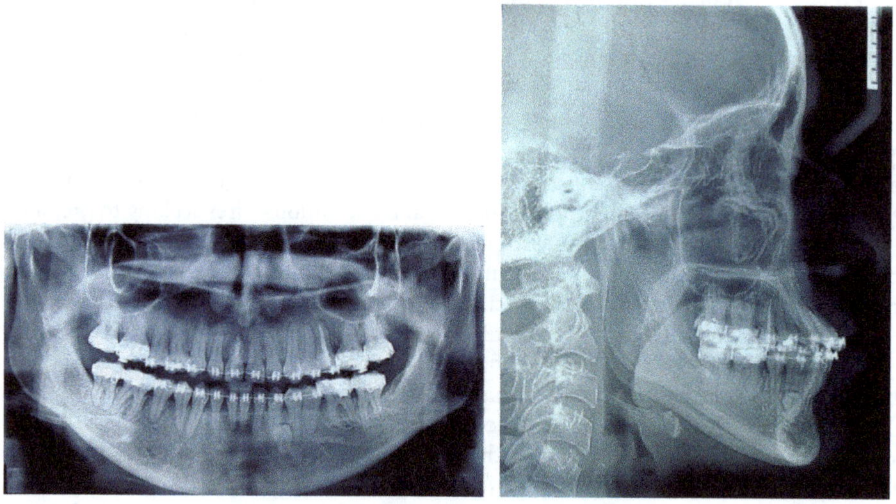

FIGURE 9: Posttreatment radiographs.

Rotation of the occlusal plane vertically in the treatment of Class III malocclusion has been reported by several authors. From studies using modern noninvasive tools such as finite element analysis proposed by Roberts et al. [13], who explained that the occlusal plane could rotate counterclockwise through a statically determined biomechanical system and without the need for premolar extractions or orthognathic surgeries. Clinical studies such as the one carried out by He et al. [23] who, in a total sample of 44 patients without growth, determined that the MEAW arch and the Class III elastics were an appropriate strategy for the management of the occlusal plane in the treatment of Class III malocclusion, even in hyperdivergent patients. The opposite rotation between the occlusal plane and the mandibular plane to return the vertical dimension to a patient with hypodivergent Class III was also highlighted by Park and Bullen [11]. The result of vertical occlusal plane management in our patients was consistent with these previous studies.

During the camouflage treatment of the Class III malocclusion, the MEAW arch can also be used in the early stages and can then be replaced by mini implants and continuous arches [24]. In the present case, it was decided to maintain the MEAW arch until the final stages of the treatment, as it was considered to have a stricter three-dimensional control of torque, tipping, extrusion, and intrusion of tooth movement.

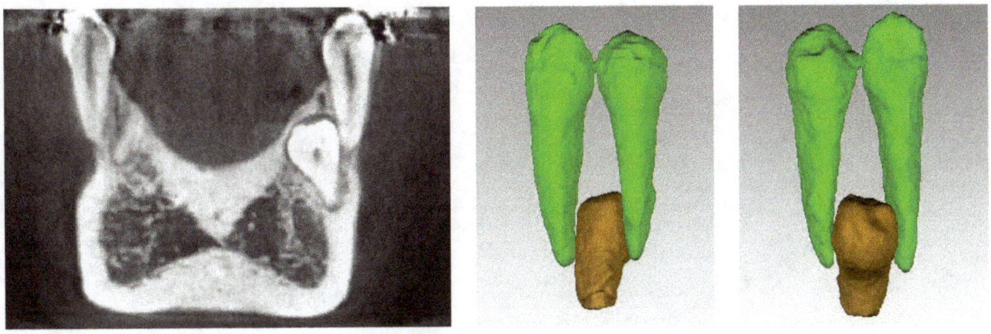

(a) (b) (c)

FIGURE 10: Final CBCT. (a) Axial view of the supernumerary tooth; 3D reconstruction of teeth: (b) vestibular view of segmented teeth, (c) lingual view.

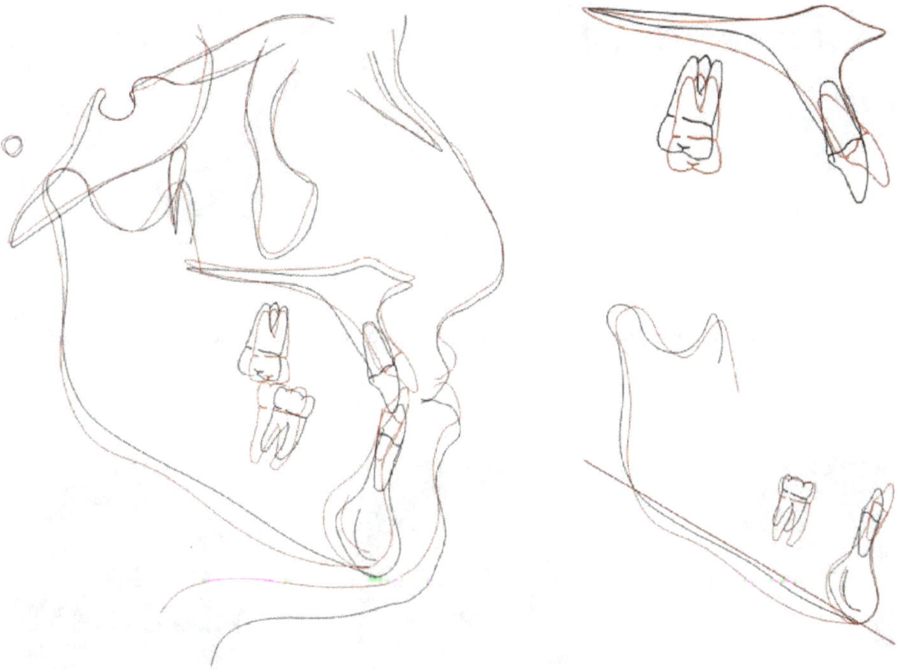

FIGURE 11: Pretreatment (black line) and posttreatment (red line).

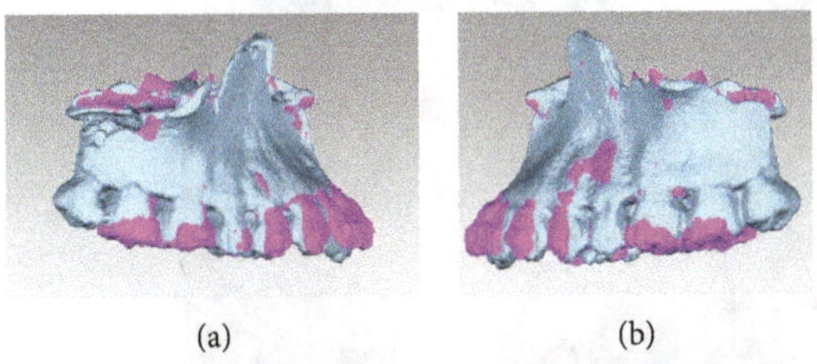

(a) (b)

(c) (d)

FIGURE 12: Initial (blue color) and posttreatment (pink color). (a) Right side, (b) left side, (c) frontal view, and (d) occlusal.

The MEAW arch can be made of 0.017 × 0.025-inch stainless steel archwire or with 0.016 × 0.022-inch "blue elgiloy" wire. In this treatment phase, second-order bends (tip-back, tip-forward, step-up, and step-down) are important for the establishment of the modified occlusal plane. Third-order bends (torque) and arch coordination should be considered during all treatment phases to avoid edge-to-edge intercuspidation of teeth [5, 13]. In our case, the relation between upper and lower right second molars was not ideal, finalizing almost in a tip-to-tip relation. The molar uprighting procedure of the molars could have caused this condition. However, it did not create any occlusal interference and the patient refused to elongate treatment to correct it. Cephalometric superimposition reveals the verticalization of the upper and lower posterior teeth, as well as the extrusion of the upper posterior teeth, enabling the counterclockwise rotation of the occlusal plane (OccPlane-SN: 14°) and the incorporation of the vertical dimension. There was also a

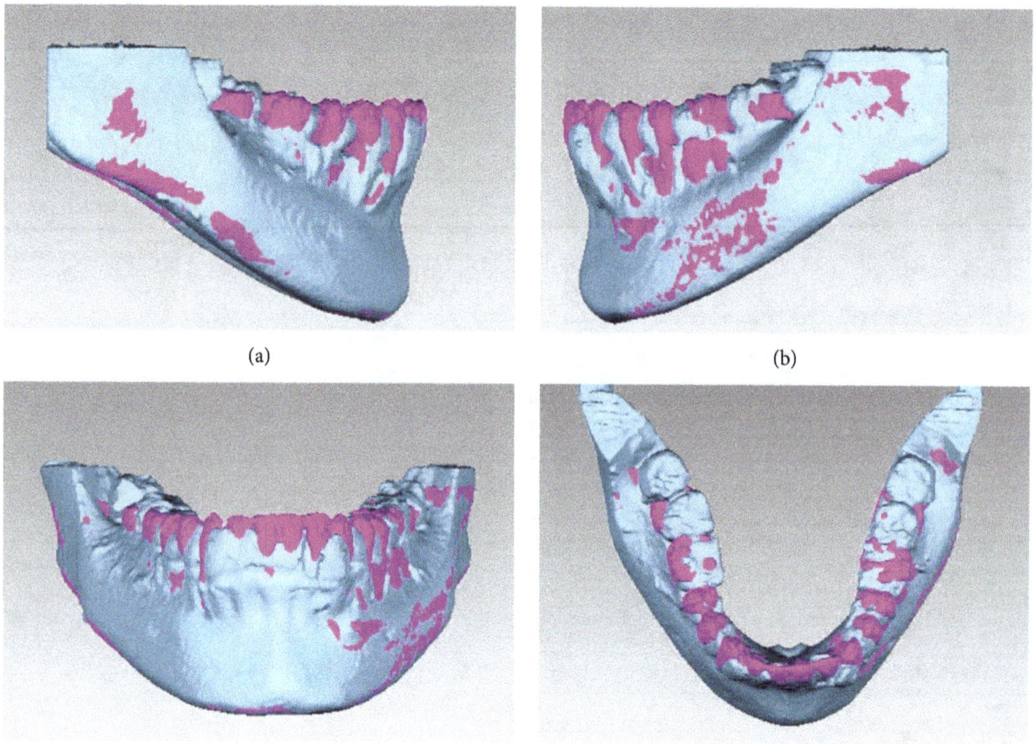

(a) (b) (c) (d)

FIGURE 13: Initial (blue color) and posttreatment (pink color). (a) Right side, (b) left side, (c) frontal view, and (d) occlusal.

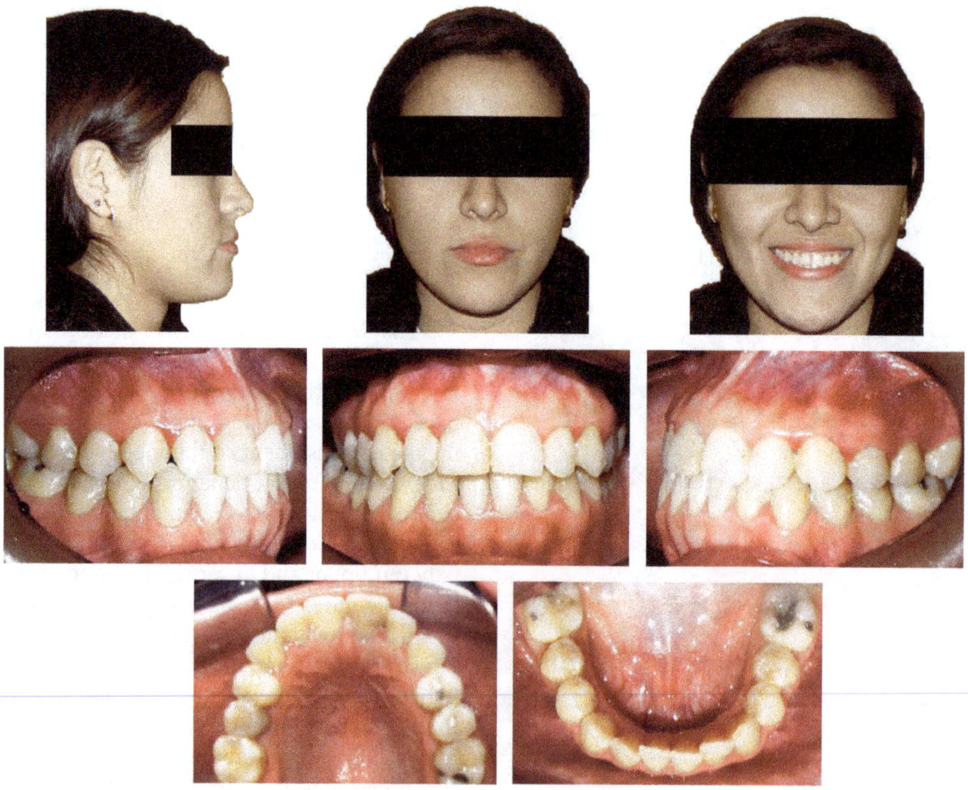

FIGURE 14: Intraoral and extraoral photographs at 3 years posttreatment.

slight clockwise rotation of the mandibular plane (FMA: 23°) and improvement of the patient's facial profile. Although there was greater proclination of the upper incisors (1-NA: 34°) than of the lower incisors (1-NB: 23°), there was no decrease in dental exposure during smile.

Thanks to the current technological management of tomographic information [25, 26], 3D superimposition of the maxilla and mandible was performed. Extrusion of the upper molars and the proclination of the upper incisors are clearly observed (Figure 12), confirming the two-dimensional results provided by the cephalometric overlays. In the 3D superimposition of the lower jaw (Figure 13), almost none extrusion and the slight verticalization of the lower molars are corroborated, as well as the slight proclination of the lower incisors. We can then suggest that the upper and posterior dentoalveolar extrusion was decisive in obtaining the balance between the mandibular ramus and maxillary height as described by previous authors [3, 4, 6, 16].

After extracting the 4 third molars, the patient was fearful of having the supernumerary extracted. The supernumerary tooth had no contact with the neighboring teeth, which was corroborated by the initial 3D segmentation performed on the compromised teeth (Figures 4 and 5). The distance between the supernumerary tooth and the canine and the premolar measured in the tomography were in a range from 0.55 to 1.30 mm, thus it was decided to follow it up during the orthodontic treatment and along periodic control appointments. The patient was alerted of the possible consequences of keeping it and of future extraction need in case the tooth contacted the neighbor teeth during the application of the mechanics or in case of any pathological development, as indicated by previous studies [27]. At the end of the treatment, a CBCT evaluation and segmentation of the supernumerary and its neighboring teeth was performed, corroborating the normal morphology of the teeth and the lack of contact with adjacent teeth (33 and 34) (Figure 10). The patient showed no discomfort in the region during treatment phases.

The MEAW technique was found effective for compensatory treatment of Class III malocclusion [28, 29], although mild discomfort was manifested by the patient at the beginning of treatment due to the presence of the bends and the use of elastics. It is critical that good quality arches are used to support the additional bends to be incorporated. These bends (tip-back, step-up, step-down, tip-forward, and torque) are incorporated into the MEAW arches in each phase of the treatment and the arches made with blue elgiloy wire should be subjected to heat treatment (470°C for approximately 3 minutes). It is vital that the patient be aware of the need to use the intermaxillary elastics since, without them, the MEAW technique will not be effective [5, 8].

Following the San Marcos University protocol, the final radiographs are registered with the brackets in position, in case there is a need to perform any additional dental movement. Three years after the end of treatment, the patient showed an adequate profile, a pleasant smile, and no sign or symptoms of temporomandibular dysfunction. The patient was followed up regularly for 2 years after treatment. Due to moving away, she did not show up during the third year. The use of retention was discontinued and she returned presenting a mild relapse of the lower incisors with a few rotations but, in general, the occlusion showed acceptable stability as described by previous authors who used the MEAW arches [19].

This case shows that, although the limitations imposed by the patient in not accepting surgery nor skeletal anchorage, it was possible to manage her chief complaint and to obtain good results through the knowledge of mechanical concepts and hand skills improving the aesthetics and occlusal conditions.

4. Conclusion

A severe skeletal Class III with a deficiency of posterior vertical dimension in the maxilla had an alternative treatment with the MEAW technique. The objectives were to obtain a counterclockwise rotation of the occlusal plane by extruding the upper molars and verticalizing the lower teeth, creating an acceptable occlusion along with a clockwise rotation of the lower jaw. Thus, the lower facial third and the patient's overall profile were improved. This MEAW technique requires some bending skills and orthodontic training, as well as an adequate compliance of the patient in the use of the intermaxillary elastics, but the results that can be obtained, in some cases, justify the attempt to overcome these difficulties.

Acknowledgments

"This article was supported in part by the *Fundação de Amparo à Pesquisa do Estado do Rio deJaneiro – FAPERJ*".

References

[1] N. R. Burns, D. R. Musich, C. Martin, T. Razmus, E. Gunel, and P. Ngan, "Class III camouflage treatment: What are the limits?," *American journal of orthodontics and dentofacial orthopedics*, vol. 137, no. 1, pp. 9.e1–9.e13, 2010.

[2] S. Sato, H. Sakai, T. Sugishita, A. Matsumoto, and Y. Kubota Susuki, "Developmental alteration of the form of denture frame in skeletal class III maloclusion and pits significance in orthodontic diagnosis and treatment," *MEAW*, vol. 1, pp. 33–46, 1994.

[3] A. Shirasu, E. Midori, and S. Sato, "Orthodontic reconstruction of occlusion in class III malocclusion with low mandibular plane angle," *The Bulletin of the Kanagawa Dental College*, vol. 35, no. 1, pp. 79–86, 2007.

[4] S. Sato and Y. Suzuki, "Relationship between the development of skeletal mesio-occlusion and posterior tooth-to-denture base discrepancy–its significance in the orthodontic reconstruction of skeletal Class III malocclusion," *Nihon Kyosei Shika Gakkai Zasshi= The Journal of Japan Orthodontic Society*, vol. 47, no. 4, pp. 796–810, 1988.

[5] S. Sato, S. Akimoto, A. Matsumoto, A. Shirasu, and Y. Junzo, "Manual for the Clinical Application of MEAW Technique," in *Bulletin Kanagawa Dental College*, Autum, 2001.

[6] S. Okuhashi, C. Basili, E. Midori et al., "Three-dimensional computer tomographic analysis of the influence of the cant of the occlusal plane in different craniofacial morphology,"

The Bulletin of the Kanagawa Dental College, vol. 39, no. 2, pp. 89–99, 2011.

[7] S. Kim, K. Kim, H. Yu, and H. Baik, "Dentoalveolar compensation according to skeletal discrepancy and overjet in skeletal Class III patients," *American Journal of Orthodontics and Dentofacial Orthopedics*, vol. 145, no. 3, pp. 317–324, 2014.

[8] Y. H. Kim, "Anterior open bite and its treatment with multiloop edgewise archwire," *The Angle Orthodontist*, vol. 57, pp. 290–321, 1987.

[9] Y. H. Kim, "A study of the regional load deflection rate of MEAW," *The Angle Orthodontist*, vol. 71, no. 2, pp. 103–109, 2001.

[10] J. L. Ackerman, T. Nguyen, and W. R. Proffit, "The decision-making process in orthodontics," in *Orthodontics, Current Principles, and Techniques*, W. L. Graber, R. L. Vanarsdall, and K. W. Vig, Eds., pp. 44-45, Mosbly Elservier, Philadelphia, 5th edition, 2012.

[11] J. H. Park and R. Bullen, "Camouflage treatment of skeletal Class III malocclusion with conventional orthodontic therapy," *American Journal of Orthodontics and Dentofacial Orthopedics*, vol. 151, no. 4, pp. 804–811, 2017.

[12] H. J. De Clerck, M. A. Cornelis, L. H. Cevidanes, G. C. Heymann, and C. J. F. Tulloch, "Orthopedic traction of the maxilla with miniplates: a new perspective for treatment of midface deficiency," *Journal of Oral and Maxillofacial Surgery*, vol. 67, no. 10, pp. 2123–2129, 2009.

[13] W. E. Roberts, R. F. Viecilli, C. Chang, T. R. Katona, and N. H. Paydar, "Biology of biomechanics: finite element analysis of a statically determinate system to rotate the occlusal plane for correction of a skeletal class III open-bite malocclusion," *American Journal of Orthodontics and Dentofacial Orthopedics*, vol. 148, no. 6, pp. 943–955, 2015.

[14] L. L. Y. Tseng, C. H. Chang, and W. E. Roberts, "Diagnosis and conservative treatment of skeletal class III malocclusion with anterior crossbite and asymmetric maxillary crowding," *American Journal of Orthodontics and Dentofacial Orthopedics*, vol. 149, no. 4, pp. 555–566, 2016.

[15] Y. H. Kim, "Treatment of severe openbite malocclusions without surgical intervention," in *Growth modifications: what works, what doesn't, and why, Craniofacial Growth Series, vol. 35, An Arbor: Center for Human Growth and Development*, J. A. Mc Namara Jr., Ed., pp. 193–212, The University of Michigan, 1999.

[16] Y. H. Kim, "Treatment of anterior openbite and deep overbite malocclusions with the multiloop edgewise archwire (MEAW) therapy," in *The enigma of the Vertical Dimension. Craniofacial Growth and Development*, J. A. Mc Namara Jr., Ed., pp. 175–202, The University of Michigan, 2000.

[17] Y. H. Kim, "Overbite depth indicator with particular reference to anterior open-bite," *American Journal of Orthodontics*, vol. 65, no. 6, pp. 586–611, 1974.

[18] Y. H. Kim and J. J. Vietas, "Anteroposterior dysplasia indicator: an adjunct to cephalometric differential diagnosis," *American Journal of Orthodontics*, vol. 73, no. 6, pp. 619–633, 1978.

[19] Y. H. Kim, U. K. Han, D. D. Lim, and M. L. Serraon, "Stability of anterior openbite correction with multiloop edgewise archwire therapy: a cephalometric follow-up study," *American Journal of Orthodontics and Dentofacial Orthopedics*, vol. 118, no. 1, pp. 43–54, 2000.

[20] S. H. Baek, S. J. Shin, S. J. Ahn, and Y. Chang, "Initial effect of multiloop edgewise archwire on the mandibular dentition in class III malocclusion subjects. A three-dimensional finite element study," *The European Journal of Orthodontics*, vol. 30, no. 1, pp. 10–15, 2008.

[21] G. L. U. Ribeiro, S. Regis, T. M. A. Cunha, M. A. Sabatoski, O. Guariza-Filho, and O. M. Tanaka, "Multiloop edgewise archwire in the treatment of a patient with an anterior open bite and a long face," *American Journal of Orthodontics and Dentofacial Orthopedics*, vol. 138, no. 1, pp. 89–95, 2010.

[22] Z. Yang, Y. Ding, and X. Feng, "Developing skeletal class III malocclusion treated nonsurgically with a combination of a protraction facemask and a multiloop edgewise archwire," *American Journal of Orthodontics and Dentofacial Orthopedics*, vol. 140, no. 2, pp. 245–255, 2011.

[23] S. He, J. Gao, P. Wamalwa, Y. Wang, S. Zou, and S. Chen, "Camouflage treatment of skeletal class III malocclusion with multiloop edgewise arch wire and modified class III elastics by maxillary mini-implant anchorage," *The Angle Orthodontist*, vol. 83, no. 4, pp. 630–640, 2013.

[24] Y. Jing, X. Han, Y. Guo, J. Li, and D. Bai, "Nonsurgical correction of a class III malocclusion in an adult by miniscrew-assisted mandibular dentition distalization," *American Journal of Orthodontics and Dentofacial Orthopedics*, vol. 143, no. 6, pp. 877–887, 2013.

[25] A. C. de Oliveira Ruellas, L. T. Huanca Ghislanzoni, M. R. Gomes et al., "Comparison and reproducibility of 2 regions of reference for maxillary regional registration with cone-beam computed tomography," *American Journal of Orthodontics and Dentofacial Orthopedics*, vol. 149, no. 4, pp. 533–542, 2016.

[26] A. C. de Oliveira Ruellas, M. S. Yatabe, B. Q. Souki et al., "3D mandibular superimposition: comparison of regions of reference for voxel-based registration," *PLoS One*, vol. 11, no. 6, article e0157625, 2016.

[27] T. Garvey, H. J. Barry, and M. Blake, "Supernumerary teeth - an overview of classification, diagnosis and management," *Journal-Canadian Dental Association*, vol. 65, no. 11, pp. 612–616, 1999.

[28] C. L. Rincon-Ducuara, "Tratamiento de maloclusión de clase III con arco multiloop edgewise arch wire (MEAW) reporte de caso clínico," *CES Odontología*, vol. 31, no. 2, pp. 76–93, 2018.

[29] G. A. Marañon-Vásquez, L. C. Soldevilla, F. A. Tolentino, C. Wilson, and F. L. Romano, "Aesthetic and functional outcomes using a multiloop edgewise archwire for camouflage orthodontic treatment of a severe class III open bite malocclusion," *Journal of Orthodontics*, vol. 44, no. 3, pp. 199–208, 2017.

17

Thermoformed Retainer: An Effective Option for Long-Term Stability

A. Giancotti, P. Mozzicato, and G. Mampieri

Department of Orthodontics, University of Rome "Tor Vergata", Rome, Italy

Correspondence should be addressed to A. Giancotti; giancotti@uniroma2.it

Academic Editor: Anastasios Markopoulos

Introduction. The concept of orthodontic retention is moving toward the idea that teeth will move unless retained indefinitely. However, permanent retention implies permanent supervision, and that is where reality clashes with stability. The cornerstone of Essix permanent retention is the complete delegation of responsibility to the patient. Essix retainers have nothing to adjust, but maximum collaboration of the patient is essential to achieve long-term stability. The purpose of this paper is to show the effectiveness of the thermoplastic appliance as a retainer, using a clinical case with a 10-year follow-up. *Case Report.* A 33-year-old male patient presented with a class II malocclusion division 2 and normal skeletal pattern. According to the patient's desire, a treatment plan was proposed to obtain the aesthetic result of the smile, maintaining the molar and canine class II relationship. The orthodontic therapy was performed by using the Invisalign System. In this case, it was possible to appreciate a posterior occlusal stability after 10 years. *Conclusion.* Currently, among orthodontists, the use of removable plastic devices is gaining popularity thanks to their capability to encapsulate and retain both posterior and anterior teeth. In this article, the technical features of thermoformed retainers will be described and one clinical case with a 10-year follow-up will be presented to emphasize the effectiveness of these retainers.

1. Introduction

In orthodontic treatment, there are some goals, and the stability of the correction achieved is one of the most important ones [1–4]. Retention of orthodontic treatment results and posttreatment stability are challenges for orthodontists. Although several factors affect stability, there are 3 major ones: time for reorganization of gingival and periodontal tissues, unstable position of the teeth after orthodontic treatment, and changes produced by growth [2, 5–8]. Our concerns about the stability of orthodontic treatment still seem to be the same as those expressed by Calvin Case in 1920: "If there is one part of orthodontia more than another that is absolutely indispensable to the success of this specialty and its establishment upon a firm foundation as one of the arts and sciences, it is the permanent retention of regulated teeth.... what does this temporary pleasure and satisfaction to ourselves and our patients amount to, if we find in a few years that the very cases which create in us the greatest pride, are going back to their former malpositions and disharmonies, in spite of everything we have been able to do with retaining appliances." [9]. Vanarsdall and White summed up the problem as follows: "Early in the development of orthodontics, a serious misconception evolved. Dentists and the public were led to believe that orthodontic treatment could result in teeth that were straight for a lifetime." [10]. For this reason, the effect of various diagnostic and treatment factors on occlusal stability in both the short term and the long term has been extensively investigated [2, 4–6, 9, 11–24]. Littlewood et al. failed to establish any reliable guidelines regarding the efficacy of various retention protocols [16]. Gianelly and others have argued that the stability of orthodontic treatment can be improved by preserving a mandibular intercanine width [19–21, 25]. This means that any increase in mandibular intercanine dimension is inherently unstable [31–33]. Along the same lines, Blake and Bibby listed six major criteria for the stability of finished orthodontic cases:

(1) The patient's pretreatment lower arch form should be maintained unaltered as much as possible

(2) The original lower intercanine width should be maintained as much as possible, because expansion of the lower intercanine width leads to the most predictable of orthodontic relapse

(3) Mandibular arch length decreases with time

(4) The most stable position of the lower incisor is its pretreatment position; advancing the lower incisors can seriously compromise stability

(5) Fiberotomy is an effective means of reducing rotational relapse

(6) Lower incisor reproximation can improve long-term posttreatment stability [4]

Little et al. have shown that only 10% of patients have a clinically stable alignment in the long term. In the study conducted at the University of Washington, the authors concluded that orthodontic results are more likely to be unstable than stable, and the only way to ensure ongoing satisfactory alignment after treatment would be to provide retention for life [13]. Also, Vaden et al. have shown that after 15 years following the end of orthodontic treatment, there was a "minimal irregularity" in the occlusal alignment [14]. Only in the study conducted by Dyer et al., researchers have shown that the correction of maxillary crowding was relatively stable in the long term [15]. However, a number of authors agree that long-term stability is closely linked to the type of removable retention appliance [1, 2, 17, 26–28].

The removable retainers show advantages and disadvantages. We know two types of removable devices for posttreatment retention: Hawley-type retainers and thermoplastic retainers. Sauget et al. noted that traditional Hawley retainers allow greater settling and thus an improvement in posterior occlusal contacts, compared to full-coverage thermoplastic retainers [29]. However, this type of retainer requires the patient's compliance, and, in addition, different from expectations, removable retainers require adequate daily cleaning in order to guarantee proper hygiene levels [30]. The major advantage of thermoplastic retainers is aesthetics. Such retainers are clear and almost invisible, so many patients prefer them to conventional Hawley devices. However, like other removable retainers, thermoplastic devices rely on patient compliance. Their material is not as durable as a Hawley type, and more replacements are needed. Finally, thermoplastic retainers do not allow occlusal settling if they are extended back to the molars, often causing anterior open bite [17, 31]. According to literature, the retainer shall be designed as comfortable and easy to wear in order to maintain occlusal stability [1, 2, 17, 26]. For this reason, Sheridan et al. in 1993 described the first invisible device [26]. The Essix appliance is an aesthetic removable plastic device, retained by the anatomy of the teeth. It is practically invisible, rapidly manufactured, and not so expensive [1, 2, 5, 6, 11–17, 26–28]. Thermoplastic retainers are generally made of two classes of material: copolyester type "A" Endure and polypropylene or ethylene copolymer type "C+" Duraforce [17]. The Essix type "A" is obtained from plastic copolyester material, in which a 1 mm thick sheet of plastic (Scheudent type A) is thermically formed on the cast reducing its thickness to 0.65 mm [26, 27]. This type "A" material is generally more aesthetic because of better clarity, although it tends to tear and crack [17, 27]. For this reason, the manufacturers are creating a new generation of thermoplastic materials, including ACE and Duraclear to improve durability, clarity, and retention [17]. Such thermoforming process guarantees the posterior stability of the appliance, providing flexibility for ease of insertion and removal, and does not interfere with speech. Therefore, it is comfortable, aesthetic, and well accepted by patients, who can easily wear the appliance full-time. However, the thermoformed appliances are limited in terms of wear resistance and fitting. A precision fit is essential in any thermoformed application, not only on initial placement but also until the appliance is worn [28]. The fit depends on the adaptation of the retentive gingival undercuts to the contact points: if they are not well defined, the appliance will be too loose; if they are excessive, it will be too tight. An incorrect fit can determine a potential demineralization of enamel and a bite alteration. Moreover, an incorrect fit can cause a loss of occlusal stability as shown by Freitas et al. [2]. In 2001, Sheridan et al. have demonstrated that the full-time use of retainers for an extensive period will cause significant premature occlusal contacts in the posterior teeth and an anterior open bite [1]. According to the "1-to-3" prosthetic concept, when a full-coverage plastic appliance is seated, the thickness of the appliance between the molars inevitably causes a hinge axis interference and thus an anterior open bite [1, 27]. Butler measured the stability of orthodontic results over the first nine months after the delivery of removable retainers. Sixty percent of the full-time patients lost or broke their retainers, as opposed to 13% of the night-only patients [32]. In a study by Lindauer and Shoff, the thermoplastic retainers were as effective as Hawley retainers in maintaining orthodontic correction, and there was an incidence of an anterior open bite in the Essix group [17, 31, 33].

The thermoformed device is a particular transparent retainer that allows better withstanding wear without causing bite alterations. According to Sheridan et al., when the thermoformed plastic is thin, the premature occlusal contacts can be easily avoided. Also, the Essix retainer is comfortable, fit, and aesthetic, thus guaranteeing the long-term stability of the occlusal alignment [2, 17, 31, 32].

In this article, we want to show how the correct characteristics of the thermoformed appliance can guarantee long-term stability. A clinical case with a 10-year follow-up in which retention was performed with an Essix worn only at night will be shown. Moreover, according to literature thanks to the technical and aesthetic characteristics of Essix, greater long-term stability and patient compliance are enhanced [1, 2, 15, 17, 26–28, 31–37].

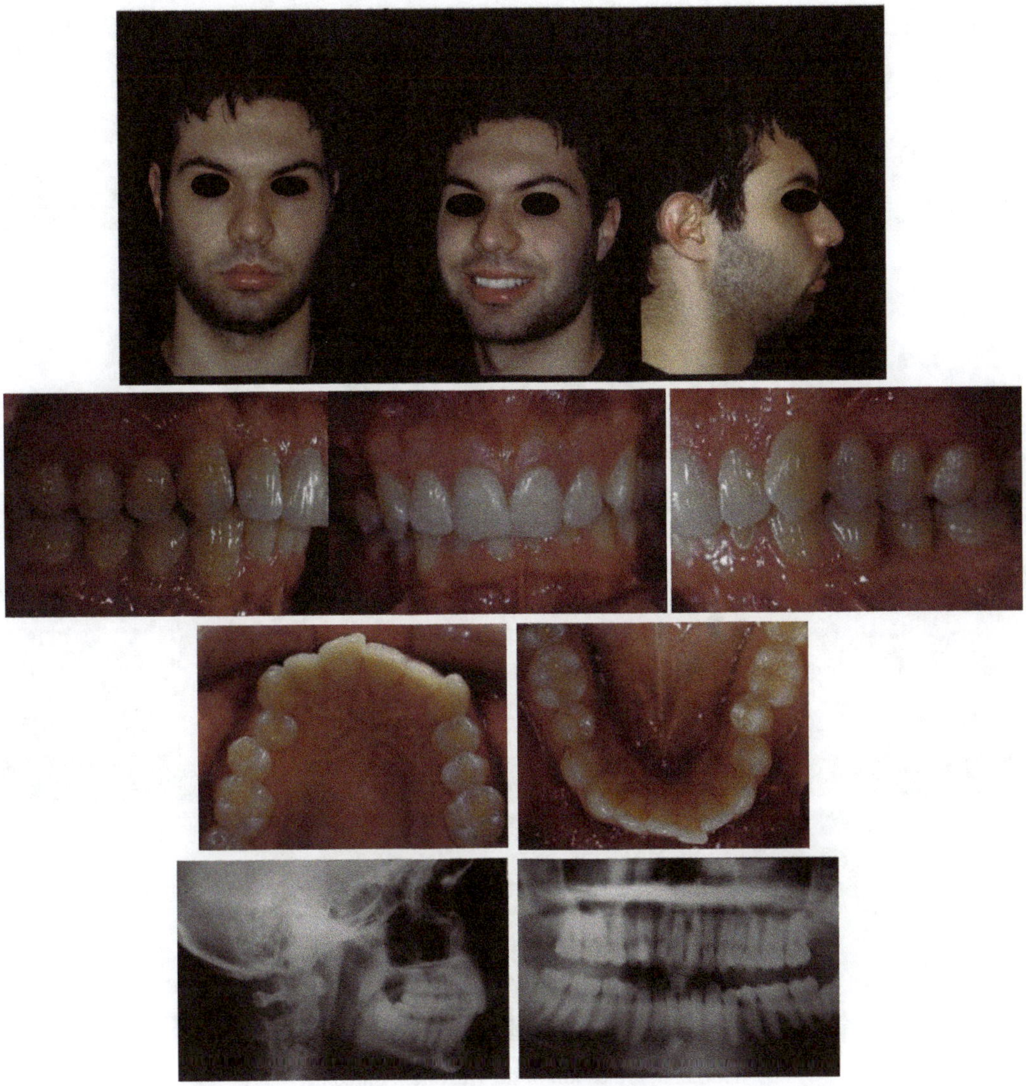

FIGURE 1: Pretreatment records.

2. Case Report

A 33-year-old male patient presented with a class II malocclusion division 2 and normal skeletal pattern. Intraoral examination showed moderate crowding both in the upper arch and in the lower arch. He presented a severe dental and skeletal deep bite (Figure 1). In order to obtain the complete correction of the malocclusion, an extractive treatment plan had been suggested. More precisely, the extraction of the first upper premolars had been proposed. However, the patient refused such therapeutic option by choosing a cosmetic treatment. So, in order to obtain an exclusively aesthetic result, the objectives of the orthodontic treatment were

(i) to improve the overbite

(ii) to align and level both arches

According to the patient's desire, a treatment plan was proposed to obtain the aesthetic result of the smile, maintaining the molar and canine class II relationship (Figure 2). The orthodontic therapy was performed using the Clear Aligners System. The Clincheck∗ treatment plan projection anticipated satisfactory resolution of dental anomalies, correction of the overbite, and alignment of the upper and lower anterior teeth (Figure 3). Twenty aligners were planned for the upper arch, and seventeen for the lower arch. The patient was seen every four to six weeks (two to four aligners) to check aligner fit, attachment stability, and cooperation. The initial phase lasted 10 months. The patient required 7 refinement aligners. After 14 months of treatment, the patient was given clear overlay retainers (Figure 4). In this case, it was possible to see a posterior occlusal stability after 10 years. The patient was monitored every year by means of photographic records, showing a correct fit of the thermoformed device without occlusal plane alteration (Figure 5).

3. Discussion

Orthodontic treatment has several objectives, and stability of the corrections achieved is one of the most important. There is consensus in the orthodontic literature that some occlusal changes will inevitably occur after treatment. It would be a

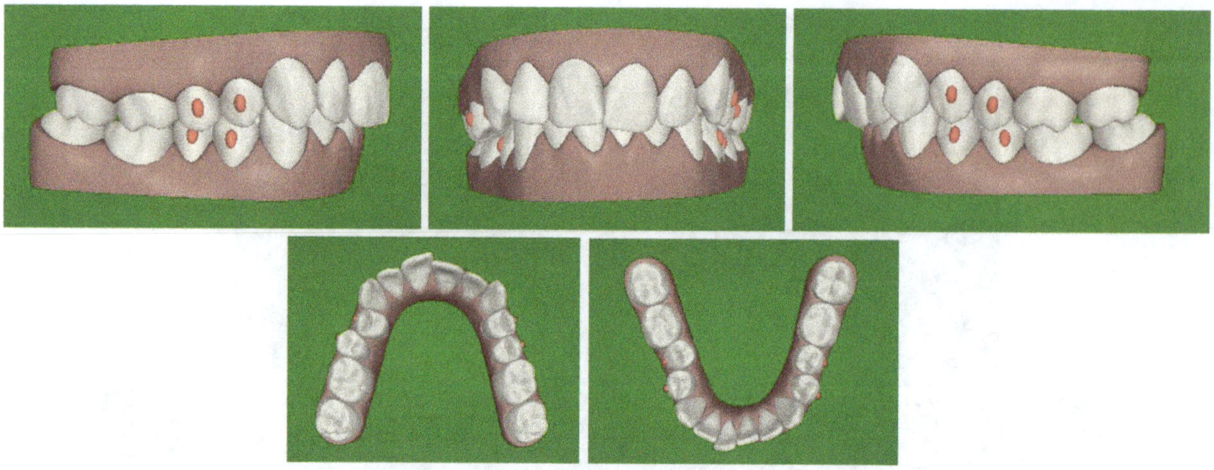

Figure 2: Initial Clincheck.

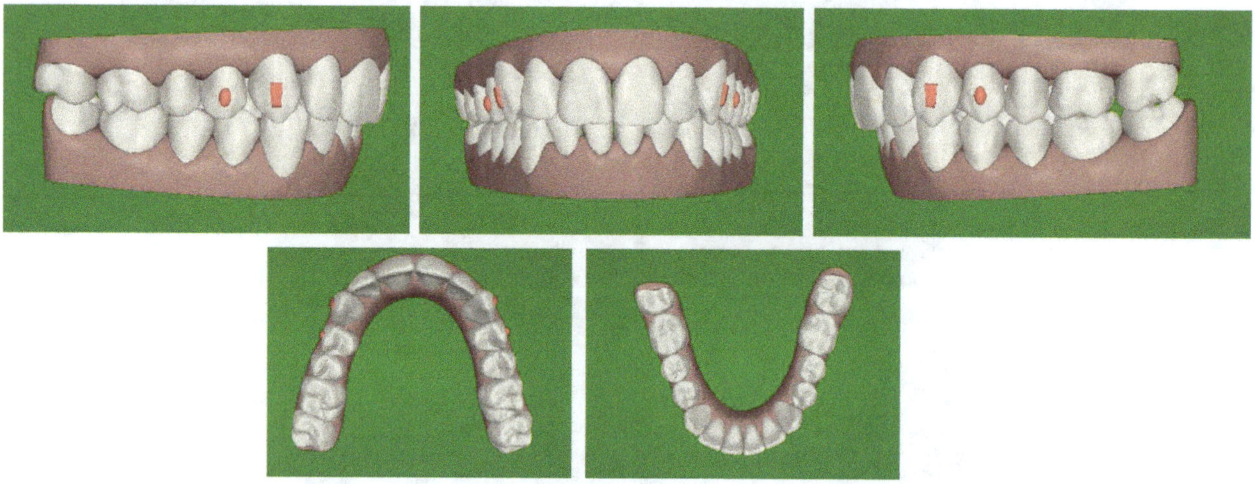

Figure 3: Projection of the treatment outcome.

great benefit to orthodontists to have a detailed prediction of these occlusal changes so that they can be prevented [18, 37, 38]. For this reason, the effects of various diagnostic and treatment factors on occlusal stability in the short and the long term have been extensively investigated [1, 11, 34]. Maintaining the arch form and new position of the teeth after orthodontic treatment is a tedious problem for orthodontists. Both fixed and removable appliances can be used for retention [17, 18, 32, 33, 39].

Essix removable retainers are gaining popularity among orthodontists, thanks to their ability to encapsulate and retain both posterior and anterior teeth. Currently, some clinicians prefer to use the clear removable device called Essix to guarantee the long-term tooth stability after the orthodontic treatment [2, 17, 26, 27, 31, 33]. Because of their minimal thickness and "U"-shaped configuration, transarch stability can sometimes be inadequate.

The removable clear device may raise some problems such as posterior instability and improper long-term fit [17, 26, 28, 33, 35]. However, orthodontists prefer to use the removable retainer because this kind of device has several advantages such as the low cost of fabrication, the minimal bulk and thickness, the durability, and the ease of clearing. [17, 26, 27]

Essix thermoplastic retainers change the rules of permanent retention, because they are thin, but stronger. However, this kind of retainer shows further disadvantages, besides the posterior instability and improper long-term fit: the presence of occlusal contacts and an anterior or lateral open bite [1, 17, 31, 39]. In a study by Littlewood et al., the authors evaluate the long-term stability of 56 patients by randomly assigning Essix and Hawley retainers [16]. The thermoplastic retainers were as effective as the Hawley retainers in maintaining orthodontic correction, but there was an incidence of an anterior open bite in the Essix group. In a prospective RTC, Profitt et al. and Hichens et al. found, after 6 months, that less incisor irregularity occurred in the group of Essix retainers; however, this group had an anterior open bite [35, 36]. In order to reduce the posterior occlusal precontacts, Rinchuse et al. suggest the use of a 3-3 Essix retainer [17]. According to literature, to guarantee long-term stability of occlusal alignment, uttermost cooperation on behalf of the patient is crucial [1, 2, 6, 13–15, 26, 28, 29, 31, 32, 36, 39, 40]. The retainer device must be comfortable,

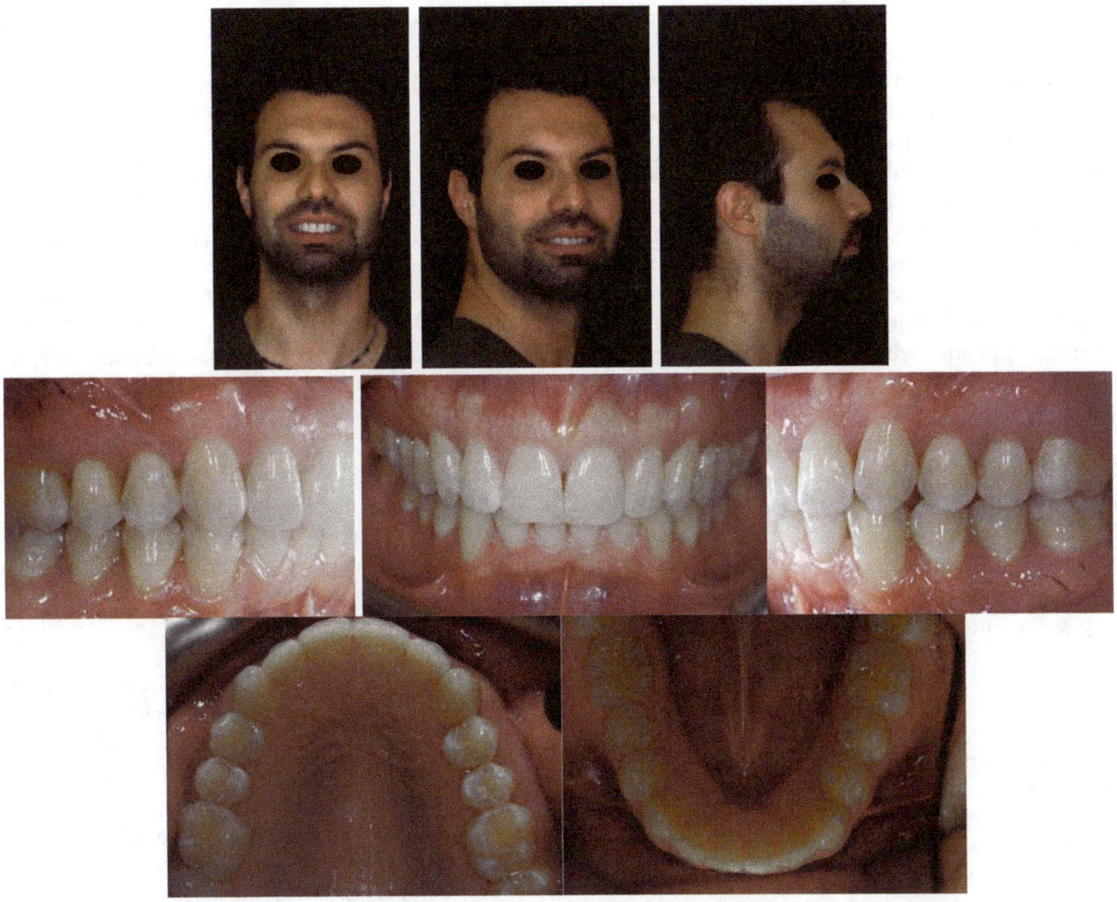

FIGURE 4: Posttreatment records.

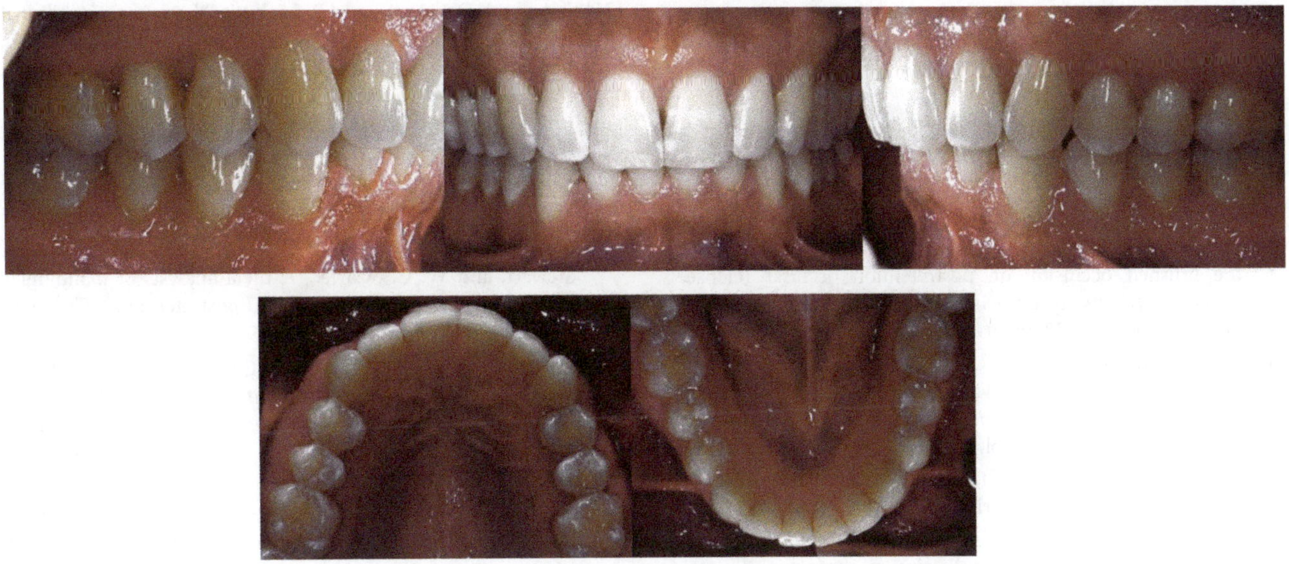

FIGURE 5: Ten-year follow-up.

aesthetic, and easy to wear. Only with the above characteristics, full patient compliance is achieved. For these reasons, patients willingly accept to wear a thermoformed appliance for a long time, showing good occlusal stability after 10 years.

4. Conclusion

Essix retainers have been proven quite versatile. Their flexibility and positioner effect make them an alternative to spring retainers in correcting minor tooth movements [26, 27].

Orthodontists' concept of retention is moving toward the idea that teeth will move unless retained indefinitely. However, permanent retention implies permanent supervision, and that is where reality clashes with stability [2, 10, 26].

We believe that it is prudent to establish a retention protocol based on the needs and concerns of each individual patient. Therefore, patient cooperation is of the utmost importance [6, 26]. Clinicians prefer to use the clear removable device called Essix to guarantee the long-term tooth stability after the orthodontic treatment [2, 17, 26, 27, 31, 33]. According to literature, in our clinical case, we opted to use a thermoformed appliance with reduced thickness to allow a perfect fit reducing the risk of a posterior open bite [2, 17, 31, 32]. The thermoplastic retainer is comfortable, aesthetic, and easy to wear, and with the above characteristics, full patient compliance can be achieved for a long time. In conclusion, it can be said that thanks to its technical properties, Essix is the effective option to use as a postorthodontic treatment retainer. Its minimum thickness and its ideal fit reduce the risk of a lateral and anterior open bite even after 10 years of follow-up as seen in this case report.

References

[1] J. J. Sheridan, P. Armbruster, E. Moskowitz, and P. Nguyen, "Avoiding demineralization and bite alteration from full-coverage plastic appliances," *Journal of Clinical Orthodontics*, vol. 35, pp. 444–448, 2001.

[2] K. M. Feritas, W. J. Guirro, D. S. De Feritas, M. R. De Feritas, and G. Janson, "Relapse of anterior crowding 3 and 33 years postretention," *American Journal of Orthodontics and Dentofacial Orthopedics*, vol. 152, no. 6, pp. 798–810, 2017.

[3] J. Yavari, M. K. Shrout, C. M. Russell, A. J. Hass, and E. H. Hamilton, "Relapse in Angle class II division 1 malocclusion treated by tandem mechanics without extraction of permanent teeth: a retrospective analysis," *American Journal of Orthodontics*, vol. 118, pp. 34–42, 2000.

[4] M. Blake and K. Bibby, "Retention and stability: a review of literature," *American Journal of Orthodontics*, vol. 114, pp. 299–306, 1998.

[5] K. M. Feritas, G. Janson, M. R. De Feritas, A. Pinzan, J. F. Henriques, and C. R. Pinzan-Vercelino, "Influece of the quality of the finished occlusion on postretention occlusal relapse," *American Journal of Orthodontics and Dentofacial Orthopedics*, vol. 132, no. 428, pp. 9–14, 2007.

[6] A. De la Cruz, P. Sampson, R. M. Little, J. Artur, and P. A. Shapiro, "Long-term chances in arch form after orthodontic treatment and retention," *American Journal of Orthodontics and Dentofacial Orthopedics*, vol. 107, pp. 518–530, 1995.

[7] N. Topouzelis and A. Diamantidou, "Orthodontic treatment in patients with reduced periodontium," *Hellenic Orthodontic Review*, vol. 6, pp. 175–195, 2003.

[8] B. U. Zachrisson, "Clinical implications of recent orthodontic-periodontic research findings," *Seminars in Orthodontics*, vol. 2, no. 1, pp. 4–12, 1996.

[9] C. S. Case, "Principles of retention in orthodontia," *International Journal of Orthodontia and Oral Surgery (1919)*, vol. 6, no. 11, pp. 627–658, 1920.

[10] R. L. Vanarsdall and R. P. White Jr., "Relapse and retention: professional and public attitudes," *American Journal of Orthodontics*, vol. 98, p. 184, 1990.

[11] P. M. Sinclair and R. M. Little, "Maturation of untreated normal occlusions," *American Journal of Orthodontics*, vol. 83, no. 2, pp. 114–123, 1983.

[12] R. M. Little, "Stability and relapse of dental arch alignment," *British Journal of Orthodontics*, vol. 17, pp. 235–241, 2019.

[13] R. M. Little, R. A. Riedel, and J. Artur, "An evaluation of changes in mandibular anterior alignment from 10 to 20 years postretention," *American Journal of Orthodontics and Dentofacial Orthopedics*, vol. 93, no. 5, pp. 423–428, 1988.

[14] J. L. Vaden, E. F. Harris, and R. L. Gardner, "Relapse revisited," *American Journal of Orthodontics and Dentofacial Orthopedics*, vol. 111, no. 5, pp. 543–553, 1997.

[15] K. C. Dyer, J. L. Vaden, and E. F. Harris, "Relapse revisited-again," *American Journal of Orthodontics and Dentofacial Orthopedics*, vol. 142, no. 2, pp. 221–227, 2012.

[16] S. J. Littlewood, D. T. Millet, B. Doubleday, D. R. Bearn, and H. V. Worthington, "Retention procedures for stabilizing tooth position after treatment with orthodontic braces," *Cochrane Database of Systematic Reviews*, vol. 25, article CD002283, 2006.

[17] D. J. Rinchuse, P. G. Miles, and J. J. Sheridan, "Orthodontic retention and stability: a clinical perspective," *Journal of Clinical Orthodontics*, vol. 61, pp. 125–132, 2007.

[18] C. A. Hawley, "A removable retainer," *Dental Cosmos*, vol. 61, pp. 449–554, 1919.

[19] A. A. Gianelly, "Rapid palatal expansion in the absence of cross-bite: added value?," *American Journal of Orthodontics*, vol. 124, pp. 362–365, 2003.

[20] A. Gianelly, "Evidence-based therapy: an orthodontic dilemma," *American Journal of Orthodontics*, vol. 129, pp. 596–598, 2006.

[21] J. Artur, J. D. GArolo, and R. M. Little, "Long-term stability of mandibular incisors following successful treatment of class II, division, malocclusion," *The Angle Orthodontist*, vol. 66, pp. 229–238, 1996.

[22] P. E. Rossouw, C. B. Preston, D. J. Lombard, and J. W. Truter, "A longitudinal evaluation of the anterior border of the dentition," *American Journal of Orthodontics*, vol. 104, pp. 146–152, 1993.

[23] S. P. Burke, A. M. Silvera, L. J. Goldsmith, J. M. Yancey, A. Van Stewart, and W. C. SCarfe, "A meta-analysis of mandibular intercanine width in treatment and postretention," *The Angle Orthodontist*, vol. 68, pp. 53–60, 1998.

[24] E. A. Al Yami, A. M. Kuijpers-Jagtman, and M. A. van't Hof, "Stability of orthodontic treatment outcome: follow-up until 10 years postretention," *American Journal of Orthodontics and Dentofacial Orthopedics*, vol. 115, no. 3, pp. 300–304, 1999.

[25] R. H. W. Strang, "The fallacy of denture expansion as a treatment procedure," *The Angle Orthodontist*, vol. 19, pp. 12–22, 1949.

[26] J. J. Sheridan, W. Ledoux, and R. McMinn, "Essix retainers: fabrication and supervision for permanent retention," *Journal of Clinical Orthodontics*, vol. 27, no. 1, pp. 37–45, 1993.

[27] M. Laboda, *The effect of Essix appliances on anterior open-bite*, Thesis, LSU Department of Orthodontics, Louisiana State University, USA, 1995.

[28] K. Hilliard and J. J. Sheridan, "Adjusting Essix appliances at

chairside," *Journal of Clinical Orthodontics*, vol. 34, no. 4, pp. 236–238, 2000.

[29] E. Sauget, D. A. Covell Jr., R. P. Boero, and W. S. Lieber, "Comparison of occlusal contacts with use of Hawley and clear overlay retainers," *The Angle Orthodontist*, vol. 67, pp. 223–230, 1997.

[30] D. Knezovic Zlataric, A. Celebic, and M. Valentic-Peruzovic, "The effect of removable partial dentures on periodontal health of abutment and non-abutment teeth," *Journal of Periodontology*, vol. 73, no. 2, pp. 137–144, 2002.

[31] D. J. Rinchuse and D. J. Rinchuse, "Active tooth movement with the Essix appliance," *Journal of Clinical Orthodontics*, vol. 31, pp. 109–112, 1997.

[32] J. Butler, *Assessment of orthodontic stability using an alternative Hawley retainer regimen of "night-time" only wear*, Thesis, Louisiana State University, New Orleans, 2002.

[33] S. J. Lindauer and R. C. Shoff, "Comparison of Essix and Hawley retainers," *Journal of Clinical Orthodontics*, vol. 32, no. 2, pp. 95–97, 1998.

[34] F. Gunay and A. Alpez Oz, "Clinical effectiveness of 2 orthodontic retainer wires on mandibular arch retention," *American Journal of Orthodontics and Dentofacial Orthopedics*, vol. 153, no. 2, pp. 232–238, 2018.

[35] W. R. Profitt, H. W. Fieldes Jr., and D. M. Sarver, *Contemporary orthodontics*, Elsevier, St. Louis, 4Th edition, 2014.

[36] L. P. Y. Hichens, S. Hollinghurst, P. Ewings, and A. C. Williams, "An RTC comparing the cost-effectiveness between Hawley and vacuum-formed retainers (abstr.)," *Journal of Orthodontics*, vol. 33, article 138, 2006.

[37] A. A. Shah, "Postretention changes in mandibular crowding: a review of the literature," *American Journal of Orthodontics and Dentofacial Orthopedics*, vol. 124, no. 3, pp. 298–308, 2003.

[38] J. Artur, A. T. Spadafora, and P. A. Shapiro, "A 3-year follow-up study of various types of orthodontic canine-to-canine retainers," *European Journal of Orthodontics*, vol. 19, pp. 501–509, 1997.

[39] J. J. Sheridan, R. McMinn, and W. LeDoux, "Essix thermosealed appliances: various orthodontic uses," *Journal of Clinical Orthodontics*, vol. 29, no. 2, pp. 108–113, 1995.

[40] E. M. Moskowitz and C. Kaner, "Predictable retention for the periodontally compromised patient," *Journal of Clinical Orthodontics*, vol. 38, pp. 14–16, 2004.

18

Correction of a Class III Malocclusion with a Functional Shift and Severe Crowding

Yahya A. Alogaibi,[1,2] **Ahmad A. Al-Fraidi**,[2] **Manar K. Alhajrasi**,[3] **and Ali A. Hassan**[4,5]

[1]*Bisha Dental Center, Ministry of Health, P.O. Box 418, Bisha 61922, Saudi Arabia*
[2]*Department of Orthodontic, King Fahad Hospital, Specialized Dental Center, Madina, Saudi Arabia*
[3]*Department of Orthodontic, North Jeddah Specialty Dental Center, MOH, Jeddah, Saudi Arabia*
[4]*Alfarabi Private College, Jeddah, Western Region, Saudi Arabia*
[5]*Department of Orthodontics, Faculty of Dentistry, King Abdulaziz University, P.O. Box 80209, Jeddah 21589, Saudi Arabia*

Correspondence should be addressed to Yahya A. Alogaibi; y1010@hotmail.com

Academic Editor: Alberto Delbem

A forward functional shift of the mandible is a significant problem that can cause both functional and aesthetic complications for many patients. This shift usually occurs in growing patients, and it is unusual to see in adult patients. This case report shows an adult patient with a forwarding functional shift that caused both anterior and posterior crossbites with a pseudo class III dental and skeletal relationship. The patient also showed severe upper arch crowding with blocked-out canines and mild crowding in the lower arch. The treatment of this patient involved extraction of the upper right and left first premolars and the lower right first premolar, followed by opening of the bite to relieve the neuromuscular reflex of the forward protrusion of the mandible during centric occlusion and to correct both the anterior and posterior crossbites. Extraction spaces were closed using class III elastics and elastomeric chains. At the end of the treatment, good functional and aesthetic results were obtained after the elimination of the forward functional shift.

1. Introduction

Class III malocclusions can be classified into three main types: pseudo class III, dental class III, and skeletal class III malocclusions. The first to suggest such classification was Tweed who, in 1966, categorized class III malocclusions into two categories: skeletal or pseudo class III [1]. The pseudo class III malocclusion was described as forward displacement of the mandible during closure accompanied by an anterior crossbite [2].

Skeletal class III malocclusions, on the other hand, have many characteristic features that may include some or all of these features: deficiency in the midface, upward and forward rotation of the mandible, prominence of the lower lip, and protruded mandible [3, 4]. The main difference between pseudo and skeletal class III malocclusions is the ability of the pseudo type to retrude the mandible in the class I relation, showing a normal appearance of the mandible without any obvious protrusion. Also, it can be diagnosed by observing the forward functional shift of the mandible during closure from the point of initial contact with the teeth, up to complete centric occlusion [5]. This is why it is sometimes called a forward functional shift as it only occurs during function (i.e., biting in occlusion) and not during rest. In most cases, these patients exhibit anterior crossbites in two or more incisors [6].

Treatment of these cases requires the correction of the neuromuscular reflex that causes this shift. This is usually done by either anterior or posterior bite-opening devices, which allow the mandible to assume its normal functional position without any forward shift [7, 8].

However, it is unusual to find this forward functional

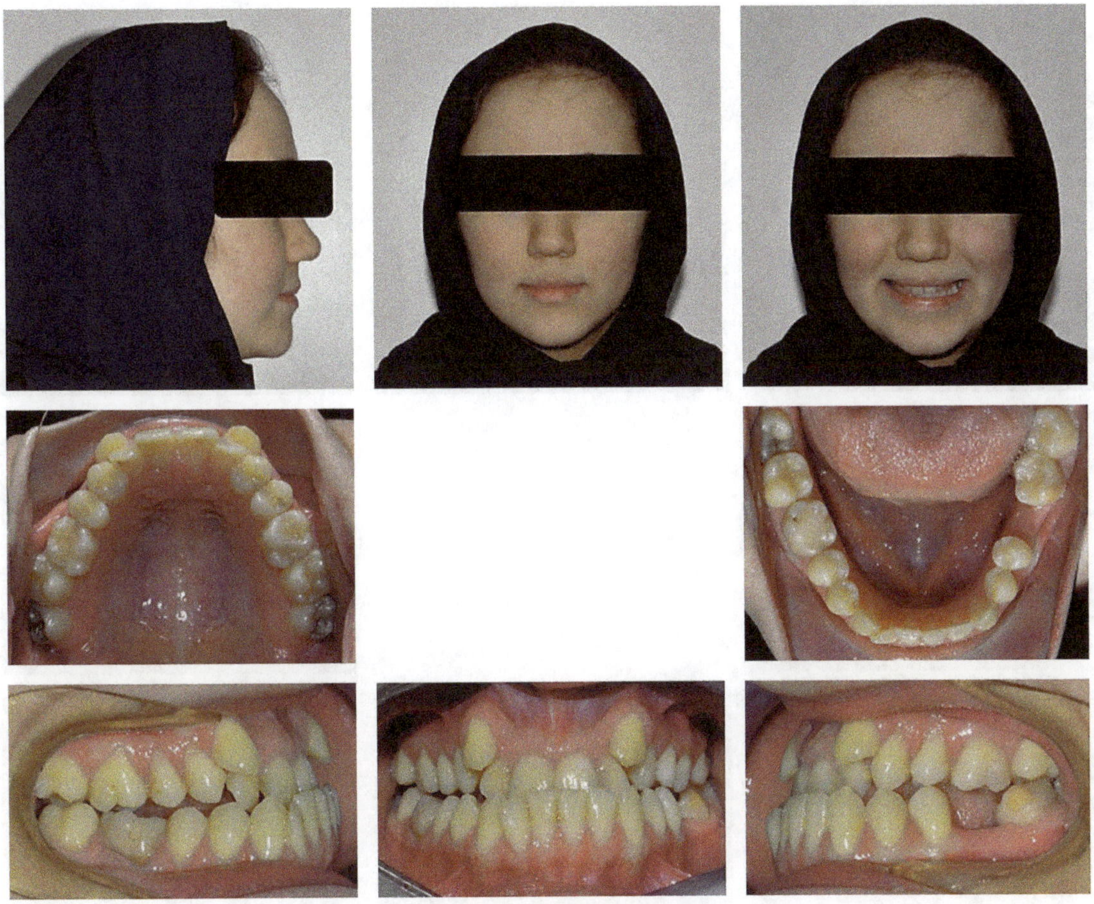

(a) Intraoral photographs in centric occlusion

Figure 1: Continued.

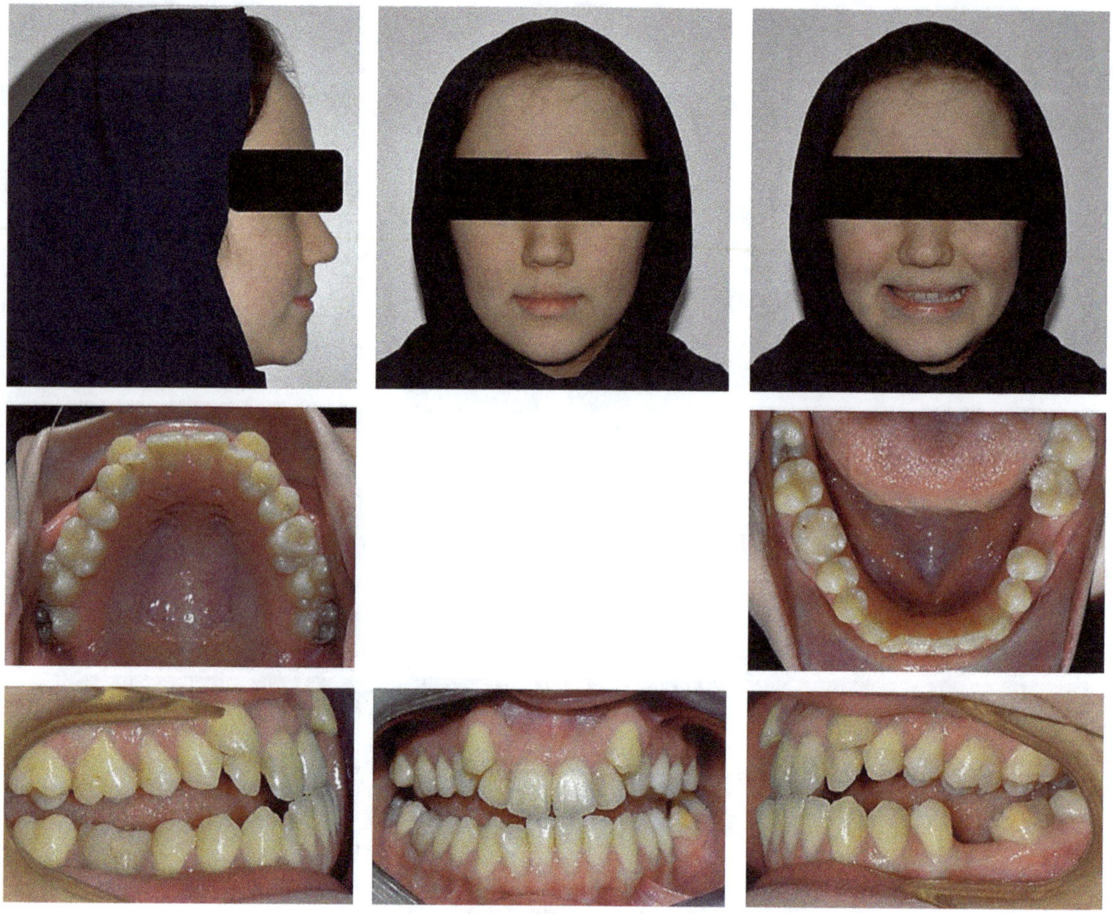

(b) Intraoral photographs in centric relation

FIGURE 1: Pretreatment extraoral and intraoral photographs of the patient.

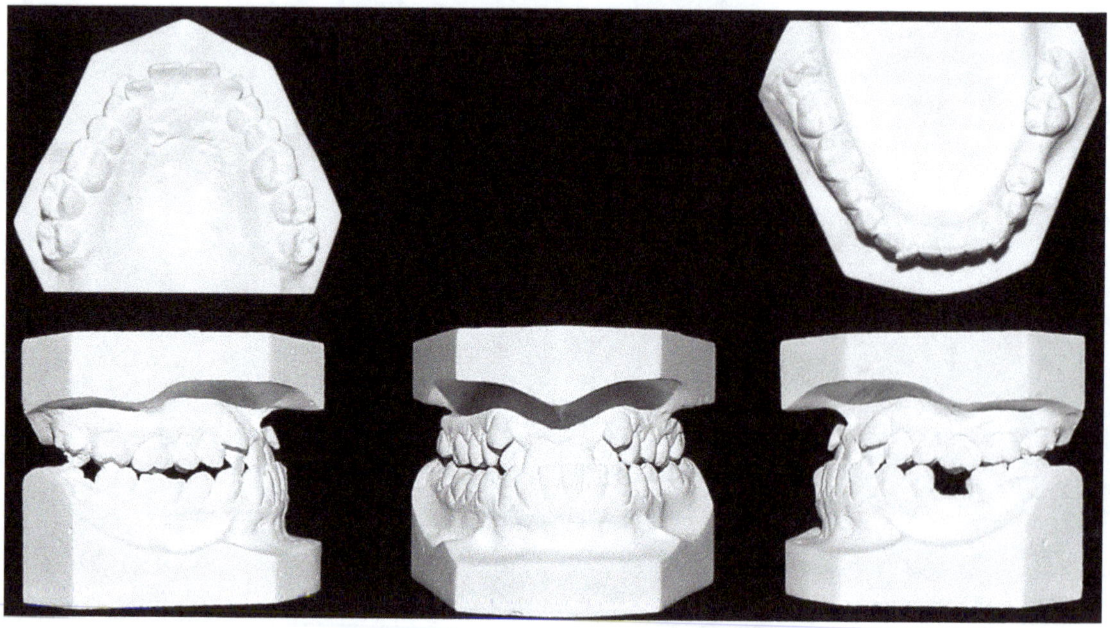

FIGURE 2: Pretreatment models.

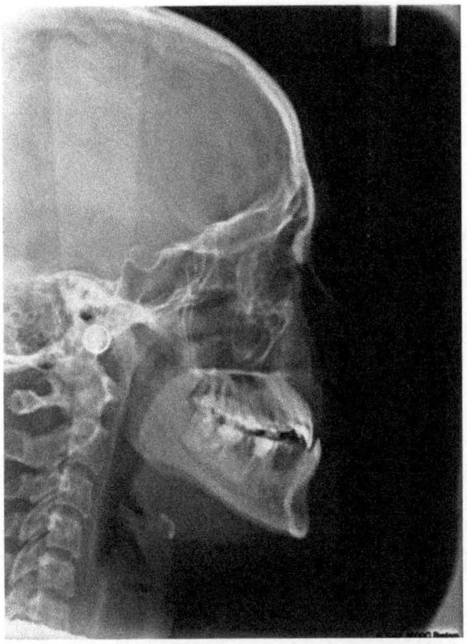

(a) Cephalometric radiograph in centric occlusion

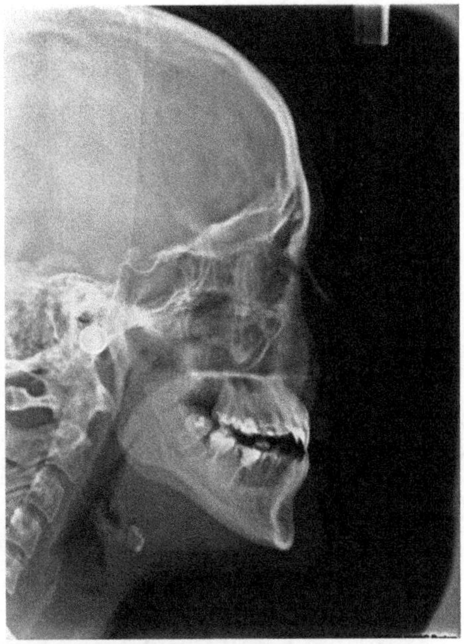

(b) Cephalometric radiograph in centric relation

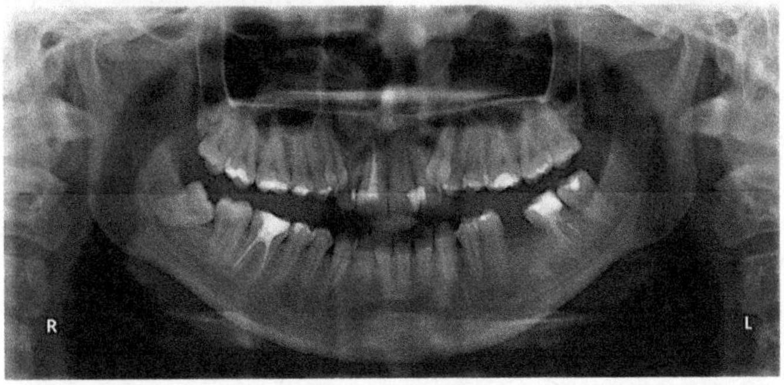

(c) Panoramic radiograph

Figure 3. Pretreatment cephalometric and panoramic radiographs

shift in adult patients as this problem usually progresses to a skeletal problem due to the effects of muscles on the growth of the mandible [2, 9, 10].

This case report describes an unusual case of an adult patient with a pseudo class III malocclusion that manifested as a forward functional shift during centric occlusion combined with retroclined upper incisors and severe upper anterior crowding.

2. Diagnosis and Treatment Planning

A 21-year-old female patient was referred to the orthodontic department with a chief complaint of inability to bite properly on her teeth. No significant problems were found in her medical history. Her dental history, on the other hand, showed a history of extraction of the lower left 1st molar and multiple restorations. Extraoral examination revealed a mesocephalic facial type, straight facial profile, and competent lips with a fairly symmetrical and well-proportioned face. Intraoral findings showed severe crowding in the upper arch that caused both upper canines to be blocked out, an anterior crossbite that included all of the upper incisors with a -3 mm reverse overjet, and a 1 mm shift to the left side in the upper midline. A posterior crossbite with cusp-to-cusp occlusion was also seen with a molar (class III) on the right side and the absence of the lower 1st molar on the left side. The lower arch showed a very mild degree of crowding and mesioangular impaction of the lower right third molar. However, when the patient assumed the rest position of the mandible, an edge-to-edge bite was obtained with a class I molar relation, which strongly suggests a forward functional shift of the mandible. Smile analysis showed an asymmetrical soft tissue smile with a flattened smile arc. No gingival tissues were exposed during smiling (low lip line), and no canting of the occlusal plane or buccal corridor was shown upon smiling. The thin periodontium was also noted (also called the washboard effect), which increases the risk of gingival recession (Figures 1 and 2).

Cephalometric analysis revealed a class III skeletal base and normal inclination of the mandibular plane with normal vertical proportions. However, when another cephalometric analysis was made in the rest position of the mandible (i.e.,

Table 1: Pre- and posttreatment cephalometric measurements.

	Measurement	Mean (±SD)	Saudi norms	Patient Initial	Patient Final
Anteroposterior	SNA (°)	82° (±3.3)	80.8 (±4.06)	77.6	78.8
	SNB (°)	80° (±3.1)	77.5 (±4.48)	79.4	77.4
	ANB (°)	2° (±1.7)	3.7 (±1.5)	-1.8	1.4
	Wits (mm)	$M = -1.17$ (±1.9) $F = -0.10$ (±1.77)	0.13 (±2.47)	-4.9	-1 mm
	Angle of convexity NA-APg (°)	0° (±5.1)	5.01 (±3.05)	11	8
	A-B plane AB:NPg (°)	-4.6° (±3.7)	-4.6° (±3.7)	4	1
Vertical	MP (Go-Gn):SN (°)	32° (±3.5)	35.9 (±5.96)	44	41
	MP (tangent lower border):FH (°)	21.9° (±3.2)	28.5 (±4.79)	41	36
	Pg:NB (mm)	4 (±2)	4 (±2)	0.1	0.1
	Y-axis (SGn:FH)	59.4° (±3.8)	69.6 (±4.2)	71	70
	LAFH (ANS to Gn ÷ N to Gn)	0.57 (±0.02)	0.57 (±0.02)	0.57	0.6
	OP:SN (°)	14° (±4.1)	14° (±4.1)	11.2	12
	OP:FH (°)	9.3° (±3.8)	9.3° (±3.8)	8.1	8.7
Dental	U1 to palatal plane (°)	109° (±6)	109° (±6)	108	112
	U1 to NA (°)	22° (±6.1)	27.3 (±7.5)	16.8	27.5
	U1 to NA (mm)	4 (±1.2)	6.8 (±2.9)	2	3
	L1 to NB (°)	25° (±4.5)	29.34 (±6.98)	31	35.5
	L1 to NB (mm)	4 (±1.5)	7.52 (±2.63)	3	4
	U1 to L1 (°) (Avg. Downs & Steiner)	131.7° (±6.5)	120 (±11.98)	124	113
	U1:APg (mm)	2.7 (±1.8)		1.3	2.5
	L1:APg (mm)	1 (±2)		3.1	3.9
	FMA (°)	25° (16-35)		50	50
	FMIA (°)	65° (60-75)		41	36
	IMPA (°)	90° (85-95)		89	94
Soft tissue	Facial convexity–G Sn Pg′ (°)	12° (±4)		9	9
	Facial angle (FH:N′Pg′) (°)	90-92°		92	91
	Nasolabial angle (°)	90-110°	80.8 (±4.06)	103	103
	Esthetic plane (E-line)—upper lip	-4 mm	77.5 (±4.48)	-2	-3
	Esthetic plane (E-line)—lower lip	-2 mm	3.7 (±1.5)	-1	0

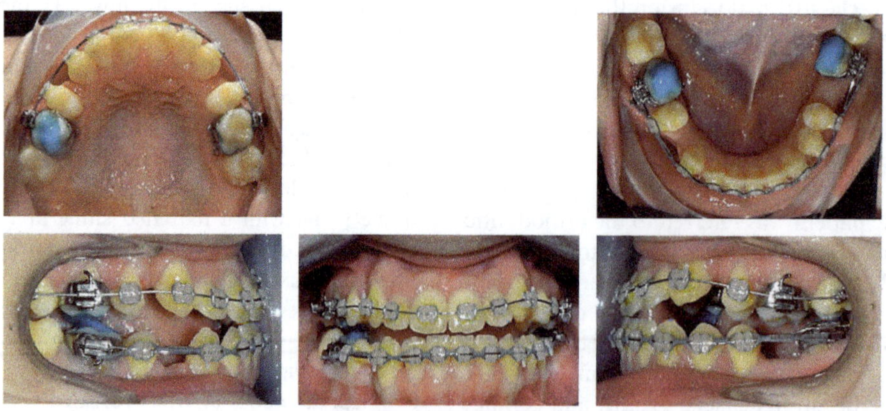

Figure 4: Progress photographs.

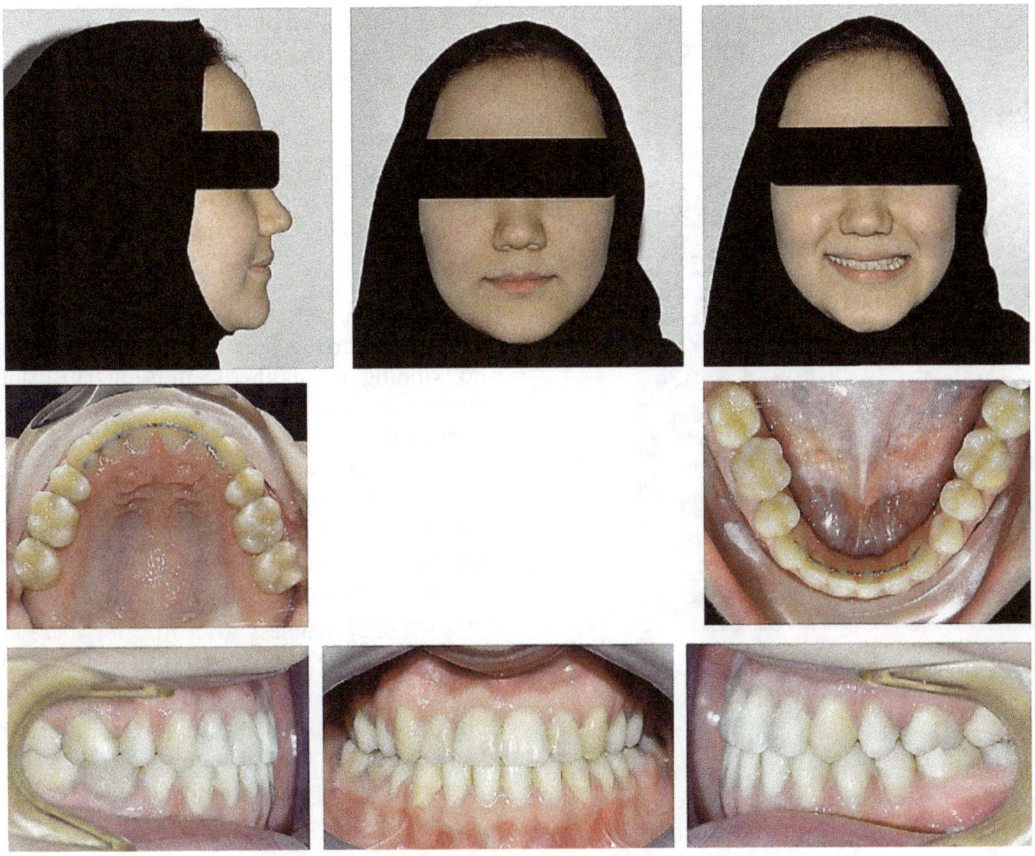

FIGURE 5: Posttreatment photographs of the patient.

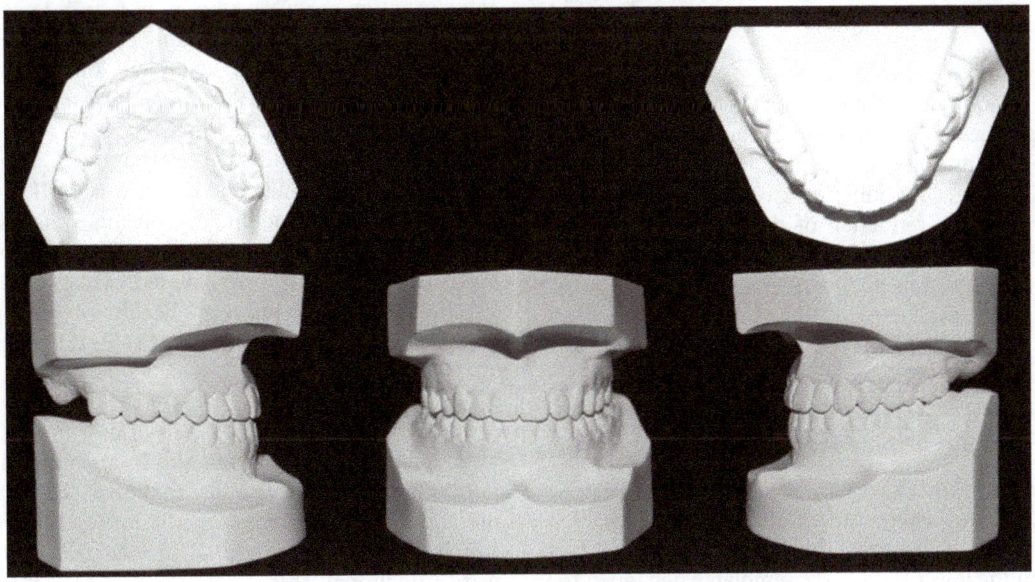

FIGURE 6: Posttreatment models.

centric relation), the skeletal relation was shown to be a normal class 1 relation. Regarding dentoalveolar measurement, it was found that the upper and lower incisors had normal inclinations (Figure 3, Table 1).

Panoramic radiography showed a missing lower first molar on the left side, multiple restorations, endodontic treatment of many teeth, and mesioangular impaction of the lower right third molar (Figure 3).

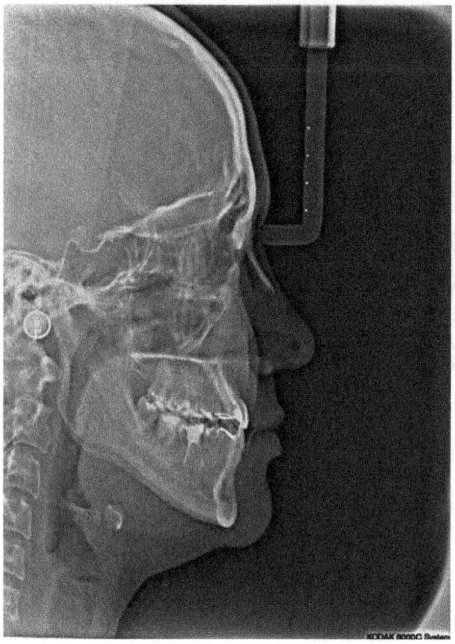

FIGURE 7: Posttreatment cephalometric radiograph.

Additionally, in the area of the lost first molar, a radiopaque shadow was noted that may signify the presence of chronic focal sclerosing osteomyelitis (also called condensing osteitis) which was related to the molar as a bone reaction to a previous periapical infection in this area. Another differential diagnosis for this radiopaque shadow includes idiopathic osteosclerosis, and both of these lesions do not require any treatment.

2.1. Treatment Objectives. The following treatment objectives were planned: (1) reinforce adequate oral hygiene and professional fluoride application before commencing treatment; (2) correct the anterior crossbite via protrusion of the upper incisors, retraction of the lower incisors, and backward shift of the mandibular arch to be enclosed inside the maxillary arch and correct the posterior crossbite via expanding the archwire; (3) achieve class I molars and canines on both sides except on the left molars, in which a class II molar relation will be achieved; (4) correct the upper midline shift and alleviate crowding; and (5) retain the achieved results.

2.2. Treatment Plan. Two treatment options were available:

The first option is to extract the upper right and left first premolars and the lower right first premolar. Then, open the bite with Build-Up composite resin on the molars followed by correction of the crossbites and space closure. The type of anchorage will be minimal in both the upper and lower arches.

The second option is to extract the upper right and left canines and the lower right first premolar and to substitute the upper canines with the upper first premolars. Then, continue with the treatment as in the first option.

After discussion of the current findings with the patient and considering the priorities of the aesthetic and functional demands for this patient, the first option was approved.

2.3. Retention Plan. The retention protocol was fixed retainers from 3-3 to wraparound retainers in the upper and lower arches in order to avoid any relapse, allow for teeth settling, maintain the expanded arch, and help in closing the band spaces.

2.4. Treatment Progress. The treatment was initiated by banding the first molars and the lower left second molar and bonding of the other teeth using 0.018 slot preadjusted edgewise ceramic brackets with Roth prescriptions. A letter for referral to extract the upper first premolars and the lower right first premolar was given to the patient, and an atraumatic extraction of these teeth was done. Build-Up composite resin was applied on both of the lower molars. Leveling and alignment were done by using a 0.012″ NiTi wire, followed by 0.014″ NiTi, 0.016″ NiTi, $0.016 \times 0.022''$ NiTi, and finally $0.016 \times 0.022''$ stainless steel wires for space closure. Space closure was done by using class III elastics and elastomeric chains. Finishing and detailing were done by using $0.016 \times 0.022''$ and $0.017 \times 0.025''$ stainless steel wires and intermaxillary elastics. All the third molars were extracted except the lower left one. The total duration of treatment was 23 months (Figure 4).

2.5. Treatment Results. Remarkable enhancement in the masticatory functions, combined with better facial aesthetics, of the patient was established. Proper and stable intercuspation between the upper and lower teeth was achieved. Both the anterior and posterior crossbites were eliminated. The forward functional shift of the mandible disappeared. However, the upper incisors were more proclined, whereas the lower incisors were more retroclined. Skeletal and dental class I relation was achieved except on the left molar side, where a firm class II molar relation was reached. Periodontal problems and several root resorptions were found; in particular, the upper incisors and buccal corridor were altered. Most importantly, the psychological and physical health of the patient was greatly enhanced (Figures 5–9) (Table 1).

3. Discussion

Functional shifts of the mandible can occur in any direction. These may be lateral functional shifts, which cause unilateral posterior crossbites, or forward functional shifts, which cause pseudo class III malocclusions [11, 12]. Forward functional shifts are usually associated with both anterior and posterior crossbites. This usually occurs for two reasons. The first reason is that the occlusal interference causes some of the upper anterior teeth (due to their lingual eruption) to interact with the lower teeth, hindering the normal closure of the mandible in the normal centric relation. The second reason, which is the main cause for the posterior crossbite, is the wider posterior width of the mandibular arch, compared to the anterior width;

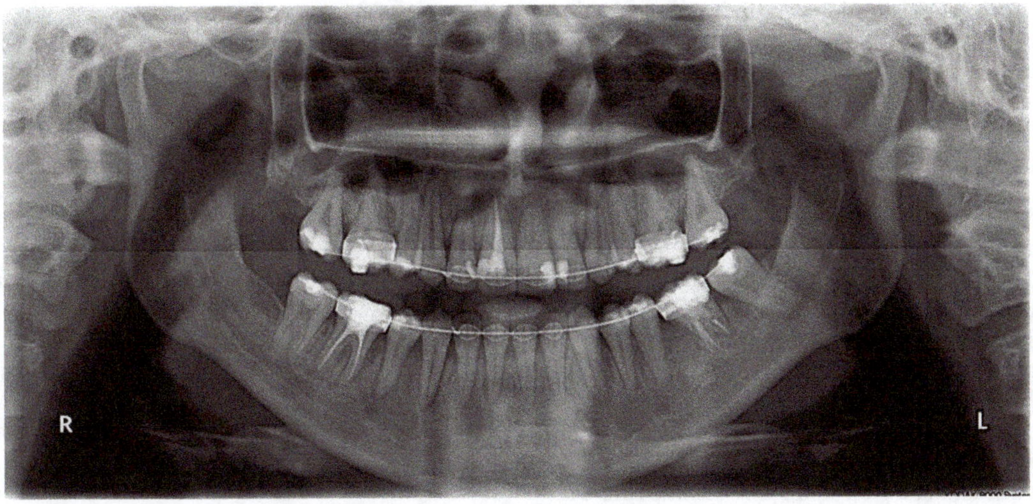

FIGURE 8: Panoramic radiograph.

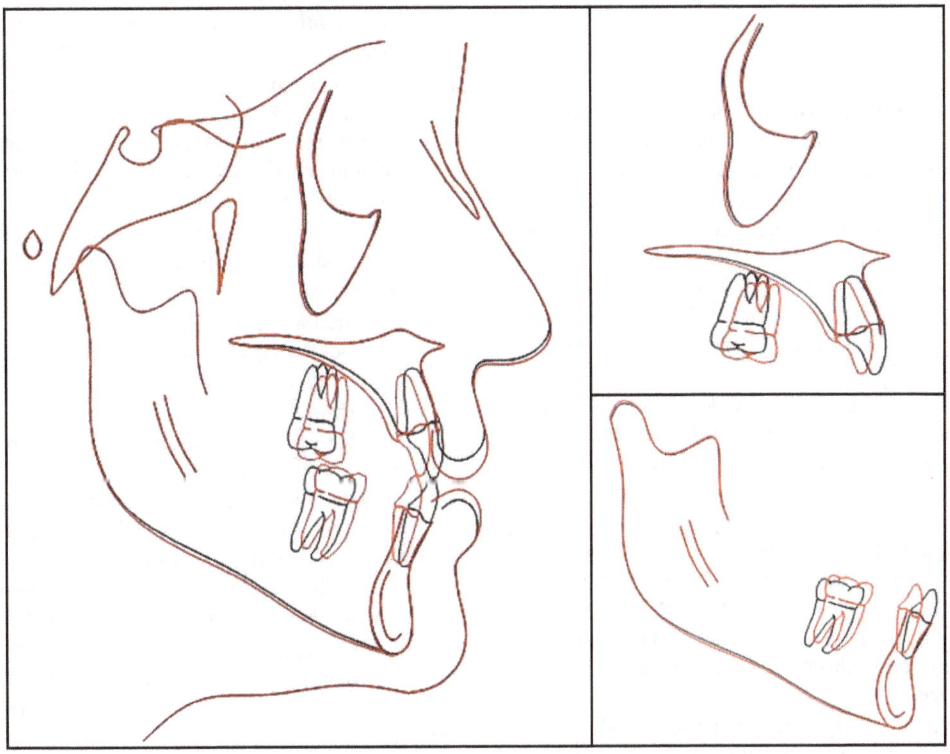

FIGURE 9: Posttreatment cephalometric superimposition. Black line: pretreatment. Red line: posttreatment.

i.e., when the mandible is advanced forward, its wider posterior arch occludes with the narrower anterior part of the maxilla, causing a posterior crossbite [6, 13–15].

The forward functional shift of the mandible was corrected by bite opening. This was done to remove the neuromuscular response that the mandible was conditioned to during the presence of the occlusal interferences. This was in agreement with a study conducted by Adly et al. who showed that all types of functional shifts totally disappeared after bite opening and the mandible assumed its normal functional position automatically, even before the removal of the occlusal interferences [5, 16, 17].

Extraction of the upper first premolars was done to relieve the severe crowding in the upper arch and allow the canine to assume its normal position. The extraction of the upper canines was avoided because of the ability of the upper canines, with their long roots, to support the bone under the nasolabial sulcus and thus to avoid deepening of this sulcus, which may contribute to an aged appearance of the face. Also, the canine is a strong tooth that is able to achieve a firm and stable canine-guided functional occlusion [18–21].

It is well known that orthodontic treatment can greatly enhance a patient's psychological and physical health [22, 23]. This is due to the better perceived self-image and the increased efficiency of mastication and digestion of food [24, 25]. This was clearly seen in this patient who had remarkable changes in her mental and physical attitudes by being more social and eating healthy foods.

4. Conclusion

In this case report, it was found that the forward functional shift of the mandible can be efficiently managed by proper diagnosis and treatment planning; however, the most important step in the treatment of such a case is to diagnose the dental and skeletal relation without this forward shift and build the treatment plan upon this condition as this condition is mostly temporary and resolved by removal of the interferences. The common error in treating these cases is the assumption of the stability of this forward functional shift and building a treatment plan upon this assumption. This may lead to dramatic results with total failure to achieve a stable occlusion.

References

[1] P. Ngan and W. Moon, "Evolution of class III treatment in orthodontics," *American Journal of Orthodontics and Dentofacial Orthopedics*, vol. 148, no. 1, pp. 22–36, 2015.

[2] A. Reyes, L. Serret, M. Peguero, and O. Tanaka, "Diagnosis and treatment of pseudo-class III malocclusion," *Case Reports in Dentistry*, vol. 2014, 6 pages, 2014.

[3] B. A. Furquim, K. M. S. de Freitas, G. Janson, L. F. Simoneti, M. R. de Freitas, and D. S. de Freitas, "Class III malocclusion surgical-orthodontic treatment," *Case Reports in Dentistry*, vol. 2014, 9 pages, 2014.

[4] F. P. C. Ferreira, M. S. Goulart, R. R. de Almeida-Pedrin, C. ACdCF, and C. MdA, "Treatment of class III malocclusion: atypical extraction protocol," *Case Reports in Dentistry*, vol. 2017, Article ID 4652685, 9 pages, 2017.

[5] M. S. Adly, A. S. Adly, and A. S. Adly, "Assessment of early orthodontic treatment on functional shifts by telemonitoring mandibular movements using a smart phone," *Journal of Telemedicine and Telecare*, vol. 26, no. 3, pp. 150–160, 2020.

[6] N. D. Kravitz, "Interceptive orthodontics with resin turbos for pseudo-class III malocclusions," *Case Reports in Dentistry*, vol. 2019, 6 pages, 2019.

[7] A. Rabie and Y. Gu, "Diagnostic criteria for pseudo–class III malocclusion," *American Journal of Orthodontics and Dentofacial Orthopedics*, vol. 117, no. 1, pp. 1–9, 2000.

[8] U. Hägg, A. Tse, M. Bendeus, and A. B. M. Rabie, "A follow-up study of early treatment of pseudo class III malocclusion," *The Angle Orthodontist*, vol. 74, no. 4, pp. 465–472, 2004.

[9] S.-P. Ad, R. Fabris Paulin, and A. C. Moreira Melo, "Pseudo-class III treatment with reverse traction: case report," *Journal of Clinical Pediatric Dentistry*, vol. 25, no. 4, pp. 267–274, 2001.

[10] Y. Gu, "The characteristics of pseudo class III malocclusion in mixed dentition," *Zhonghua kou qiang yi xue za zhi= Zhonghua kouqiang yixue zazhi= Chinese Journal of Stomatology*, vol. 37, no. 5, pp. 377–380, 2002.

[11] D. B. Kennedy and M. Osepchook, "Unilateral posterior crossbite with mandibular shift: a review," *Journal-Canadian Dental Association*, vol. 71, no. 8, pp. 569–573, 2005.

[12] P. H. Nerder, M. Bekke, and B. Solow, "The functional shift of the mandible in unilateral posterior crossbite and the adaptation of the temporomandibular joints: a pilot study," *The European Journal of Orthodontics*, vol. 21, no. 2, pp. 155–166, 1999.

[13] P. Ngan, "Early treatment of class III malocclusion: is it worth the burden?," *American Journal of Orthodontics And Dentofacial Orthopedics*, vol. 129, no. 4, pp. S82–S85, 2006.

[14] K. Negi and K. Sharma, "Treatment of pseudo class III malocclusion by modified Hawleys appliance with inverted labial bow," *Journal of Indian Society of Pedodontics and Preventive Dentistry*, vol. 29, no. 1, pp. 57–61, 2011.

[15] B. Akan and I. Veli, "Comparison of dental arch and mandibular-maxillary base widths between true and pseudo-class III malocclusions," *American Journal of Orthodontics and Dentofacial Orthopedics*, vol. 151, no. 2, pp. 317–323, 2017.

[16] R. Showkatbakhsh, A. Jamilian, M. Behnaz, M. Ghassemi, and A. Ghassemi, "The short-term effects of face mask and fixed tongue appliance on maxillary deficiency in growing patients–a randomized clinical trial," *International Journal of Orthodontics (Milwaukee, Wis.)*, vol. 26, no. 1, pp. 33–38, 2015.

[17] R. Showkatbakhsh, L. Toumarian, A. Jamilian, A. Sheibaninia, M. Mirkarimi, and T. Taban, "The effects of face mask and tongue plate on maxillary deficiency in growing patients: a randomized clinical trial," *Journal of Orthodontics*, vol. 40, no. 2, pp. 130–136, 2013.

[18] R. M. Cruz, "Orthodontic traction of impacted canines: concepts and clinical application," *Dental Press Journal of Orthodontics*, vol. 24, no. 1, pp. 74–87, 2019.

[19] R. Miralles, "Canine-guide occlusion and group function occlusion are equally acceptable when restoring the dentition," *Journal of Evidence Based Dental Practice*, vol. 16, no. 1, pp. 41–43, 2016.

[20] O. Schierz and D. Reissmann, "Influence of guidance concept in complete dentures on oral health related quality of life–canine guidance vs. bilateral balanced occlusion," *Journal of Prosthodontic Research*, vol. 60, no. 4, pp. 315–320, 2016.

[21] M. Farret and M. M. FARRET, "Practical and esthetic considerations in adult canine-extraction treatment," *Journal of Clinical Orthodontics*, vol. 47, pp. 353–360, 2013.

[22] R. J. Klima, J. K. Wittemann, and J. E. McIver, "Body image, self-concept, and the orthodontic patient," *American Journal of Orthodontics*, vol. 75, no. 5, pp. 507–516, 1979.

[23] A. Ukra, F. Bennani, and M. Farella, "Psychological aspects of orthodontics in clinical practice. Part one: treatment-specific variables," *Progress in Orthodontics*, vol. 12, no. 2, pp. 143–148, 2011.

[24] S. J. Cunningham and N. P. Hunt, "Quality of life and its importance in orthodontics," *Journal of Orthodontics*, vol. 28, no. 2, pp. 152–158, 2014.

[25] W. Hickory and R. Nanda, "Nutritional considerations in orthodontics," *Dental Clinics of North America*, vol. 25, no. 1, pp. 195–201, 1981.

19

Class III Orthodontic Camouflage: Is the "Ideal" Treatment Always the Best Option? A Documented Case Report

Lorenzo Rustico,[1] **Vincenzo Ronsivalle**,[1] **Flavia Iaculli**,[2] **Gianrico Spagnuolo**,[2] **Gaetano Isola**,[1] **and Antonino Lo Giudice**[1]

[1]*Department of Medical-Surgical Specialties, School of Dentistry, University of Catania, Policlinico Universitario "G. Rodolico", Via Santa Sofia 78, 95123 Catania, Italy*
[2]*Department of Neurosciences, Reproductive and Odontostomatological Sciences, University of Naples "Federico II", Via Pansini 5, 80131 Naples, Italy*

Correspondence should be addressed to Gianrico Spagnuolo; gspagnuo@unina.it

Academic Editor: Sivakumar Nuvvula

Angle's Class III is one of the most complex malocclusions to treat. In nongrowing skeletal class III malocclusions, the choice between orthognathic surgery and camouflage treatment remains a challenge to the orthodontist. In class III borderline cases, clinicians are called to find the best compromise between functional and aesthetics outcomes, with the latter which often turns in avoiding worsening of profile characteristics, which makes the treatment of these patients quite challenging. This case report describes a borderline nongrowing patient with skeletal class III malocclusion, upper incisor proclination and spacing, lower crowding, and arch width discrepancy, which has already undergone previous orthodontic treatment. The orthodontic treatment involved the mandibular first premolar extraction, resulting in class I canine relation with good overjet and overbite as well as good arch coordination. The orthodontic camouflage improved the dental relationship with normalization of upper incisor inclination without a relevant retroclination of lower incisors; the skeletal facial pattern of the patient experienced a slight improvement. The tendency to skeletal class III has remained nearly unaffected. Treatment outcomes were stable after 1-year posttreatment follow-up.

1. Introduction

Angle's Class III is one of the most complex malocclusions to treat, and it is usually characterized by combined skeletal and dentoalveolar features [1–3].

The combination of a normal maxilla with a prognathic mandible has been identified by Jacobson et al. as the most frequent class III malocclusion pattern [4].

Angle's Class III correction can be accomplished by growth modification [5, 6], orthodontic camouflage [7], or orthodontic surgery [8].

Adult nongrowing Class III patients are even more challenging to treat due to the limited availability of treatment options. The decision between orthodontic camouflage and orthognathic surgery remains a trial for the orthodontist [9].

The best treatment option for nongrowing skeletal class III patients is represented by orthognathic surgery; however, this option is often refused by the patients due to finances or the invasiveness related to the procedure. Class III patients who refuse orthognathic surgery can be treated, with an orthodontic camouflage, extractions, utilising multibrackets and class III elastics, multiloop edgewise archwire treatment, or skeletal anchorage devices (TADs) for mandibular distalization [9–14]. In class III borderline cases, clinicians are called to find the best compromise between functional and aesthetic outcomes, with the latter which often turns in avoiding worsening of profile characteristics, which makes the treatment of these patients quite challenging.

Lower tooth extraction is sometimes indicated in moderate class III skeletal cases and may implicate first premolar or incisor extractions. The choice is influenced by many

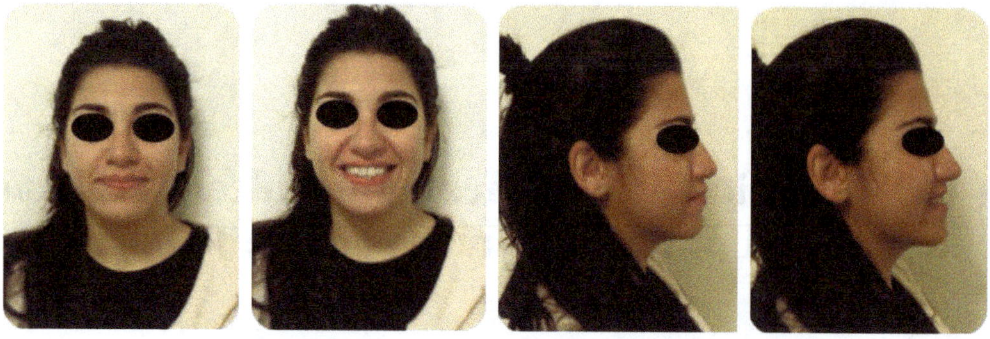

FIGURE 1: Pretreatment extraoral photographs.

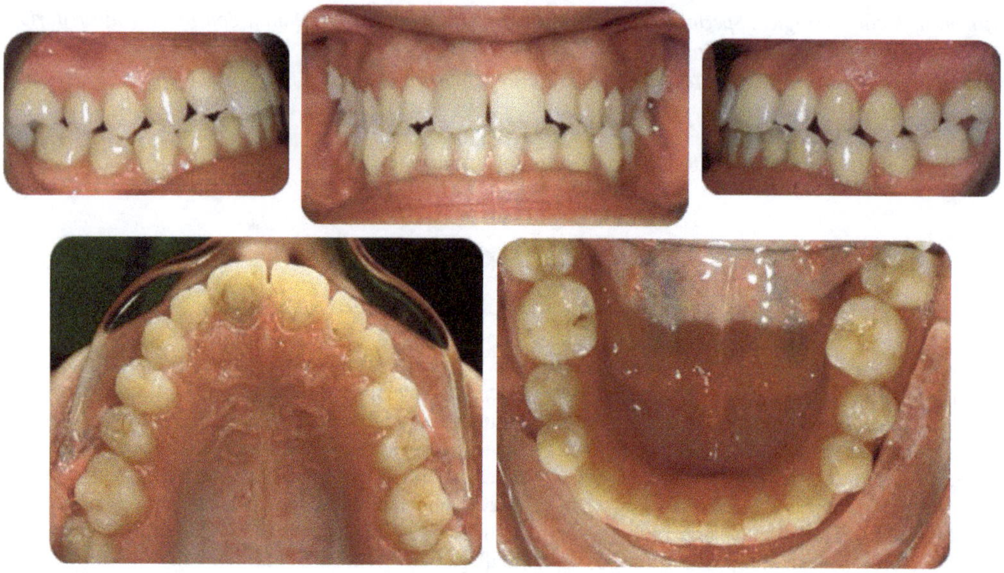

FIGURE 2: Pretreatment intraoral photographs.

factors, such as the severity of the mandibular anterior crowding, the Bolton discrepancy, and negative overjet and overbite intensity [15].

This case report presents a skeletal class III orthodontic camouflage in an adult patient, illustrating the diagnostic process and the therapeutic options evaluated before opting for the lower first premolar extraction.

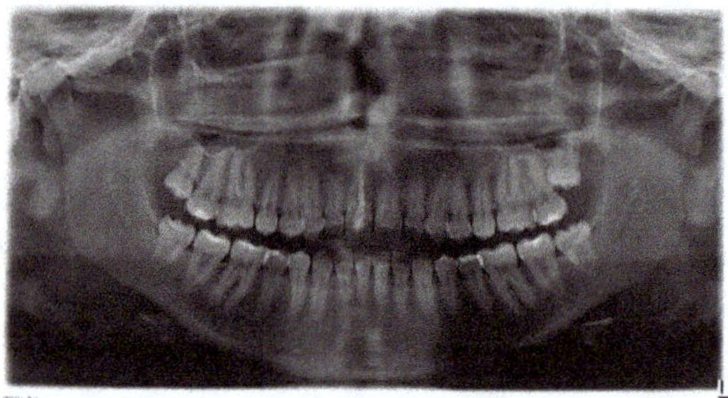

FIGURE 3: Pretreatment orthopantomogram.

2. Case Report

2.1. Diagnosis and Etiology. A 19-year-old female has come to orthodontic consultation with a chief complaint about the relapse of her occlusion after previous orthodontic treatment and the aesthetics of her smile. The patient had a moderate skeletal class III malocclusion with a flat profile, normal facial vertical dimension, and an adequate soft tissue projection with a slight lip strain (Figure 1). In the frontal view, the face had a good symmetry. The intraoral examination and the orthopantomogram showed spacing in the maxillary arch and severe crowding in the mandibular arch, with crossbite of 1.3 and 2.3 and edge-to-edge relationship of upper and lower premolars, with a discrepancy in upper and lower arch form (Figures 2 and 3). The spacing in the upper arch, with the crowding in the lower arch, could indicate an alteration of the Bolton index; however, this is not the case, as has been shown by the analysis of the plaster models. It seems more likely that this discrepancy is linked to the failure of the compensation carried out during the previous orthodontic treatment. The teleradiography and the consequent cephalometric analysis highlight the class III skeletal malocclusion in a subject tended to hyperdivergence, with an importance of upper incisor proclination and normal

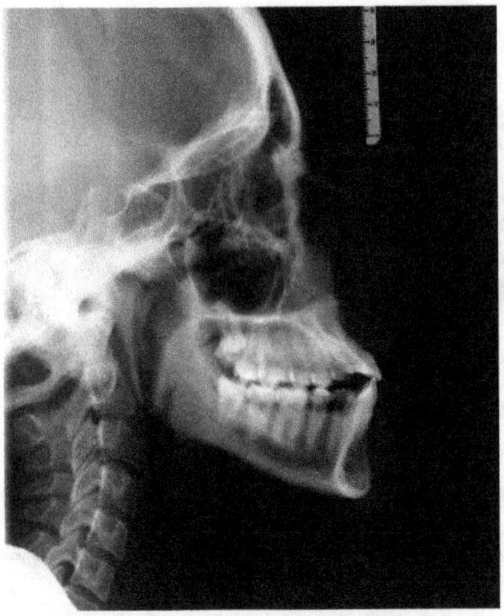

	Value	Norm	Std Dev	Dev Norm
SNA (°)	88.0	82.0	3.5	1.7 *
SNB (°)	87.8	80.9	3.4	2.0 **
ANB (°)	0.1	1.6	1.5	-1.0 *
Wits Appraisal (mm)	-6.4	-1.0	1.0	-5.4 *****
SN - GoGn (°)	35.7	32.9	5.2	0.5
SGo/NGn (%)	57.6	100.0	10.0	-4.2 ****
Mandibular length (Go-Gn) (mm)	82.8	65.9	5.5	3.1 ***
Length of Mand Base (Go-Pg) (mm)	76.3	73.0	3.0	1.1 *
Mx anterior height (Sn'-Mx1) (mm)	22.6	25.7	2.1	-1.5 *
Occ Plane to SN (°)	11.9	14.4	2.5	-1.0 *
U1 - SN (°)	117.4	102.8	5.5	2.7 **
U1 - Palatal Plane (°)	128.2	110.0	5.0	3.6 ***
IMPA (L1-MP) (°)	89.4	95.0	7.0	-0.8
L1 - SN (°)	52.9	57.8	8.5	-0.6
subnasale (Sn') (mm)	0.0			
soft tissue A Point' (A') (mm)	-1.9	-0.1	1.0	-1.8 *
upper lip anterior (ULA) (mm)	-1.7	3.7	1.2	-4.5 ****
lower lip anterior (LLA) (mm)	-4.0	1.9	1.4	-4.2 ****
soft tissue B point (B') (mm)	-10.0	-5.3	1.5	-3.1 ***
soft tissue Pogonion (Pog') (mm)	-11.2	-2.6	1.9	-4.6 ****

FIGURE 4: Pretreatment cephalometric analysis.

position of lower incisors (Figure 4). During anamnestic and clinical evaluation, no signs or symptoms of temporomandibular disorder (TMD) were described.

2.2. Treatment Objectives. The aims of the orthodontic treatment were the correction of maxillary spacing and mandibular crowding, normalization of upper incisors inclination, and coordination of the upper and lower arch form in order to correct the crossbite of teeth 1.3 and 2.3; moreover, improve the smile aesthetics without worsening the facial profile achieving those occlusal outcomes.

2.3. Treatment Alternatives. The first option was orthognathic surgery; however, the patient and her parents refused any surgical approach.

The second option was to treat the patient with four-premolar extraction (both upper and lower first or second premolars). This strategy would have permitted to correct both maxillary incisor proclination and mandibular crowding; however, this option would have probably worsened patients' facial aesthetics since the elimination of dental compensation would have accentuated the class III profile.

The third alternative was an orthodontic camouflage; this option could be achieved with class III elastics, with distalization of the lower arch through the use of TADs, or with mandibular first premolar extraction; however, the first two options for orthodontic camouflage were not suitable for this case: the first one because of the needs to correct the upper incisor proclination, which would surely be worsened by the use of class III elastics, and the second one because of the important and not very predictable lower distalization required which in any case would have required lower third molar extraction.

Consequently, the camouflage with first mandibular premolar extraction is the most reasonable option, capable of allowing the normalization of upper incisor inclination and the correction of mandibular crowding. This option would lead to a predictable improvement of facial aesthetics with a biological cost comparable to the lower arch distalization option.

Both patients' parents and the orthodontists preferred the latter option.

2.4. Treatment Progress. A 0.22 fixed appliance with preadjusted Roth prescription (American Orthodontics) has been bonded to all the erupted teeth on the buccal surface, except 3.4 and 4.4 that were extracted during treatment early stages. The same sequence of archwire was used for both arches: 0.014 heat-activated NiTi; 0.014×0.025 heat-activated NiTi; 0.019×0.025 heat-activated NiTi; and 0.019×0.025 SS. By the means of this archwire sequence alignment, leveling and the coordination of the maxillary and mandibular arch were achieved.

After 20 months of orthodontic therapy, the appliance was removed, lingual-bonded fixed retainers were applied to both maxillary and mandibular front teeth, and removable retainers were provided to the patient for the upper and lower arch [16].

2.5. Results. The posttreatment photographs show the substantial improvement in the aesthetics of the patient (Figures 5 and 6). The posttreatment orthopantomogram displayed the good root parallelism achieved without root resorption (Figure 7). The posttreatment cephalometric analysis and the tracing superimposition illustrate the modifications obtained with the treatment (Figures 8 and 9). The posttreatment intraoral view shows the achievement of a functional canine class I canine relation with the normalization of overjet and overbite. The maxillary spacing correction has determined a normalization of upper incisor position; the lower crowding correction by means of extractions allowed correcting lower arch form and the crossbite of teeth 1.3 and 2.3. Furthermore, this extractive treatment option allowed compensating for the class III skeletal discrepancy improving the dental support of both upper and lower lips. Labial competence was improved with a reduction of the lip strain. Looking at the posttreatment lateral

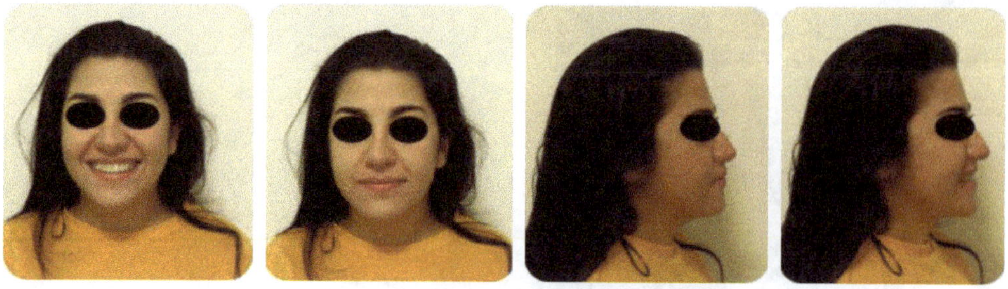

FIGURE 5: Posttreatment extraoral photographs.

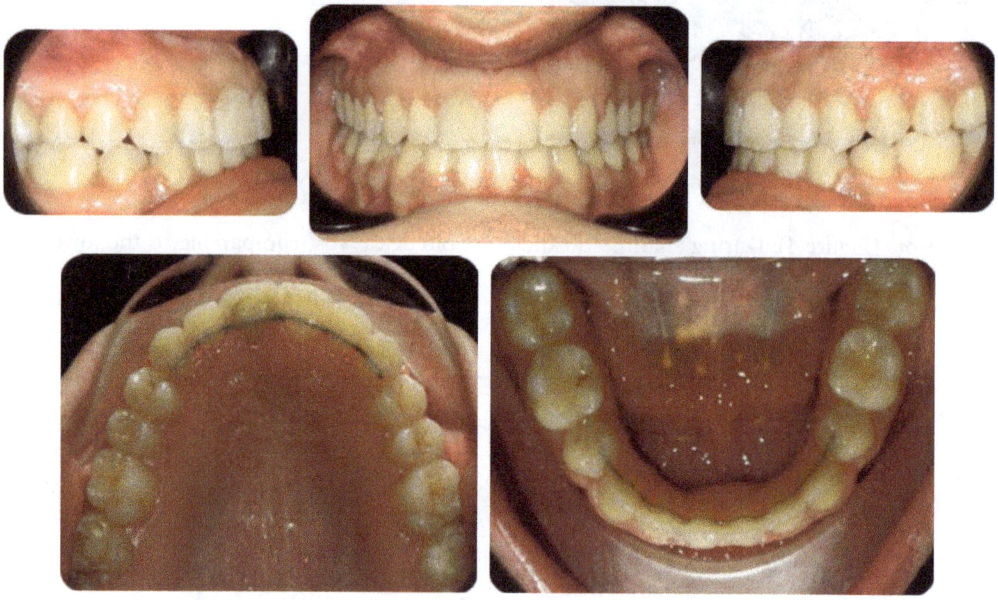

FIGURE 6: Posttreatment intraoral photographs.

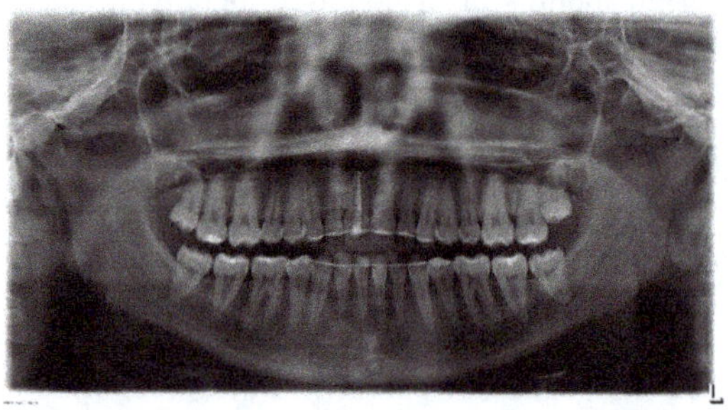

FIGURE 7: Posttreatment orthopantomogram.

cephalogram, the orthodontic camouflage improved the dental relationship with a normalization of upper incisor inclination without a relevant lingualization of lower incisors; the skeletal facial pattern of the patient experienced a slight improvement.

Facial and intraoral view after 12 months of retention shows the stability of the results and the improvement of dental aesthetics thanks to the maturation of the tissues in the retention period. Tooth 1.1, which was dyschromic since the beginning of the treatment, due to a previous endodontic treatment, has been treated with the walking bleach technique (Figures 10 and 11) [17].

3. Discussion

Angle's Class III is notoriously one of the most complex malocclusions to understand, and it is also one of the most challenging malocclusions for which to develop an optimal treatment plan avoiding overtreatment or undertreatment [18–20].

The present case reports shows a borderline class III patient treated with an orthodontic camouflage achieved by lower first premolar extraction. As previously mentioned, this case left room for various therapeutic options, but the will to improve as much as possible the patient's aesthetics without resorting to orthognathic surgery led us to the decision to extract only lower first premolars. Since avoiding the extraction of upper first premolars would have allowed to achieve and maintain a good soft tissue balance, compensating for the lower lip protrusion; on the contrary, upper first premolar extraction and the consequent upper incisor retroclination would have worsened the upper lip projection, revealing the class III relationship. This aspect was crucial

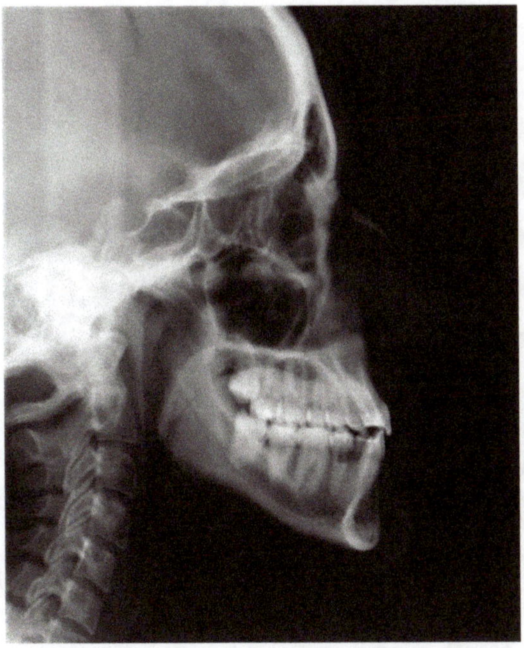

	Value	Norm	Std Dev	Dev Norm
SNA (°)	89.4	82.0	3.5	2.1 **
SNB (°)	87.1	80.9	3.4	1.8 *
ANB (°)	2.3	1.6	1.5	0.5
Wits Appraisal (mm)	-5.7	-1.0	1.0	-4.7 ****
SN - GoGn (°)	36.5	32.9	5.2	0.7
SGo/NGn (%)	56.7	100.0	10.0	-4.3 ****
Mandibular length (Go-Gn) (mm)	82.8	65.9	5.5	3.1 ***
Length of Mand Base (Go-Pg) (mm)	76.3	73.0	3.0	1.1 *
Mx anterior height (Sn'-Mx1) (mm)	22.4	25.7	2.1	-1.6 *
Occ Plane to SN (°)	15.9	14.4	2.5	0.6
U1 - SN (°)	104.3	102.8	5.5	0.3
U1 - Palatal Plane (°)	114.7	110.0	5.0	0.9
IMPA (L1-MP) (°)	83.1	95.0	7.0	-1.7 *
L1 - SN (°)	58.0	57.8	8.5	0.0
subnasale (Sn') (mm)	0.0			
soft tissue A Point' (A') (mm)	-1.3	-0.1	1.0	-1.2 *
upper lip anterior (ULA) (mm)	0.3	3.7	1.2	-2.9 **
lower lip anterior (LLA) (mm)	-4.3	1.9	1.4	-4.4 ****
soft tissue B point (B') (mm)	-10.8	-5.3	1.5	-3.7 ***
soft tissue Pogonion (Pog') (mm)	-10.6	-2.6	1.9	-4.2 ****

FIGURE 8: Posttreatment cephalometric analysis.

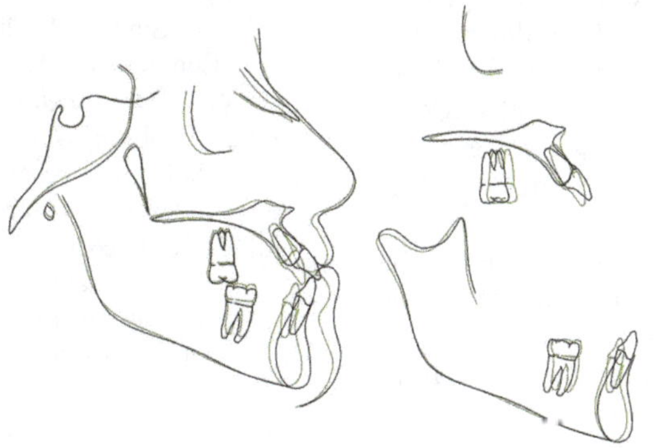

FIGURE 9: Pretreatment and posttreatment tracing superimposition.

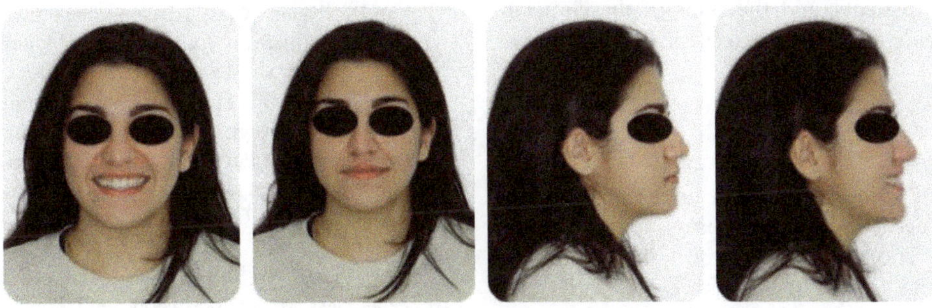

FIGURE 10: 12-month follow-up, extraoral photographs.

in the therapeutic choice, especially considering the patient's request not to excessively modify her facial aesthetics.

Furthermore, the extraction of lower first premolars, which were already in crossbite, allowed the clinician to correct the transversal discrepancy between upper and lower arches, achieving correct arch coordination.

In terms of treatment plan strategy, the class III malocclusion orthodontic camouflage by the means of the extraction of lower first premolars could be considered specular to upper premolar extraction in class II malocclusion orthodontic camouflage. The latter is a common therapeutic option in those situations in which class II relationship and

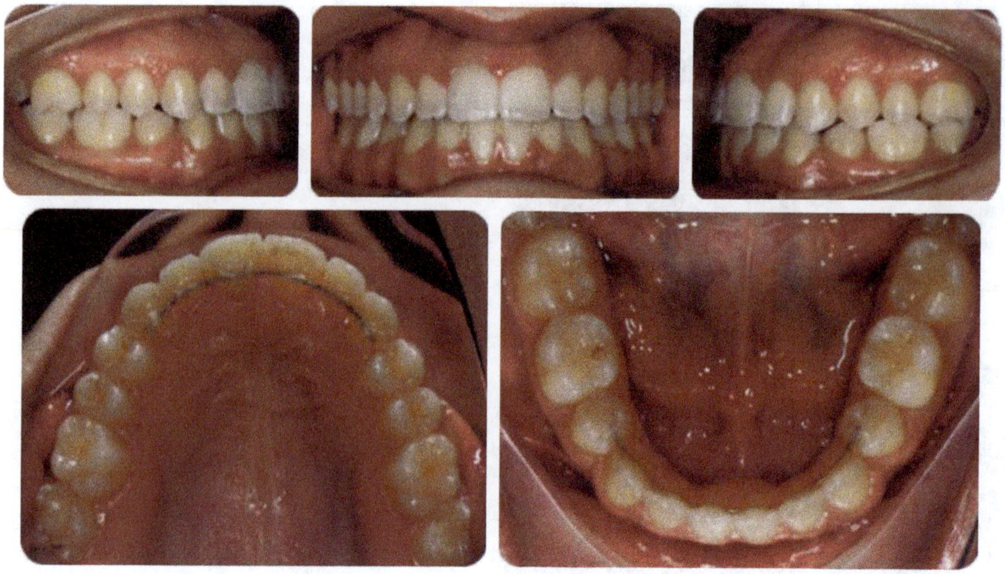

FIGURE 11: 12-month follow-up, intraoral photographs.

increased overjet are accompanied by the need not to worsen the position of the lower teeth, as it could instead happen using class II mechanics; long-term evaluation of patients treated with orthodontic class II camouflage did not highlight any functional damage [21, 22]. Similarly, for class III orthodontic camouflage, there is no evidence that single arch extraction could lead to functional damage, not even with molar class III relationship if canine class I relationship is achieved.

What prompted us to share this clinical case is the need to review the concept of excellence in the orthodontic field, since in this case, notwithstanding the many valid therapeutic options and despite not having achieved all the standard canons of excellence [23], the biological sacrifice of two premolars made it possible to correct the malocclusion and significantly improve the patient's facial aesthetics. Therefore, orthodontic excellence should always be reviewed according to the initial clinical conditions, the needs and possibilities of the patients, and the skills of the clinician, aiming at tailor-made orthodontic excellence.

4. Conclusion

To date, there are no guidelines that can guide the orthodontist through the decision-making process for borderline orthodontic cases. The present case report shows how the choice of an effective treatment plan must necessarily take into account numerous clinical and extraclinical factors, aiming at orthodontic excellence, with a tailor-made treatment plan for each patient.

References

[1] F. Mackay, J. A. Jones, R. Thompson, and W. Simpson, "Craniofacial form in class III cases," *British Journal of Orthodontics*, vol. 19, no. 1, pp. 15–20, 1992.

[2] J. M. Battagel, "The aetiological factors in class III malocclusion," *European Journal of Orthodontics*, vol. 15, no. 5, pp. 347–370, 1993.

[3] E. C. Guyer, E. E. Ellis, J. A. McNamara Jr., and R. G. Behrents, "Components of class III malocclusion in juveniles and adolescents," *The Angle Orthodontist*, vol. 56, no. 1, pp. 7–30, 1986.

[4] A. Jacobson, W. G. Evans, C. G. Preston, and P. L. Sadowsky, "Mandibular prognathism," *American Journal of Orthodontics*, vol. 66, no. 2, pp. 140–171, 1974.

[5] G. Cordasco, G. Matarese, L. Rustico et al., "Efficacy of orthopedic treatment with protraction facemask on skeletal class III malocclusion: a systematic review and meta-analysis," *Orthodontics & Craniofacial Research*, vol. 17, no. 3, pp. 133–143, 2014.

[6] P. Ngan, B. Wilmes, D. Drescher, C. Martin, B. Weaver, and E. Gunel, "Comparison of two maxillary protraction protocols: tooth-borne versus bone-anchored protraction facemask treatment," *Progress in Orthodontics*, vol. 16, no. 1, p. 26, 2015.

[7] N. R. Burns, D. R. Musich, C. Martin, T. Razmus, E. Gunel, and P. Ngan, "Class III camouflage treatment: what are the limits," *American Journal of Orthodontics and Dentofacial Orthopedics*, vol. 137, no. 1, pp. 9.e1–9.e13, 2010.

[8] R. Trauner and H. Obwegeser, "The surgical correction of mandibular prognathism and retrognathia with consideration of genioplasty: Part I. Surgical procedures to correct mandibular prognathism and reshaping of the chin," *Oral Surgery, Oral Medicine, and Oral Pathology*, vol. 10, no. 7, pp. 677–689, 1957.

[9] J. H. Park, J. Yu, and R. Bullen, "Camouflage treatment of skeletal class III malocclusion with conventional orthodontic therapy," *American Journal of Orthodontics and Dentofacial Orthopedics*, vol. 151, no. 4, pp. 804–811, 2017.

[10] A. Lo Giudice, I. Brewer, R. Leonardi, N. Roberts, and G. Bagnato, "Pain threshold and temporomandibular function in systemic sclerosis: comparison with psoriatic arthritis," *Clinical Rheumatology*, vol. 37, no. 7, pp. 1861–1867, 2018.

[11] Y. A. Kook, J. H. Park, M. Bayome, S. K. Kim, E. Han, and C. H. Kim, "Distalization of the mandibular dentition with a ramal plate for skeletal class III malocclusion correction,"

American Journal of Orthodontics and Dentofacial Orthopedics, vol. 150, no. 2, pp. 364–377, 2016.

[12] H. Liu, X. Wu, J. Tan, and X. Li, "Safe regions of miniscrew implantation for distalization of mandibular dentition with CBCT," *Progress in Orthodontics*, vol. 20, no. 1, pp. 1–8, 2019.

[13] K. Tai, J. H. Park, M. Tatamiya, and Y. Kojima, "Distal movement of the mandibular dentition with temporary skeletal anchorage devices to correct a class III malocclusion," *American Journal of Orthodontics and Dentofacial Orthopedics*, vol. 144, no. 5, pp. 715–725, 2013.

[14] A. Lo Giudice, V. Ronsivalle, M. Lagravere, R. Leonardi, S. Martina, and G. Isola, "Transverse dentoalveolar response of mandibular arch after rapid maxillary expansion (RME) with tooth-borne and bone-borne appliances," *The Angle Orthodontist*, vol. 90, no. 5, pp. 680–687, 2020.

[15] P. Ngan and W. Moon, "Evolution of class III treatment in orthodontics," *American Journal of Orthodontics and Dentofacial Orthopedics*, vol. 148, no. 1, pp. 22–36, 2015.

[16] Y. Kartal and B. Kaya, "Fixed orthodontic retainers: a review," *Turkish journal of Orthodontics*, vol. 32, no. 2, pp. 110–114, 2019.

[17] G. Plotino, L. Buono, N. M. Grande, C. H. Pameijer, and F. Somma, "Nonvital tooth bleaching: a review of the literature and clinical procedures," *Journal of Endodontia*, vol. 34, no. 4, pp. 394–407, 2008.

[18] A. Stellzig-Eisenhauer, C. J. Lux, and G. Schuster, "Treatment decision in adult patients with class III malocclusion: orthodontic therapy or orthognathic surgery," *American Journal of Orthodontics and Dentofacial Orthopedics*, vol. 122, no. 1, pp. 27–37, 2002.

[19] R. Leonardi, S. Muraglie, A. Lo Giudice, K. S. Aboulazm, and R. Nucera, "Evaluation of mandibular symmetry and morphology in adult patients with unilateral posterior crossbite: a CBCT study using a surface-to-surface matching technique," *European Journal of Orthodontics*, vol. 42, no. 6, pp. 650–657, 2020.

[20] A. Lo Giudice, L. Rustico, A. Caprioglio, M. Migliorati, and R. Nucera, "Evaluation of condylar cortical bone thickness in patient groups with different vertical facial dimensions using cone-beam computed tomography," *Odontology*, vol. 108, no. 4, pp. 669–675, 2020.

[21] C. A. Mihalik, W. R. Proffit, and C. Phillips, "Long-term follow-up of class II adults treated with orthodontic camouflage: a comparison with orthognathic surgery outcomes," *American Journal of Orthodontics and Dentofacial Orthopedics*, vol. 123, no. 3, pp. 266–278, 2003.

[22] R. Scott Conley and C. Jernigan, "Soft tissue changes after upper premolar extraction in class II camouflage therapy," *The Angle Orthodontist*, vol. 76, no. 1, pp. 59–65, 2006.

[23] L. F. Andrews, "The six keys to normal occlusion," *American Journal of Orthodontics*, vol. 62, no. 3, pp. 296–309, 1972.

20

Direct Anterior Tracks: Early and Functional Management of Class III Malocclusions—Case Report and Literature Review

Echeverry Juan Carlos[1] **and Barbosa-Liz Diana**[2]

[1]*Faculty of Dentistry, University of Antioquia, Calle 70 #52-21 Medellín, Colombia*
[2]*Orthopedic Maxillary and Orthodontic Postgraduate Program, Faculty of Dentistry, Universidad de Antioquia, Calle 70 #52-21 Medellín, Colombia*

Correspondence should be addressed to Barbosa-Liz Diana; dimabarbosa@gmail.com

Academic Editor: Hüsamettin Oktay

The prevalence of class III malocclusion ranged from 0 to 26% in different populations. Many types of treatments have been described in dental literature. The results of early treatment have been positive. The purpose of this report is to describe the case of a four-year-old patient with class III malocclusion who received an innovative treatment using direct anterior tracks. This therapy efficiently obtained immediate improvement of profile and occlusal relationships.

1. Introduction

The development and establishment of class III malocclusions can occur from the early stages of life, and the establishment of early functional alterations can permanently affect the growth of craniofacial structures [1–3].

Dentofacial changes achievable with maxillary orthopedics can induce harmonic growth when an early approach of these maxillofacial alterations is made [4].

1.1. Etiopathogenesis. Multiple factors can influence the presence of a class III malocclusion and its etiology has a multifactorial origin. The influence of inheritance on the appearance of this dysplasia and its primary etiological role have been widely reported [5, 6].

Class III malocclusion can be skeletal, dental, or functional. Alterations in the size and/or position of the maxilla and mandible may favor the establishment and development of skeletal class III malocclusion. On the other hand, the premature contact between the anterior incisors at early ages or the inadequate inclination of these teeth could be etiological factors of functional and dental class III malocclusion [4]. Likewise, other functional and epigenetic factors, such as lingual anterior lower position, oral breathing, and the absence of teeth on upper arch, among others, have been identified as environmental etiological factors of class III [4].

Altered eruption can induce an unfavorable incisal guide, generating an anterior crossbite. The anterior displacement of the mandible and its condyle as a consequence of unfavorable incisal guidance can produce a pseudo-class III or class III malocclusion. Likewise, the premature loss of primary molars can cause mandibular anterior displacement due to the change in the occlusal guide of the teeth that are in malposition or to the lingualization of the maxillary incisors [3]. The prevalence of class III malocclusion varies from 0.6 to 1.2% depending on the population studied. In Colombia, there is a prevalence of 5.8% of functional and pseudo-class III alterations in children of 5-17 years. The prevalence of true or skeletal class III in the same population was 3.7% [7].

Graber et al.'s recognition of the condyle's ability to adapt to different stimuli received from the growth of the mandible in malocclusions with anterior crossbite makes the functional orthopedics of the jaws a relevant value for early management of sagittal skeletal alterations [3].

The differential diagnosis of true class III, functional class III, and class I with anterior crossbite is important and it takes into account the profile, posterior dental relationships, dental inclinations, the presence or absence of anterior mandibular deflection, and the complete evaluation of the functional aspect [8].

If possible and the lateral cephalic radiograph exists, the evaluation of maxillomandibular position and size is useful. Likewise, the anterior crossbite can be a sign of different combinations of skeletal and dental discrepancies [9].

The orthopedic-orthodontic treatment will depend on the etiology and the specific characteristics of the malocclusion. The age of the patient also influences the treatment decision. Therapeutic approaches range from maxillary advance with facial mask, progenie mechanical devices, functional orthopedic appliances like Bionator and Frankel, to functional myo-dynamic orofacial orthopedics among others.

As the transversal width of the maxilla is usually affected, the treatment must take into account this aspect, using rapid maxillary expanders [10].

The systematic review of De Toffol et al. evaluated the scientific evidence of the effectiveness of orthopedic treatment with the use of facial mask, chip cup, Frankel 3, and Bionator, among others. The results described over 75% of success of treatment with rapid maxillary expansion (RME) and facial mask therapy at a follow-up observation 5 years after the end of orthopedic therapy. Regarding other therapies, they could not find enough evidence about the success and stability of the treatment [11]. Other authors have found similar findings [5, 12]. Recently, with the advance of skeletal anchorage using miniscrews, the combined treatments using bone anchorage and mechanic appliances have showed positive results [13]. However, this kind of treatments is used to be indicated for mixed dentition patient.

1.2. Early Vision of the Therapeutics of Anterior Crossbites. It is important that parents have children checked early for anterior crossbite treatment. Therapy should be directed toward the elimination of the etiological and conditioning factors that can contribute to anterior crossbite [14] since it interferes with the down and forward growth and displacement of the maxilla [5]. This early correction can reduce the need for further treatments (maxillary orthopedics, orthodontics, and/or maxillofacial surgery) and can allow for more optimal psychological and social development [15]. In anterior crossbites, the occlusal plane tends toward convergence with respect to the Camper plane, causing a more open angle between these planes and upsetting the balance of one of the laws of Planas in craniofacial growth.

1.3. Therapeutic Objectives in Early Treatment of Anterior Crossbite. The objectives of the treatment of anterior crossbites are (1) to achieve a normal overjet and generate changes in the neuromuscular activity of the chewing muscles while at rest and in function, (2) to influence the position of the condyle in the glenoid cavity, (3) to restore the posture and position of the craniocervical-hyoid complex, (4) to produce changes in the control of the morphogenetic and tissue rotation of the maxilla [16] and the mandible [17], (5) to control the position and pressure of the tongue in the orofacial apparatus, (6) to allow homeostasis in the maxillomandibular growth when there are discrepancies between them, (7) to make the centric occlusion coincide with the centric relation, thereby eliminating the occlusal or functional deflection, and (8) to attempt to parallelize the occlusal plane to the Camper plane [18]. To achieve this, we must try to achieve ideal function by changing the position of the mandible and the pattern of mandibular movements and by improving masticatory muscle activity and mandibular dynamics [19]. The clinician can explore therapeutic variables to reestablish a harmonic occlusion, such as selective cutting and/or the use of direct tracks.

Direct tracks, designed and developed by Dr. Pedro Planas [20], are a good therapeutic option in deciduous dentition and have been used in the molar sector to therapeutically restore the occlusal plane [21]. They are made with resins or acrylic of resins or acrylic of lesser and greater consistencies and strengths. Therapeutically, it is designed to generate a physiological occlusal plane with movements of laterality with freedom that allows neural excitation, rehabilitating the maxillofacial growth vectors and the function of the temporomandibular joint in the mandibular dynamics.

Contact surfaces are created between the upper and lower arches to occlude in the usual position and allow the most appropriate mandibular sliding. They aid in the anterior or posterior reposition of the mandible (depending on the inclination of the tracks) in retroposition, laterognatism, or in mandibular protrusion, and they allow rotation of the jaw in a clockwise direction. Additionally, they prevent the establishment of morphological and positional asymmetries in the maxillofacial complex in children [22]. These tracks are preserved until the molars are replaced.

Likewise, flat tracks, according to Simoes [18], rehabilitate the masticatory function and improve the contact surfaces and rub at the posterior level, stimulating growth at the transverse level of the jaws and allowing sagittal synchronized growth between the jaws. The following clinical case shows the development and use of the direct tracks proposed by Dr. Planas and clinically adapted by Dr. Simoes for the early treatment of anterior and posterior crossbites with one modification: they are placed on the anterior teeth.

There is no scientific data regarding the use of direct tracks in the anterior deciduous teeth as part of early treatment of anterior crossbites. The clinical approach of this type of therapy can contribute to the early management of these alterations as an option in the prevention of skeletal class III malocclusions.

2. Case Presentation

Patient, four years old, was brought to consultation for presenting anterior crossbite that, according to the mother, began with the eruption of deciduous incisors.

During clinical evaluation, the patient presented a concave profile (Figure 1). Complete deciduous dentition with molar and canine class III relationships at 1 mm, an OJ of -1.5 mm, and an OB of 50% were observed (Figure 2).

The lateral cephalometric radiograph was taken in maximum intercuspidation and a hyperdivergent class III

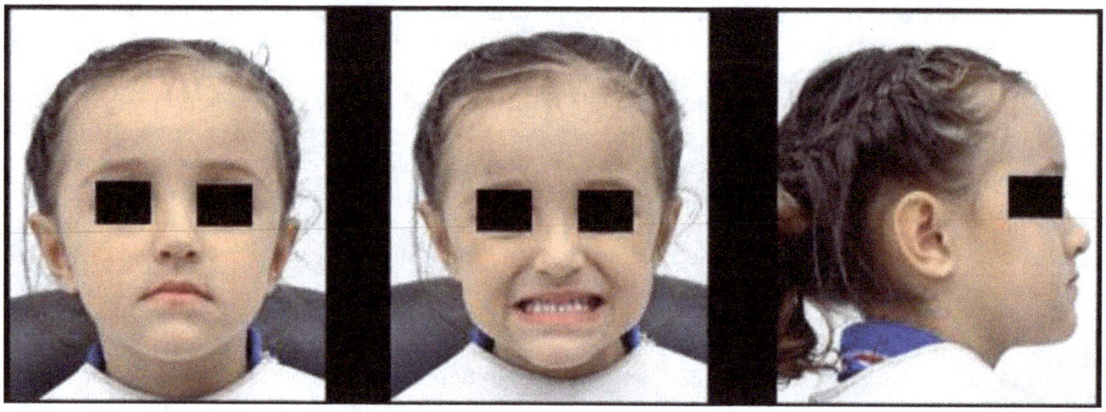

FIGURE 1: Extraoral photos.

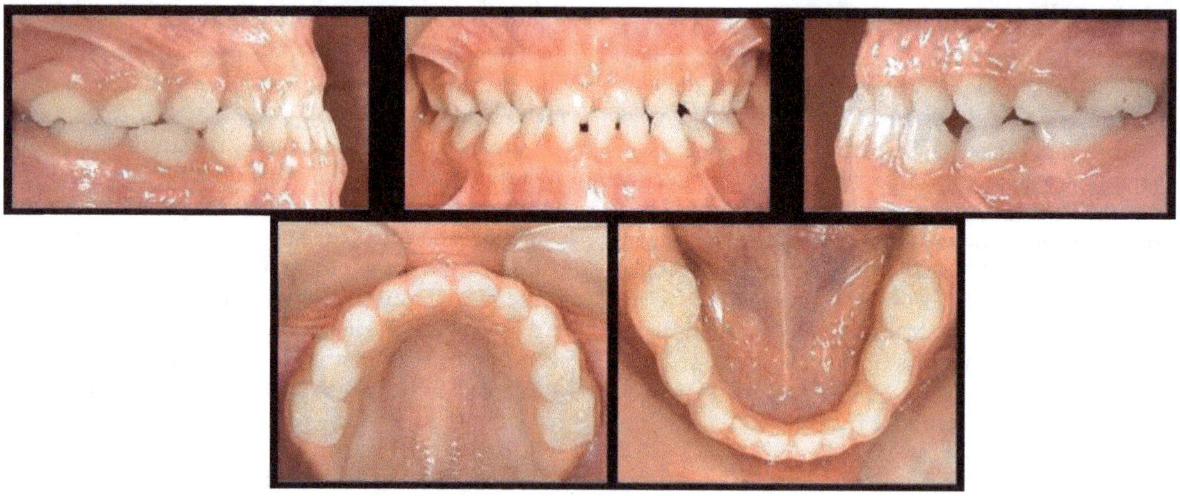

FIGURE 2: Intraoral findings.

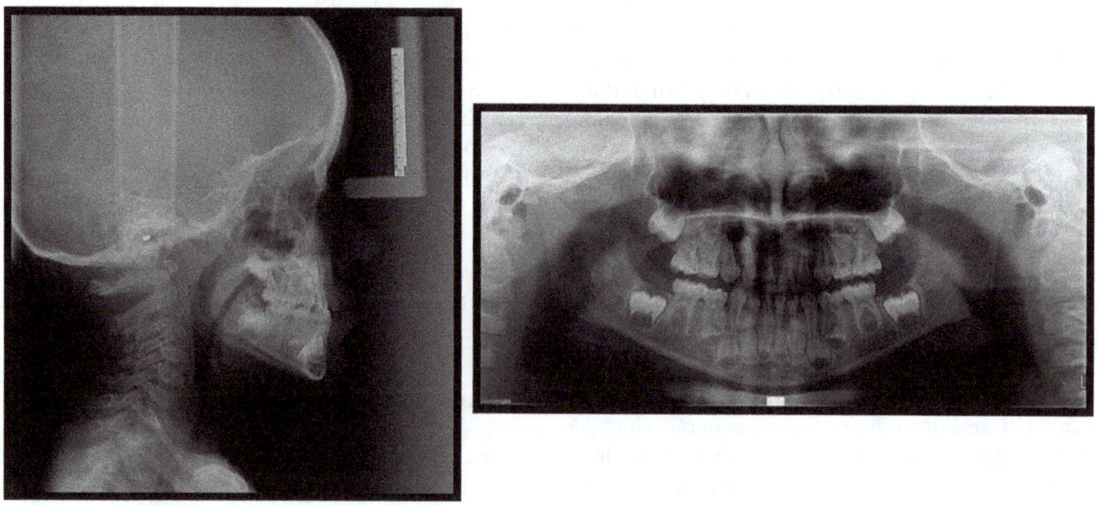

FIGURE 3: Extraoral X-rays.

relationship with decreased ANB angle and increased mandibular body length was found. The findings of panoramic radiography were normal (Figure 3).

After a functional evaluation, the patient mandible was manipulated and carried to the front edge-to-edge relationship, and an anterior deflection with a left side deviation of

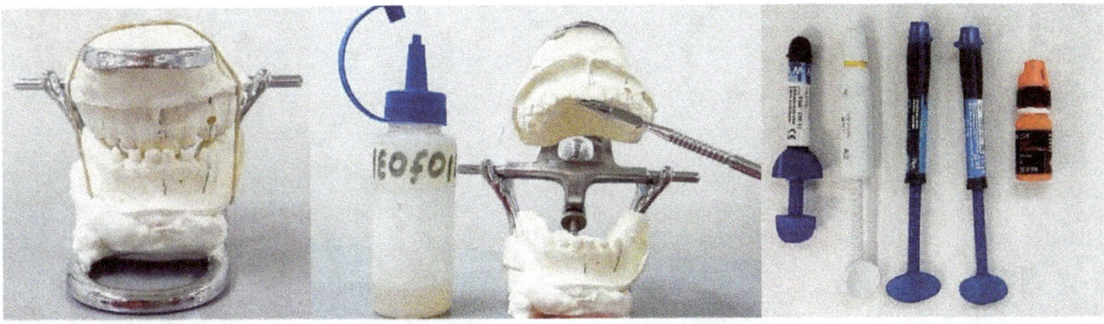

FIGURE 4: Preparing the track construction.

the lower midline of 2 mm was observed. A diagnosis of pseudo-class III was made, as well as a decision to use cemented anterior direct tracks.

2.1. Impression, Bite Register, and Laboratory Procedures. For the construction of the tracks, upper and lower impressions must be taken. The bite registration must be as retrusive as the mandible can be. Then, it must be mounted on a hinge articulator. Once assembled on the articulator, the buccal and palatal surface of the anterior superior teeth must be isolated with insulating material (neo foil) (Figure 4).

On the vestibular surface of the four upper incisors, individual veneers are made on each of the anterior teeth with hybrid resin with microfiller with the following specifications:

1. The incisal edge should have a thickness of 2.5 to 4 mm to prevent the closing path from being anterior. Its thickness depends on the previous slip between centric relation and centric occlusion
2. Extend 1-2 mm on the incisal in the model to create the closure guide, thickening it more towards the buccal and, at the same time, taking the incisal third towards the palatal covering with resin with a minimum possible thickness depending on the patient's closure to give a larger surface of retention to the veneer. On the laterals, make a rounded distoincisal angle to allow the patient's lateroprotrusive to be free
3. Cover the interproximal surfaces as far as the buccal surface with a razor-edge finish between the tooth surface and the resin without generating dental plaque entrapment and creating the risk of interproximal caries
4. At the gingival level, there should be a thickness of 0.5 mm, finished with a chamfer or knife edge to avoid the accumulation of dental plaque and the risk of cervical caries
5. Evaluate the closing trajectory in the articulator so that the four upper anterior teeth are left with a determinate area (DA) constructed, as much as possible, so that the patient is left without anterior crossbite (Figure 5)

2.2. Clinical Procedure: Cementation. The clinical procedure is described as follows:

1. Use prophylaxis with bicarbonate on the surfaces of the anterior teeth to remove impurities at the level of the enamel of the teeth that will serve as anchorage
2. Demineralize the surfaces of the deciduous that will serve as receptors for direct tracks with orthophosphoric acid for 30 seconds. Wash demineralized areas profusely
3. Dry the surfaces of the anterior teeth and check that the surface is white with chalk and matt tone
4. Apply bonding agent according to the manufacturer's instructions required to make the veneers on the surfaces that will serve as receptors, pass the dental floss through the interproximal surfaces, and apply the light of the curing lamp according to the manufacturer's specifications to polymerize the bonding agent
5. Apply fluid resin to each of the veneers and treat each tooth individually according to tracks designed for each tooth. Remove the excess resin from surfaces, including palatal extensions with tracks and light cures
6. Verify excess material resins at both incisal, interproximal, and cervical areas, and polish any excess resin with a finishing bur. Use metal sandpaper on the interproximal area and polish the remaining points. Keep the anatomy as similar as possible to the natural receiving teeth. Remember that the endings of the resin with the dental surfaces must be razor-sharp and have no sites that can retain dental plaque
7. Examine the lateral, protrusive, and lateroprotrusive movements. In the protrusive, the four anterior teeth should make contact to prevent fracture or the failure of the direct tracks. When doing lateral movements, there should be a disocclusion canine or group, guided by the canine and molars, that does not interfere with the anterior teeth. In lateroprotrusive movements, the distoincisal angle should be rounded to avoid interference in movement

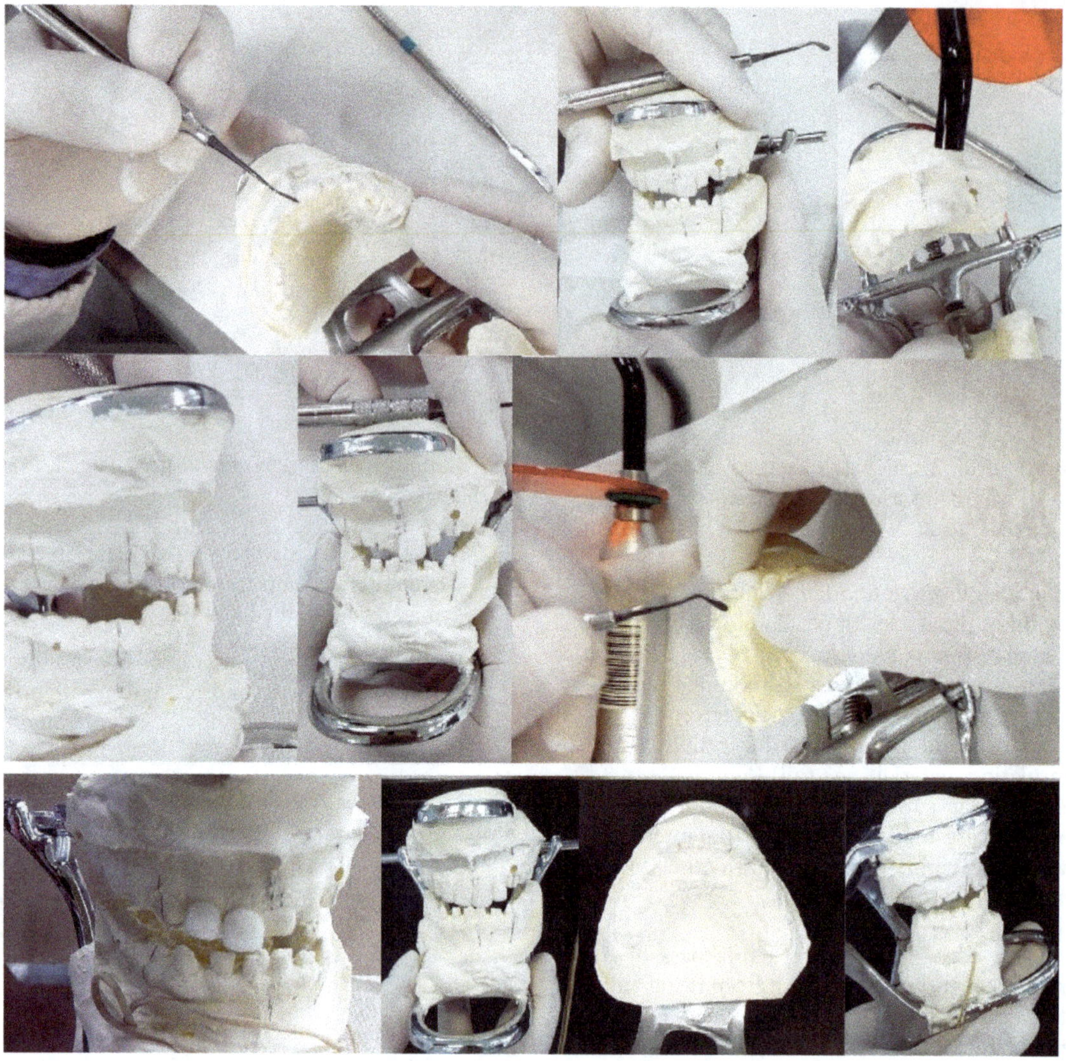

Figure 5: Laboratory procedures.

8. An angular carving of 15 degrees or more should be made between the incisal edge towards the palatal if the occlusion allows for a posterior closure guide, so that the lower anterior teeth slide behind the upper anterior teeth when making the closure and achieve the DA necessary to provide the principles of neural excitation at the dental level (Figures 6(a)–6(f))

2.3. Controls. It should be made clear that during the first week the patient will have nocturnal bruxism because the vertical dimension has been increased and there is little, if any, contact in the posterior part to allow the eruption of the molars to generate a new therapeutic occlusal plane and let the jaw slide later.

Further treatment begins with periodic review appointments, the first 2-3 weeks later, and then every month. If the tracks are restored, and if necessary, the inclination of the incisal edge track towards the palatal should be prolonged and the incisal edge of the enamel can be worn to guarantee the maintenance of the DA and the mandibular position behind the maxilla.

Verify oral hygiene and reinforce oral preventive measures.

As therapeutic results and patient responses to treatment are evaluated, therapy can be reinforced with functional and orthopedic appliances.

With time, the posterior teeth will become extruded, there will be a correction in the occlusion, and the open bite will be closed. The overjet will be improved with stable and acceptable functional and aesthetic results. From the aesthetic point of view, there will be improvement in the smile line and in the exposition of incisors at rest and in sleep, and from the functional point of view, the anterior deflection will be eliminated and the appropriate occlusal function will be restored (Figures 7 and 8). The anterior direct tracks are left in position until the anterior deciduous teeth are exfoliated, controlling so that a posterior occlusion is established promoting occlusal stability. The time for the new occlusal relationships to be established was 6 months.

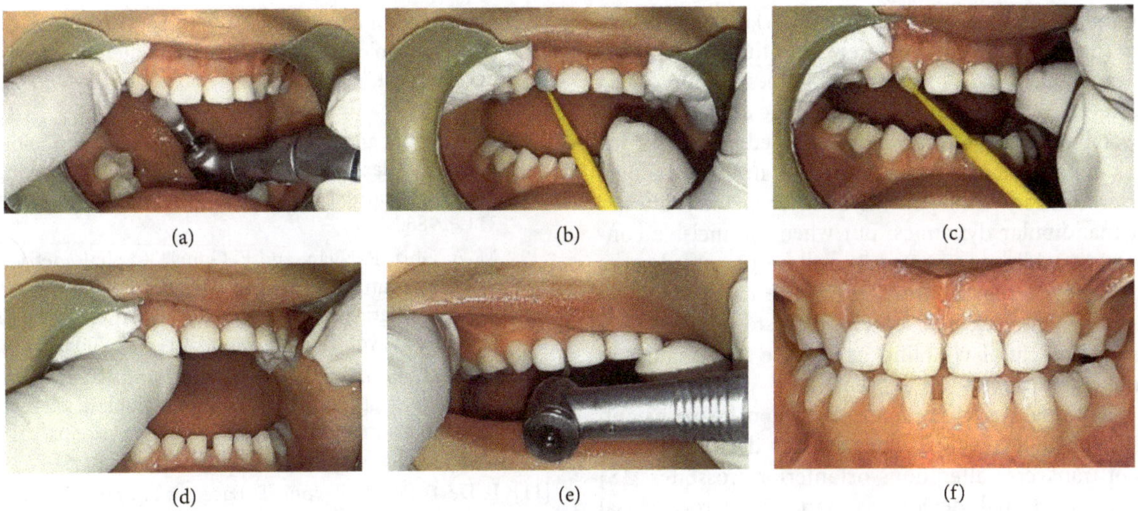

FIGURE 6: Cementation and immediate track intraoral photos.

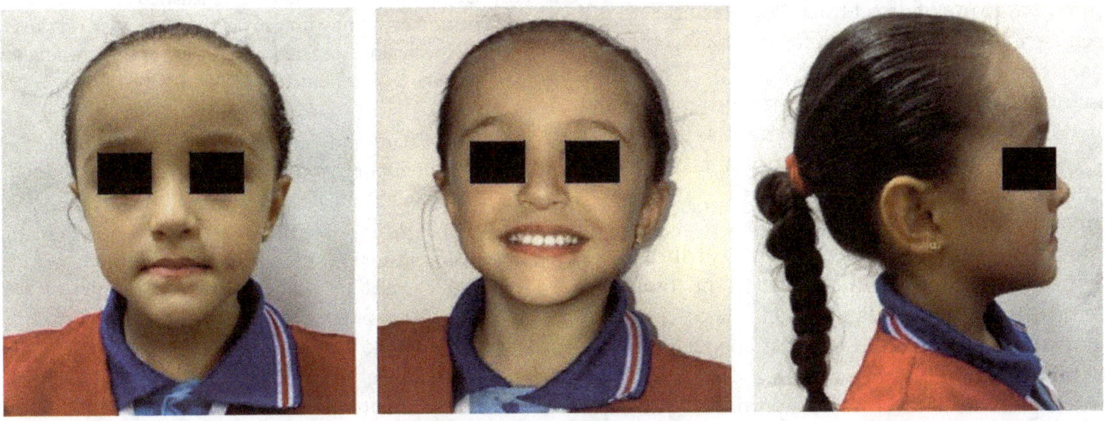

FIGURE 7: Three-month posttreatment extraoral photo.

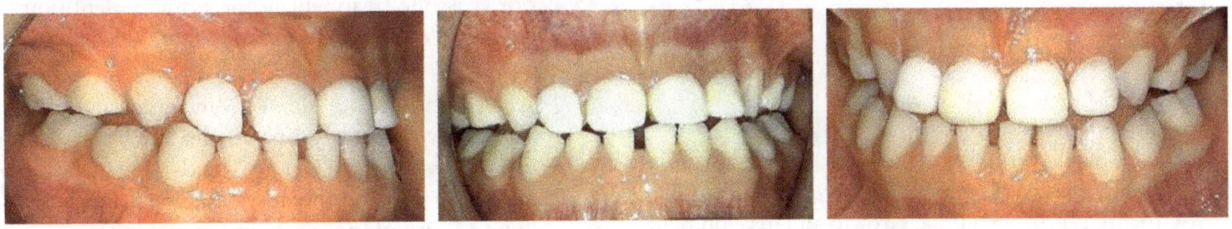

FIGURE 8: Three-month posttreatment intraoral photo.

3. Discussion

Early management of class III malocclusions has been shown to have substantial influence on long-term outcome and treatment prognosis, and it has been suggested that there are short-term effects as well [23]. The sooner that results are obtained, the more efficient and stable the treatment will bc [24]. This case describes the management of a class III malocclusion in a patient with deciduous dentition with the goal of creating a new occlusal plane, an adequate determinate area (DA) incisor contact, and the promotion of mandibular rotation by means of anterior direct tracks [18].

Although management with removable orthopedic appliances is effective, fixed treatment that promotes the establishment of a new mandibular position is another good therapeutic option.

Balance of the stomatognathic system structures is achieved through the aforementioned neural excitation and physiological or therapeutic mandibular posture changes [25], principles on which the techniques developed by researchers of functional appliances, such as Balters [26], Planas, Bimler, and Frankel [27], are based. These techniques act as bimaxillary by modifying the position of the jaw to obtain better and faster clinical results. Functional orthopedic devices can modify the nociceptive reflexes, favoring the development of new circuits of neuronal reflexes [18]. The results are most effective when initiating position change and when contact between deciduous incisors or between permanent teeth in the determined area (DA) are established. However, the change must be made within the physiological limits of each individual. According to Simoes, if this contact is not achieved, it makes the evolution of the chosen therapy less predictable and produces a more reserved prognosis due to the lack of neural excitement. Alterations in closure trajectory can produce instability in the condyle in the joint and deficient mandibular dynamics. But when the incisive contact (DA) is established, the results will be perceived more quickly in the efferent neuronal response component. In early management, selective carvings must be made that interfere with occlusal coupling or achieve this change in therapeutic posture [18].

The traditional tracks are made of composite resins and cemented with fluid resins in the posterior deciduous teeth in cases of transverse alterations or anterior crossbites [18] and act as functional devices as part of neuro-occlusal rehabilitation, allow returning functionality to the patient, and improve their aesthetic appearance.

Based on this, the use of direct tracks in anterior teeth is a novel and efficient therapeutic option for the management of class III malocclusions.

The use of previous direct tracks allows better marginal adaptation, visibility, and patient management, as well as better oral hygiene. Likewise, the aesthetic impact is immediate, restoring confidence and facial harmony to the patient.

It is important to remark that since upper posterior collapse and posterior crossbite problems are usually presented in class III, the evaluation and management of the transverse plane are fundamental in the treatment. In this case, specifically, the upper transversal width was just adequate but the progress of this finding needs supervision.

This article presents a novel way of approaching occlusal therapy, solving class III functional malocclusion in a simple, fast, and economical way. It may be an adequate therapeutic alternative for clinicians.

References

[1] A. Bjork and V. Skieller, *Informationen aus Orthodontie und Kieferorthopadie : mit Beitragen aus der internationalen Literatur*, vol. 16, no. 1, pp. 9–52, 1984, Growth and development of the maxillary complex.

[2] A. Bjork, "Prediction of mandibular growth rotation," *American Journal of Orthodontics*, vol. 55, no. 6, pp. 585–599, 1969.

[3] T. Graber, T. Rakosi, and A. Petrovic, *Ortopedia dentofacial con aparatos funcionales, Segunda*, Mosby, Madrid, 1998.

[4] P. Ngan and W. Moon, "Evolution of Class III treatment in orthodontics," *American Journal of Orthodontics and Dentofacial Orthopedics*, vol. 148, no. 1, pp. 22–36, 2015.

[5] S. C. Woon and B. Thiruvenkatachari, "Early orthodontic treatment for Class III malocclusion: A systematic review and meta-analysis," *American Journal of Orthodontics and Dentofacial Orthopedics*, vol. 151, no. 1, pp. 28–52, 2017.

[6] P. Ngan, "Early Timely Treatment of Class III Malocclusion," *Seminars in Orthodontics*, vol. 11, no. 3, pp. 140–145, 2005.

[7] B. Thilander, L. Pena, C. Infante, S. S. Parada, and C. de Mayorga, "Prevalence of malocclusion and orthodontic treatment need in children and adolescents in Bogota, Colombia. An epidemiological study related to different stages of dental development," *European Journal of Orthodontics*, vol. 23, no. 2, pp. 153–168, 2001.

[8] S. Williams and C. E. A. Aarhus, "The morphology of the potential Class III skeletal pattern in the growing child," *American Journal of Orthodontics*, vol. 89, no. 4, pp. 302–311, 1986.

[9] M. A. Ghiz, P. Ngan, and E. Gunel, "Cephalometric variables to predict future success of early orthopedic Class III treatment," *American Journal of Orthodontics and Dentofacial Orthopedics*, vol. 127, no. 3, pp. 301–306, 2005.

[10] C. Maspero, G. Galbiati, L. Giannini, and G. Farronato, "Sagittal and vertical effects of transverse sagittal maxillary expander (TSME) in three different malocclusion groups," *Progress in Orthodontics*, vol. 16, no. 1, 2015.

[11] L. De Toffol, C. Pavoni, T. Baccetti, L. Franchi, and P. Cozza, "Orthopedic Treatment Outcomes in Class III Malocclusion," *Angle Orthodontist*, vol. 78, no. 3, pp. 561–573, 2008.

[12] G. Cordasco, G. Matarese, L. Rustico et al., "Efficacy of orthopedic treatment with protraction facemask on skeletal Class III malocclusion: a systematic review and meta-analysis," *Orthodontics & Craniofacial Research*, vol. 17, no. 3, pp. 133–143, 2014.

[13] H. P. Chang and Y. C. Tseng, "Miniscrew implant applications in contemporary orthodontics," *Kaohsiung Journal of Medical Sciences*, vol. 30, no. 3, pp. 111–115, 2014.

[14] I. Tollaro, T. Baccetti, V. Bassarelli, and L. Franchi, "Class III malocclusion in the deciduous dentition: a morphological and correlation study," *European Journal of Orthodontics*, vol. 16, no. 5, pp. 401–408, 1994.

[15] E. Zere, P. K. Chaudhari, J. Saran, K. Dhingra, and N. Tiwari, "Developing Class III malocclusions: Challenges and solutions," *Clinical, Cosmetic and Investigational Dentistry*, vol. - Volume 10, pp. 99–116, 2018.

[16] H. C. F. Pereira da Silva, J. B. de Paiva, and J. Rino Neto, "Anterior crossbite treatment in the primary dentition: Three case reports," *International Orthodontics*, vol. 16, no. 3, pp. 514–529, 2018.

[17] T. Deguchi, T. Kuroda, Y. Minoshima, and T. M. Graber, "Craniofacial features of patients with Class III abnormalities: Growth-related changes and effects of short-term and long-term chincup therapy," *American Journal of Orthodontics and Dentofacial Orthopedics*, vol. 121, no. 1, pp. 84–92, 2002.

[18] W. A. Simoes, *Ortopedia funcional de los maxilares a travès de la rehabilitaciòn neuro-oclusal*, Artes Médicas, 3rd ed. edition, 2004.

[19] S. E. Bishara and R. R. Ziaja, "Functional appliances: a review," *American Journal of Orthodontics and Dentofacial Orthopedics*, vol. 95, no. 3, pp. 250–258, 1989.

[20] P. Planas, *Rehabilitación Neuro-Oclusal (RNO)*, pp. 179–194, 2008, 2a ed..

[21] J. Hernandez, D. Gaviria, E. Londoño, C. Llano, and M. C. Llano, "Dimensional changes of the deciduous dental arch class I with crowding, using direct planas tracks. Medellin 2012-2013," *CES Odontología*, vol. 27, no. 2, pp. 26–35, 2014.

[22] G. O. Ramirez-Yañez, "Planas direct tracks for early crossbite correction," *Journal of clinical orthodontics : JCO*, vol. 37, no. 6, pp. 294–298, 2003.

[23] R. S. D. Smyth and F. S. Ryan, "Early treatment of class III malocclusion with facemask," *Evidence-Based Dentistry*, vol. 18, no. 4, pp. 107-108, 2017.

[24] K. Kajiyama, T. Murakami, and A. Suzuki, "Comparison of orthodontic and orthopedic effects of a modified maxillary protractor between deciduous and early mixed dentitions," *American Journal of Orthodontics and Dentofacial Orthopedics*, vol. 126, no. 1, pp. 23–32, 2004.

[25] P. Ngan, A. M. Hu, and H. W. Fields Jr, "Treatment of Class III problems begins with differential diagnosis of anterior crossbites," *Pediatric Dentistry*, vol. 19, no. 6, pp. 386–395, 1997.

[26] P. Cozza, A. Marino, and M. Mucedero, "An orthopaedic approach to the treatment of Class III malocclusions in the early mixed dentition," *European Journal of Orthodontics*, vol. 26, no. 2, pp. 191–199, 2004.

[27] X. Yang, C. Li, D. Bai et al., "Treatment effectiveness of Fränkel function regulator on the Class III malocclusion: A systematic review and meta-analysis," *American Journal of Orthodontics and Dentofacial Orthopedics*, vol. 146, no. 2, pp. 143–154, 2014.

21

A New Appliance for Class III Treatment in Growing Patients: Pushing Splints 3

Stefano Martina,[1] Roberto Martina,[2] Lorenzo Franchi,[3] Vincenzo D'Antò,[2] and Rosa Valletta[2]

[1]*Department of Medicine, Surgery and Dentistry, "Scuola Medica Salernitana", University of Salerno, Via Allende, 84081 Baronissi, Italy*
[2]*School of Orthodontics, Department of Neurosciences, Reproductive Sciences and Oral Sciences, University of Naples Federico II, Via Pansini 5, 80131 Naples, Italy*
[3]*Department of Experimental and Clinical Medicine, University of Florence, Largo Brambilla 3, 50134 Florence, Italy*

Correspondence should be addressed to Stefano Martina; smartina@unisa.it

Academic Editor: Wasiu L. Adeyemo

Several orthopedic procedures have been used in early treatment to reduce the need for orthognathic surgery in skeletal Class III. The most used treatment is Rapid Maxillary Expansion and Facemask. This procedure also determines a clockwise rotation of the mandible, increasing the vertical dimensions of the lower third of the face. Therefore, the control of vertical dimension appears to be a key objective in Class III hyperdivergent patients. This article shows two skeletal Class III patients treated with a new appliance (Pushing Splints 3), that is able to correct sagittal discrepancy with a good control of the vertical growth. In both cases, Class I relationship with a proper Overjet and Overbite was achieved with improvement of profile. The final cephalometric values demonstrated a stable sagittal relationship and a good control of the vertical growth. The specific biomechanic features of the PS3 appliance permit the improvement of the sagittal jaw relationship, delivering at the same time vertical vectors that are able to control the alveolar and skeletal components of the vertical growth. This could be useful in the treatment of Class III hyperdivergent patients.

1. Introduction

Skeletal Class III is one of the most challenging malocclusions for the orthodontist. The skeletal and dental components of Class III malocclusions are usually present since early childhood [1], and an early treatment is usually suggested to avoid or to reduce the need for an orthognathic surgery [2].

Several orthopedic procedures have been used to reach this purpose in early treatment such as Fränkel III [3], chin cup [4], mandibular reverse headgear, and bone-anchored maxillary protraction [5].

Currently, the most frequently used treatment procedure involves the combination of Rapid Maxillary Expansion and Facemask [6, 7], but there is still a need of high-quality evidence about the effectiveness of this treatment, particularly regarding long-term stability [8]. On the contrary, many authors demonstrated that the desired forward movement of the maxilla is accompanied by a downward mandibular movement which also determines a clockwise rotation of the mandible. The overall effect appears to be an increase in vertical dimensions of the lower third of the face that is obviously inappropriate for patients with increased vertical skeletal relationships [8].

Therefore, the control of vertical dimension appears to be a key objective in Class III hyperdivergent patients.

This article describes the use of a modified version of the SEC appliance originally presented by Ferro et al. [9].

2. Appliance Design

The appliance (Pushing Splints 3, PS3) consists of three components: two acrylic splints and a Forsus™ L-pin module per side.

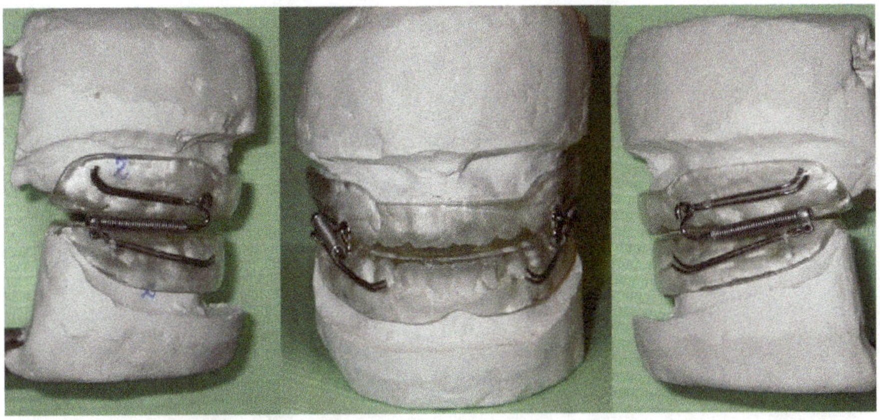

FIGURE 1: PS3 appliance.

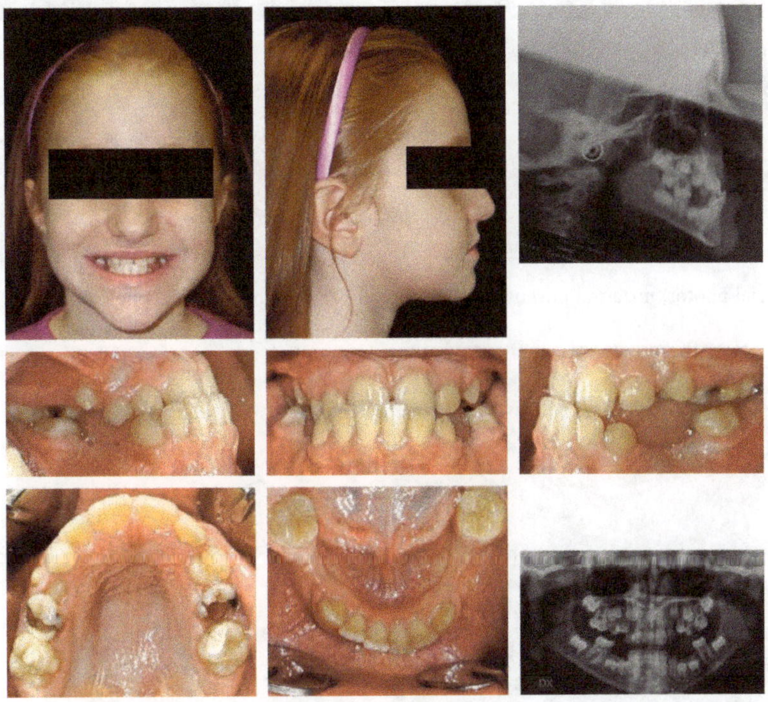

FIGURE 2: Case no. 1 facial photos, intraoral photos, panoramic radiograph, and lateral cephalogram at T_0 (pretreatment).

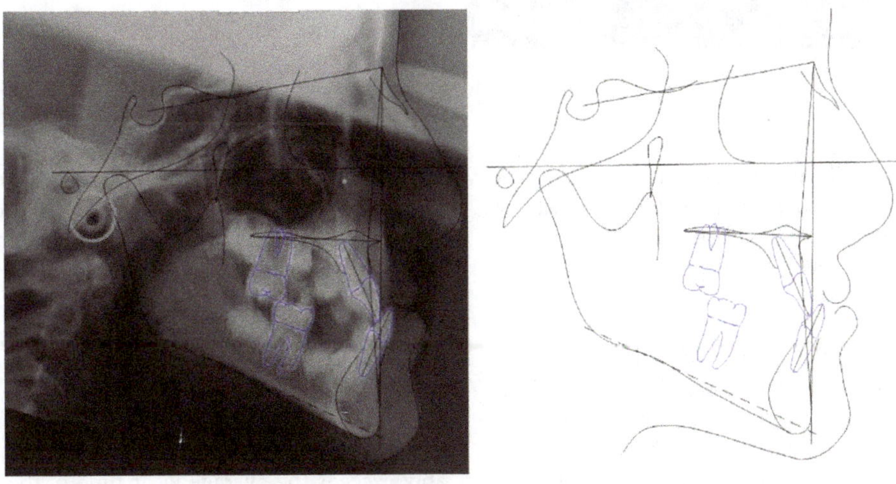

FIGURE 3: Case no. 1 tracings (pretreatment).

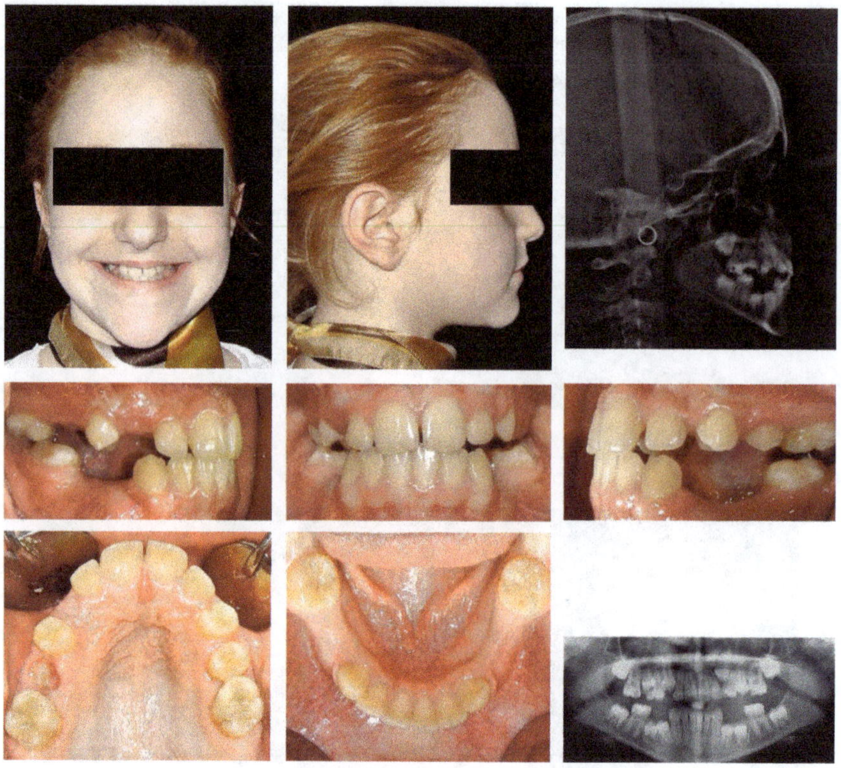

FIGURE 4: Case no. 1 facial photos, intraoral photos, panoramic radiograph, and lateral cephalogram at T_1 (after PS3 treatment).

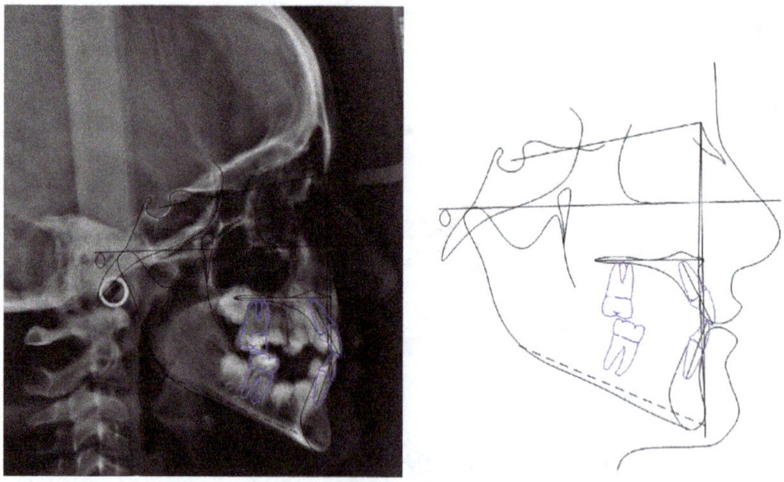

FIGURE 5: Case no. 1 tracings at T_1.

The two splints are built-up through a traditional acrylic appliance construction procedure by a dental technician. A 2 mm high construction bite is used in order to leave the space necessary to have a flat occlusal plane on both of the splints.

The two splints cover all the tooth crowns—usually from the left first permanent molar to the right first permanent molar 6 to 6—in both arches. The Forsus™ L-pin modules are used in order to deliver a force of 200 g per side in a forward direction to the upper splint and in a backward direction to the lower splint. In an opposite way from Class III elastics, the vertical component of the force delivered by the Forsus™ L-pin module is directed upward and forward in the maxilla and downward and backward in the mandible (Figure 1). Working with a pushing system is important to obtain a good retention of the splint even if some grinding is needed now and then to avoid interference with the eruption of permanent teeth.

However, the really important advantage of PS3's force system is the control of the vertical growth.

Patients are instructed to use the splints as much as possible, with a minimum time of 14 hours per day, which probably exceeds the average wear time of the Facemask, whose wearing is certainly more invasive than the intraoral splints.

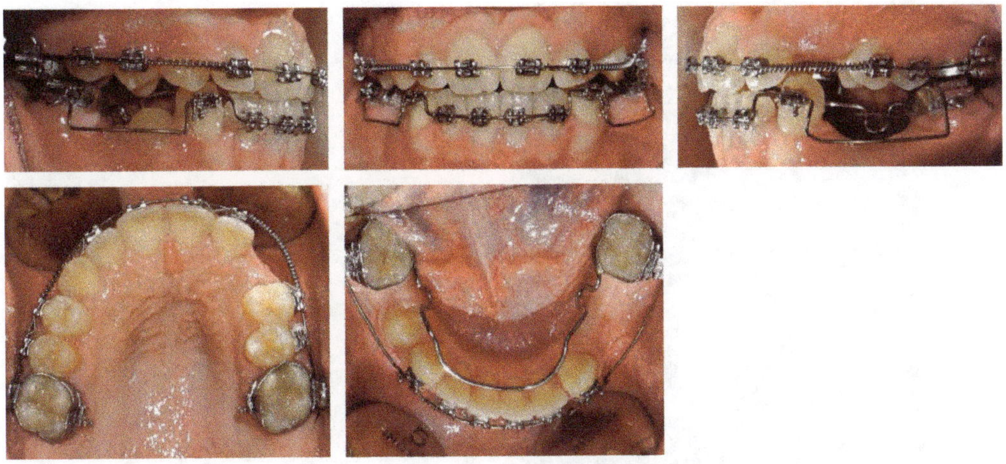

FIGURE 6: Case no. 1 fixed appliance phase.

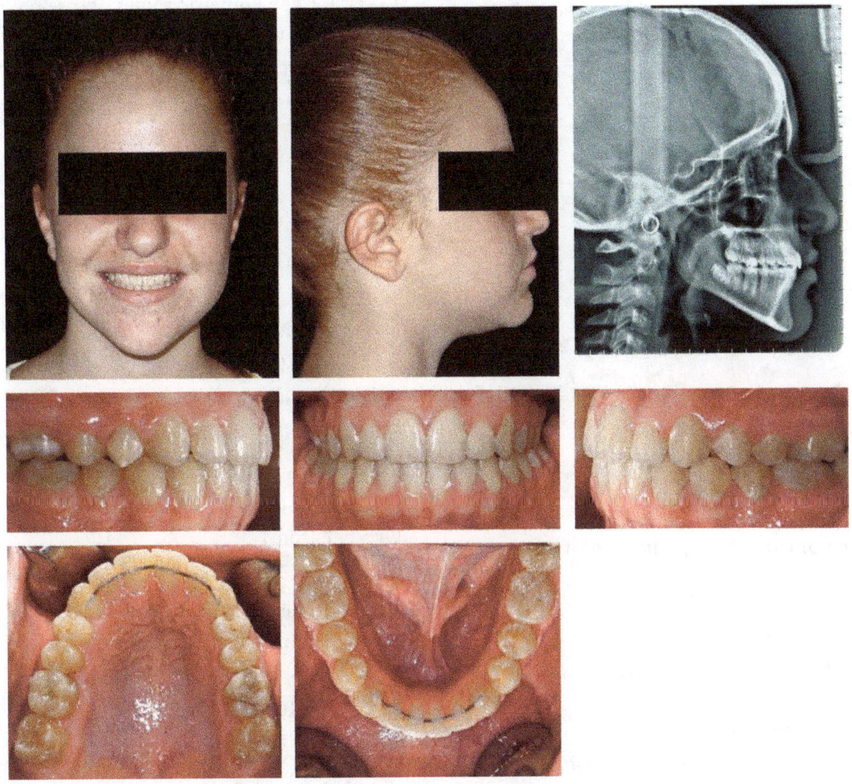

FIGURE 7: Case no. 1 facial photos, intraoral photos, and lateral cephalogram at T_2 (posttreatment).

3. Case Report No. 1

The patient was an 8.0-year-old female with a Class III dental and skeletal (A-N-Pg = −4.5°) malocclusion. A bilateral posterior crossbite and a midline discrepancy were also present. Due to decay, 7.4, 7.5, 8.4, and 8.5 were extracted (Figure 2).

The increased value of the Sn-GoGn angle (33 degrees) showed a tendency to a hyperdivergent vertical skeletal relationship that was also demonstrated by the condyle neck morphology (Figure 3).

The main treatment objective was to correct the Class III growth pattern. Because of the increased vertical growth, an important treatment objective was also to control the hyperdivergency.

In order to control the vertical growth usually increased by this kind of treatment, a PS3 appliance was used in the orthopedic phase.

The treatment time with the PS3 was 13 months. The appliance was reactivated after 6 months adding a split crimp (1.5 mm) to the push rod bilaterally. The upper splint was once relined to increase its stability.

After the orthopedic phase of the treatment, the profile greatly improved. Normal values of Overjet and Overbite were also achieved. A tendency to a Class III molar relationship was

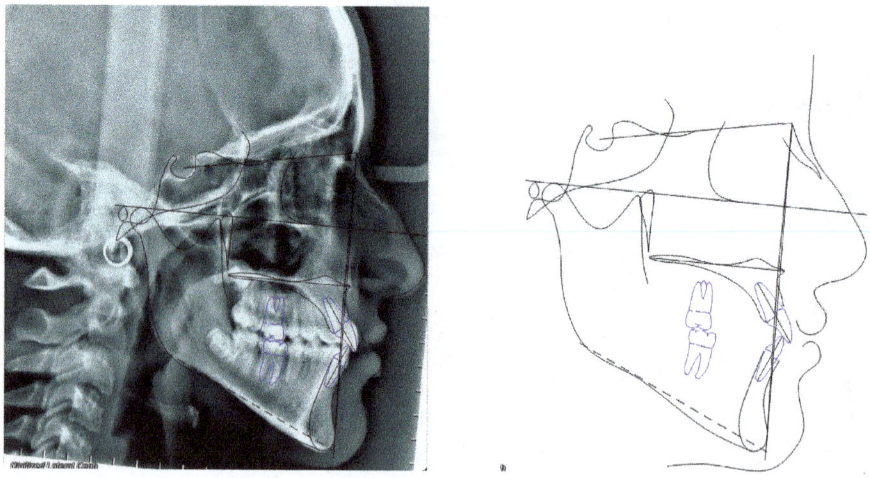

FIGURE 8: Case no. 1 tracings at T_2.

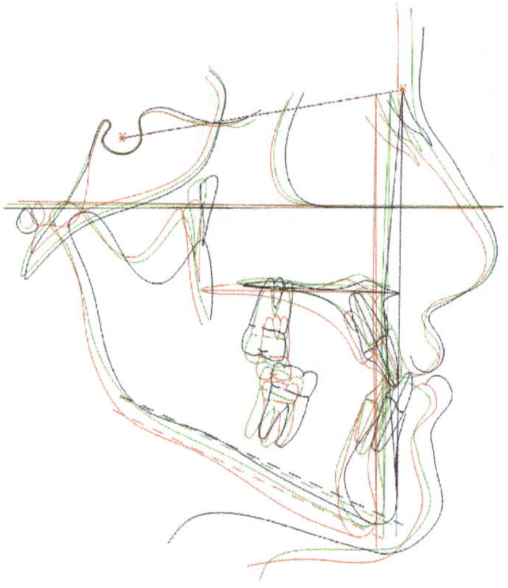

FIGURE 9: Case no. 1 tracing superimpositions.

TABLE 1: Cephalometric values of case no. 1 before treatment, after PS3 treatment, and at the end of fixed appliance treatment.

Values	Initial	Progress	Final
SNA (°)	75.2	77.9	79.8
S-N-Pg (°)	79.7	79.6	80.6
A-N-Pg (°)	-4.5	-1.7	-0.8
Co-Gn (mm)	113.6	115.9	117.6
Co-Go (mm)	48.6	51.9	54.9
Co-Go-Me (°)	131.9	136.3	134.3
S-N/ANS-PNS (°)	12.2	10.6	10.1
S-N/Go-Gn (°)	33.0	33.6	34.0
ANS-PNS/Go-Gn (°)	23.3	25.8	26.0
U1-ANS-PNS (°)	117.5	115.9	125.0
L1-Go-Gn (°)	92.1	87.7	90.7
Overjet (mm)	-3.9	2.0	2.7
Overbite (mm)	4.2	0.6	1.7

still present on the right side due to the lower first molar mesial shift because of the early extraction of deciduous molars (Figure 4).

The sagittal relationship improved (A-N-Pg angle value from -4.5 to -1.7 degrees) and the hyperdivergent growth pattern was under control (Sn-GoGn angle 33.6 degrees) (Figure 5).

Fixed appliances were progressively bonded to both arches with MBT prescription. Bilateral Class III elastics and box elastics with a Class III component were shortly used in the last phase to reach the final occlusion. The fixed appliance phase lasted 24 months as a consequence of the delayed time of 3.4 and 3.5 eruption (Figure 6).

A Class I relationship with a proper Overjet and Overbite was achieved. A straight nice profile with a good vertical proportion was also maintained after the pubertal growth spurt (Figure 7).

The final cephalometric values demonstrated a stable sagittal relationship (ANPg angle -0.8 degree), a good control of the vertical growth also in this phase of treatment (Sn-GoGn angle 34 degrees), and nearly no dental compensation of the lower incisors (Figures 8 and 9) (Table 1).

4. Case Report No. 2

The patient was an 8.9-year-old female with a Class III dental and skeletal (A-N-Pg = −1.0 degree) malocclusion. A negative Overjet (-1.4 mm) and Overbite (-3.7 mm) were present. A bilateral posterior crossbite was also present (Figure 10).

The increased value of the Sn-GoGn angle (43.7 degrees) showed a severe vertical growth pattern. The mandible morphology confirmed a severe structural hyperdivergency (Figure 11).

The profile also corroborates both the skeletal component of the Class III malocclusion and the increased vertical skeletal relationship.

As in the previous case, the treatment objective was to improve the skeletal Class III relationship and to control the hyperdivergency.

An interceptive orthopedic treatment plan with PS3 was proposed with the aim of improving the sagittal skeletal

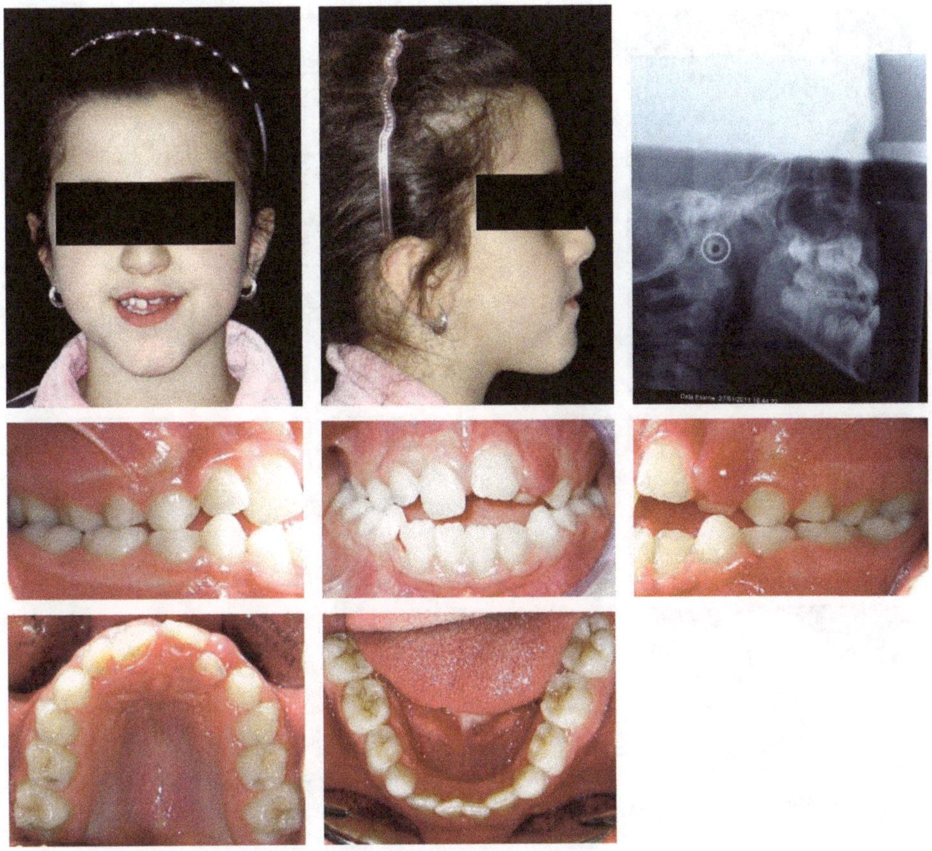

FIGURE 10: Case no. 2 facial photos, intraoral photos, panoramic radiograph, and lateral cephalogram at T_0 (pretreatment).

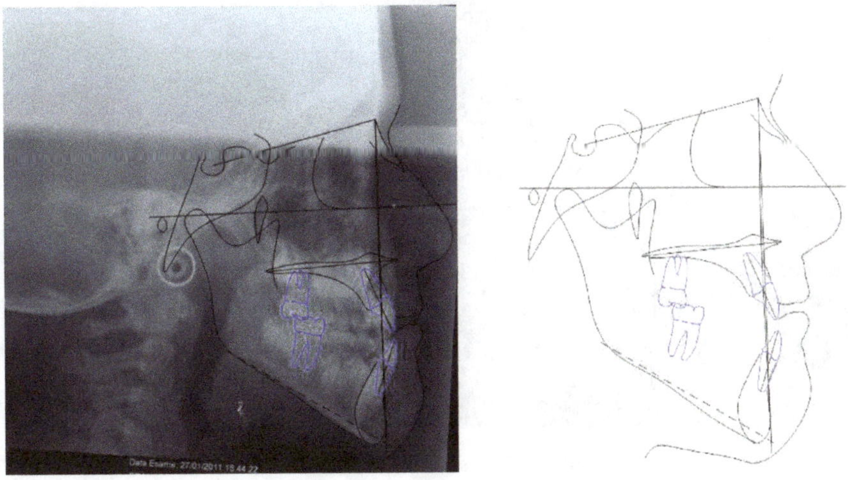

FIGURE 11: Case no. 2 tracings (pretreatment).

relationship and to control at the same time the vertical dimension.

The treatment time with the PS3 was 16 months. The appliance was reactivated after 6 and 12 months adding a split crimp (1.5 mm) to the push rod bilaterally. The upper splint was once relined to increase its stability.

After the orthopedic phase of treatment, the profile greatly improved. An overcorrection of the Overjet was obtained (6.7 mm) while the open bite was still present (-2.0 mm). A full Class II molar relationship was reached on the left side, while an edge-to-edge relationship was present on the right side (Figure 12).

The sagittal relationship improved (ANPg angle value from -1 to 1.3 degrees). The mandibular inclination decreased (Sn-GoGn from 43.7 to 39.5 degrees) (Figure 13).

A fixed appliance was progressively bonded to both arches with MBT prescription. Bilateral Class III elastics and box elastics with a Class III component were shortly used in the last phase to refine the occlusion. The fixed appliance phase lasted 23 months.

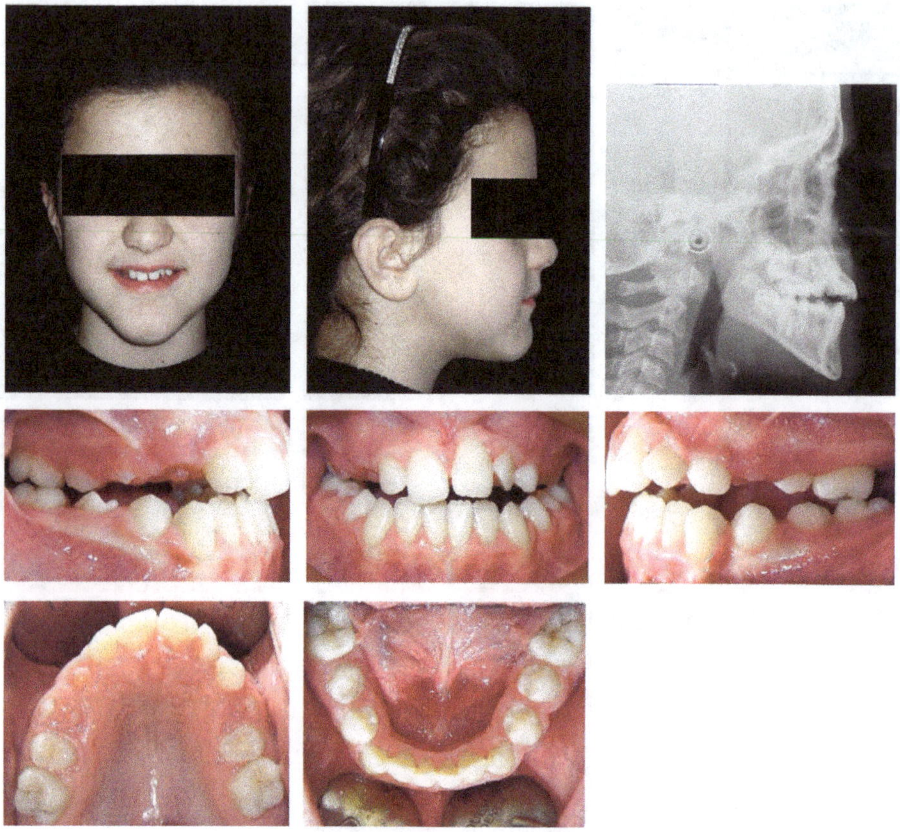

FIGURE 12: Case no. 2 facial photos, intraoral photos, panoramic radiograph, and lateral cephalogram at T_1 (after PS3 treatment).

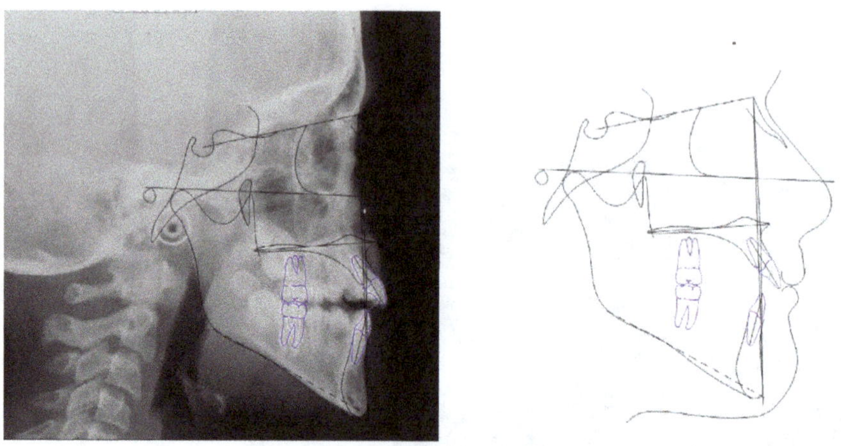

FIGURE 13: Case no. 2 tracings at T_1.

A very good Class I intercuspation with a proper Overjet and Overbite eventually was achieved (Figure 14).

The final ANPg angle was 0.9 degree keeping stable a good correction of the sagittal jaw relation. The mandibular inclination increased again to 41.3 degrees (Table 2), but considering the very severe hyperdivergent growth pattern, the final value should be considered as a quite favorable result (Figures 15 and 16).

The profile, however, was affected by the mandibular inclination and morphology. A chin surgery could be considered in case of an esthetic request from the patient.

5. Discussion

As widely recognized, Facemask and RPE are still the most utilized treatment procedure for a Class III malocclusion. Some limits should be considered in this protocol: (1) the need for a huge cooperation, (2) space lost in the upper arch due to upper posterior teeth mesial shifting, and (3) the increase in the vertical dimension.

Point (1) is obvious, due to the invasiveness of the use of FM. Furthermore, a more significant orthopedic result is usually obtained with a very early treatment, which generally also

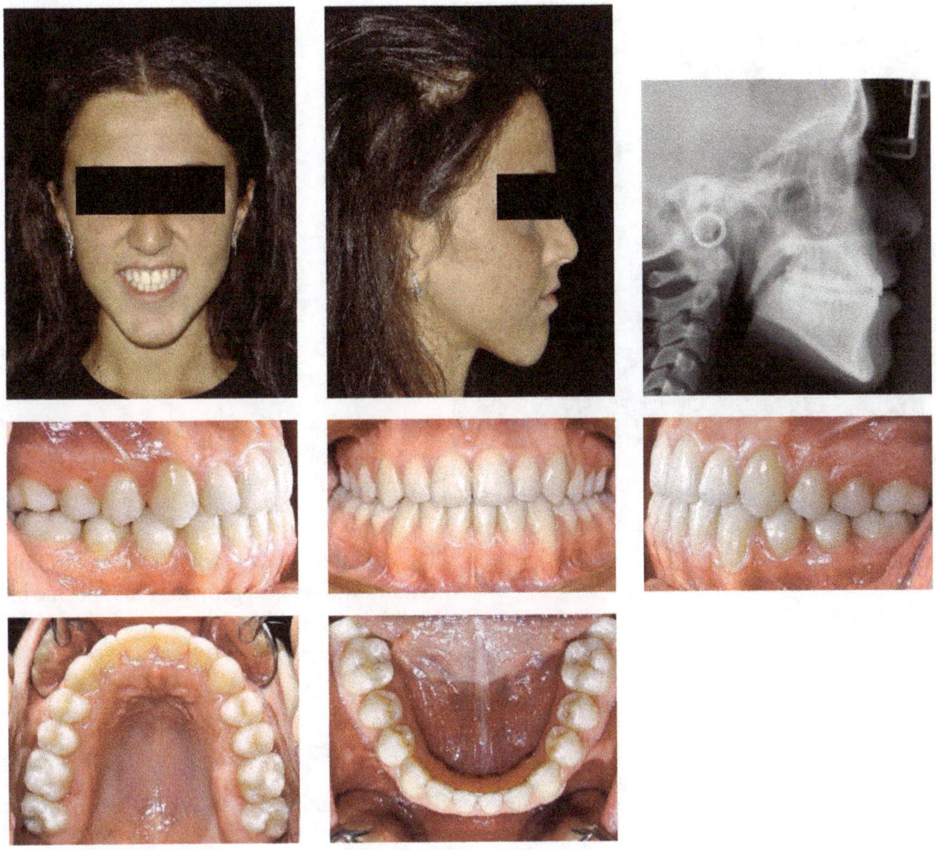

Figure 14: Case no. 2 facial photos, intraoral photos, and lateral cephalogram at T_2 (posttreatment).

Table 2: Cephalometric values of case no. 2 before treatment, after PS3 treatment, and at the end of fixed appliance treatment.

Values	Initial	Progress	Final
SNA (°)	76.7	81.7	81.6
S-N-Pg (°)	77.6	80.5	80.7
A-N-Pg (°)	-1.0	1.3	0.9
Co-Gn (mm)	114.9	118.7	121.5
Co-Go (mm)	55.4	56.8	62.2
Co-Go-Me (°)	138.2	136.2	136.9
S-N/ANS-PNS (°)	9.0	7.4	10.8
S-N/Go-Gn (°)	43.7	39.5	41.3
ANS-PNS/Go-Gn (°)	37.7	34.3	32.7
U1-ANS-PNS (°)	109.5	118.3	113.9
L1-Go-Gn (°)	77.7	76.4	82.0
Overjet (mm)	-1.4	6.7	2.0
Overbite (mm)	-3.7	-2.0	0.3

corresponds to an even lower level of cooperation. PS3, not needing an extra oral appliance, could facilitate cooperation.

Point (2) is connected to the FM/RPE biomechanics that determines a mesial movement of posterior teeth covered by the acrylic splints. The PS3 splints cover the whole arch, offering a good control of the arch length.

Point (3) is specifically related to the peculiar biomechanics of the FM/RPE protocol whose sagittal activation modality facilitates at the same time a vertical movement of the upper jaw and the upper arch [7]. Rongo et al. [8] showed that FM therapy determined a clockwise rotation of the lower jaw that leads to an increase in vertical skeletal relationships; hence, even if Class III early orthopedic treatment has been demonstrated effective in sagittal correction, it may produce unfavorable side effects in hyperdivergent patients.

The most important advantage of PS3 pushing biomechanics is the good control of upper jaw vertical growth, which is extremely important in hyperdivergent cases, such as those reported in the present article.

Finally, data from a recent paper [10] confirmed that the PS3 protocol is able to improve the sagittal relationship (ANPg $T_1 - T_0 = 2.8$ degrees, $p < 0.001$) and to preserve clockwise mandibular rotation (Sn-GoGn $T_1 - T_0 = 0.6$ degrees, $p > 0.05$).

This is a crucial point of difference also with the treatment performed with Class-III elastics in a fixed appliance, since even the elastics biomechanics has the effect of increasing the vertical dimension.

According to Fränkel and Fränkel [3], FR-3 is "an orthopedic exercise device that is capable of overcoming the faulty spatial disorders as well as the faulty postural performances of the orofacial musculature associated with Class III malocclusions" but a long treatment time—at least 5 years—is necessary for the appliance to be effective, which greatly reduces the efficiency of the treatment.

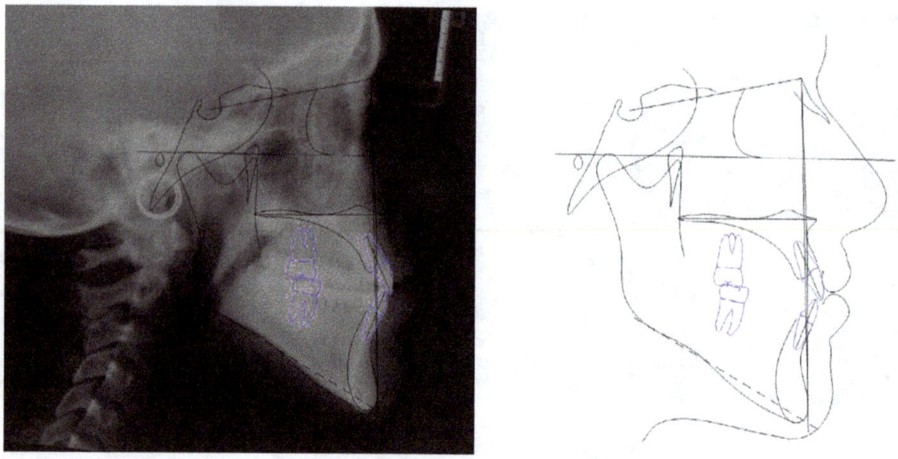

FIGURE 15: Case no. 2 tracings at T_2.

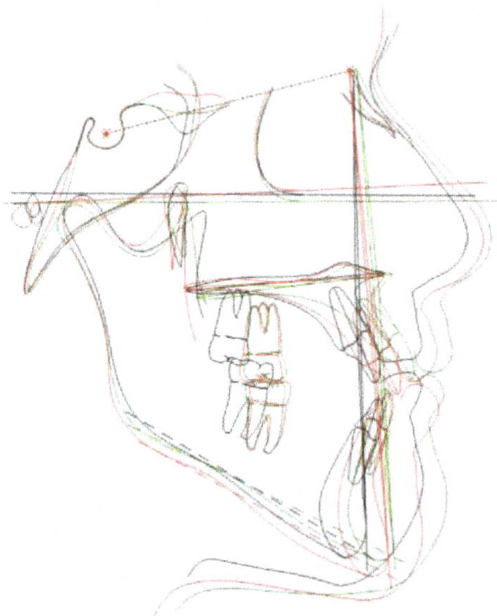

FIGURE 16: Case no. 2 tracing superimpositions.

Some other protocols have been suggested in the last years, but they require invasive surgery and some cooperation [5] or some surgery and important cooperation [11]. None of these treatments could anyway guarantee the certainty of avoiding relapse and the need for surgery.

Two systematic reviews [12, 13] reported that Facemask and chin cup did not constitute a risk factor of TMD. Since both these appliances use higher forces than PS3 compressing the TMJ, it could be assumed that PS3 should not cause TMD. This assumption seems to be confirmed by the observation of over a hundred treated cases.

6. Conclusions

The control of the vertical dimension appears to be a key objective in Class III hyperdivergent patients.

The specific biomechanic features of the PS3 appliance permit the use of forces useful to improve the sagittal jaw relationship, delivering at the same time vertical vectors that are able to control the alveolar and skeletal components of the vertical growth. This specific biomechanic feature should be considered as a useful benefit in the treatment of severe hyperdivergent patients.

References

[1] W. Proffit, H. Fields, and B. Larson, *Contemporary Orthodontics*, Mosby, 6th Edition edition, 2018.

[2] T. Baccetti and I. Tollaro, "A retrospective comparison of functional appliance treatment of Class III malocclusions in the deciduous and mixed dentitions," *European Journal of Orthodontics*, vol. 20, no. 3, pp. 309–317, 1998.

[3] R. Fränkel and C. Fränkel, *Orofacial Orthopedics with the Function Regulator*, Karger, 1989.

[4] M. I. Chatzoudi, I. Ioannidou-Marathiotou, and M. A. Papadopoulos, "Clinical effectiveness of chin cup treatment for the management of Class III malocclusion in pre-pubertal patients: a systematic review and meta-analysis," *Progress in Orthodontics*, vol. 15, no. 1, p. 62, 2014.

[5] H. J. De Clerck, M. A. Cornelis, L. H. Cevidanes, G. C. Heymann, and C. J. F. Tulloch, "Orthopedic traction of the maxilla with miniplates: a new perspective for treatment of midface deficiency," *Journal of Oral and Maxillofacial Surgery*, vol. 67, no. 10, pp. 2123–2129, 2009.

[6] T. Baccetti, L. Franchi, and J. A. McNamara Jr., "Treatment and posttreatment craniofacial changes after rapid maxillary expansion and facemask therapy," *American Journal of Orthodontics and Dentofacial Orthopedics*, vol. 118, no. 4, pp. 404–413, 2000.

[7] R. S. D. Smyth and F. S. Ryan, "Early treatment of class III malocclusion with facemask," *Evidence-Based Dentistry*, vol. 18, no. 4, pp. 107-108, 2017.

[8] R. Rongo, V. D'Antò, R. Bucci, I. Polito, R. Martina, and A. Michelotti, "Skeletal and dental effects of Class III orthopaedic treatment: a systematic review and meta-analysis," *Journal of Oral Rehabilitation*, vol. 44, no. 7, pp. 545–562, 2017.

[9] A. Ferro, L. P. Nucci, F. Ferro, and C. Gallo, "Long-term stability of skeletal class III patients treated with splints, Class III elastics, and chincup," *American Journal of Orthodontics*, vol. 123, no. 4, pp. 423–434, 2003.

[10] R. Martina, V. D'Antò, V. De Simone, A. Galeotti, R. Rongo, and L. Franchi, "Cephalometric outcomes of a new orthopaedic appliance for Class III malocclusion treatment," *European Journal of Orthodontics*, vol. 17, 2019.

[11] M. Nienkemper, B. Wilmes, L. Franchi, and D. Drescher, "Effectiveness of maxillary protraction using a hybrid hyrax-facemask combination: a controlled clinical study," *The Angle Orthodontist*, vol. 85, no. 5, pp. 764–770, 2015.

[12] M. A. Zurfluh, D. Kloukos, R. Patcas, and T. Eliades, "Effect of chin-cup treatment on the temporomandibular joint: a systematic review," *European Journal of Orthodontics*, vol. 37, no. 3, pp. 314–324, 2015.

[13] X. Huang, X. Cen, and J. Liu, "Effect of protraction facemask on the temporomandibular joint: a systematic review," *BMC Oral Health*, vol. 18, no. 1, p. 38, 2018.

22

Canine Rise Method: A Conservative Approach for Worn Teeth Rehabilitation with Different Adhesive Restorative Materials

Hamid Kermanshah[1] **Aws Alzwghaibi**[2] **Maitham Al-Tufaili**[3]
and Sholeh Ghabraei[4]

[1]*Dental Research Center, Dentistry Research Institute, Department of Restorative Dentistry, School of Dentistry, Tehran University of Medical Sciences, Tehran, Iran*
[2]*Department of Orthodontics, School of Dentistry, Shahid Beheshti University of Medical Sciences, Tehran, Iran*
[3]*Department of Restorative Dentistry, School of Dentistry, Tehran University of Medical Sciences, Tehran, Iran*
[4]*Department of Endodontics, School of Dentistry, Tehran University of Medical Sciences, Tehran, Iran*

Correspondence should be addressed to Maitham Al-Tufaili; maithamy788@gmail.com

Academic Editor: Maria Beatriz Duarte Gavião

Background. In this article, two cases with generalized dental wear and four cases with localized dental wear are reported. In some of the cases, the worn teeth were restored with direct composite techniques with no mock-up and articulator mounting according to the canine rise method. This method is used without any change in the intercuspation of posterior teeth without a muscle relaxation appliance. It introduces a stable occlusal condition that can alter neuromuscular reflex activity, leading to improvements in certain muscle pain disorders. It is also used to protect the teeth and supporting structures from abnormal forces that might create a further breakdown and/or tooth wear. *Methods.* The first step of treatment in all the cases was a composite build-up for maxillary and mandibular canines to restrict and guide the horizontal and vertical jaw movements and create adequate space for restorations. The second step was the placement of direct or indirect restorations on upper and lower anterior teeth efficiently and accurately. *Results.* This method enhanced the esthetic outcomes in a conservative approach with no reduction in tooth material or time-consuming treatments. *Conclusions.* This technique can be suggested for the treatment of worn teeth in patients with Angle's Cl I and Cl II classifications of malocclusion based on the follow-up results. It is not applicable for the treatment of worn teeth in patients with Angle's class III because occlusion is reversed, and canine teeth do not have guidance role. *Practical Implications.* This method significantly reduces the overall treatment time, and additional steps are required to restore the worn-out teeth and/or occlusion using the canine rise method.

1. Introduction

One of the well-established occlusal diseases (masticatory dysfunction) is dental wear. It is one of the common destructive dental disorders due to several etiological factors. Usually, this disease is progressive without intervention, and the eventual outcome is tooth loss [1]. Dawson, a pioneer in occlusal disease, has described the condition as follows: the process resulting in the noticeable loss of the occluding surfaces of the teeth [2]. However, Dowson has defined it as "deformation or disturbance of function of any structures within the masticatory system that are in disequilibrium with a harmonious interrelationship between the TMJs, the masticatory musculature, and the occluding surfaces of the teeth [2]. Therefore, we can draw a simple conclusion that dental wear is associated with neuromuscular and/or TMJ disorders.

Crown length and tooth general appearance changes are caused by a multifactorial disease; dental wear, attrition, erosion, and abrasion are the responsible factors [3, 4].

Generally, dental wear is associated with several biological, functional, and esthetic problems [5].

Tooth wear is a significant dental problem caused by various factors, including mechanical, physical, chemical, or trauma. Based on the Adult Dental Health Survey (ADHS), tooth wear is found in approximately 77% of adults, with 15% exhibiting moderate wear and 2% having severe tooth wear [6]. Loomans et al. defined severe tooth wear as "tooth wear with substantial loss of tooth structure, with dentin exposure and significant loss (≥1/3) of the clinical crown" [1], while pathological tooth wear was defined as "tooth wear which is atypical for the age of the patient, causing pain or discomfort, functional problems, or deterioration of esthetic appearance," which if it progresses, might give rise to undesirable complications of increasing complexity [1].

Thornton defined canine guidance as disocclusion of all the teeth by the contact of unilateral maxillary and mandibular canines only in lateral excursion movement; it is also known as "canine-protected occlusion, mutually protected occlusion, canine disocclusion, canine-lift, and canine rise" [7]. Canine rise occlusion, compared to the group function occlusion, is more efficient in reducing tooth surface friction. Another advantage of canine rise occlusion is the reduction of masticatory muscle activities. Many electromyography (EMG) studies [8–11] and intraoral bite splint studies [12–15] have shown that canine rise occlusion leads to more reductions in masticatory muscle activity compared to the group function occlusion. Numerous clinical studies have indicated that the lack of canine guidance can damage the dentition [16]. The strategic location of the canines away from the fulcrum was effective in reducing compression on the TMJ [10].

Since one of the mechanisms for the occlusal disease is friction, [2] reducing the friction on the tooth surface can be a strategy to control it. It seems that the involvement of the incisal edge of canine teeth in lateral excursion movement reduces friction; therefore, a reduction in tooth wear is expected. Canine teeth are an excellent choice for decreasing tooth occlusal friction because of their dome-shaped morphology. New technologies and advances nowadays allow us to use composites to treat dental wear since the technology of dental adhesives has had an accountable advancement in recent years. Several studies have shown the accountability of composite restorations as a treatment choice for worn teeth with acceptable results [17, 18]. A systematic review of treatment options by Muts et al. recommended conventional ceramic restorations and composite resins as a choice for generalized dental wear treatment [5]. The use of direct composite restorations is conservative and relatively easy to maintain compared to other applicable restorative techniques for dental wear [19].

Minimally invasive treatment strategies are recommended according to the dynamic restorative treatment concept, which is based on new guidelines regarding the treatment of patients with severe dental wear [1]. The present report presents six cases of dental wear treated by the canine rise method. The treatment plan for all the cases was based on adhesive, conservative, and esthetic principles. The first stage of treatment was building up the maxillary and mandibular canines by composite restorations without the mock-up and articulator stages, as mentioned before. It was carried out to restrict and guide the horizontal and vertical jaw movements and create adequate space between the upper and lower incisors, while the posterior teeth are still in contact. Therefore, the mandible can move backward to the centric relation position without increasing the vertical dimension.

2. Cases Presentation

2.1. Case 1. The patient suffered from generalized severe dental wear involving both the anterior and posterior teeth, as seen in Figures 1(a)–1(c). Her chief complaint involved esthetic problems. The teeth were too short and discolored with a diastema between them. The first stage of treatment was started by composite restoration for maxillary and after mandibular canines with direct restorative technique without any need for mock-up, wax-up, and an articulator to restrict and guide the horizontal jaw movements. The canine teeth were built up to the original shape after two weeks' recall, and the restriction of jaw movements, relaxation of the masticatory muscles, and rotation and backward movement of the mandible to centric relation were achieved. Therefore, adequate occlusal space between maxillary and mandibular anterior teeth was created with the same intercuspation of posterior teeth, as seen in Figures 1(d)–1(f). As shown in Figures 1(d)–1(f), the contact between 17, 47, 27, and 37 (FDI tooth numbering system), confirms that space has been created with the same intercuspation of posterior teeth. At the two weeks' recall appointment, the impression of maxillary and mandibular teeth was taken to mock up and construct provisional composite restorations. After a few weeks, the patient was evaluated for esthetic, phonetic, and function before definitive treatment. The patient was not satisfied with the color of the teeth; therefore, the treatment plan was shifted to laminate veneers. The first step was to place indirect ceramic veneers (IPS e.max Press, Ivoclar Vivadent) on 11, 12, 13, 21, and 22, as seen in Figures 1(g) and 1(h). Then, indirect ceramic veneers were placed on 23. After restoring the anterior guidance of the patient, restorations of posterior teeth (except the second molars) were constructed by conservative indirect ceramic veneers or a porcelain-fused-to-metal bridge on 25, 26, 27, and 28 or crown on 46, as seen in Figures 1(i)–1(m). In this case, the canine rise method was used by indirect restorations. The follow-up photography, after three years, is presented in Figures 1(n)–1(p); while, Figures 1(q) and 1(r) showed the case before and after treatment, respectively.

2.2. Case 2. The patient suffered from generalized severe dental wear involving both the anterior and posterior teeth, as seen in Figures 2(a)–2(e). The chief complaint was the poor esthetic appearance of the anterior teeth and tooth sensitivity. Based on clinical and radiographic examinations of worn teeth, there was no evidence of necrosis or irreversible pulpitis. Thus, the conservative approach, "canine rise method," was adopted through a direct restorative technique without mock-up. First, a build-up by composite restorations was

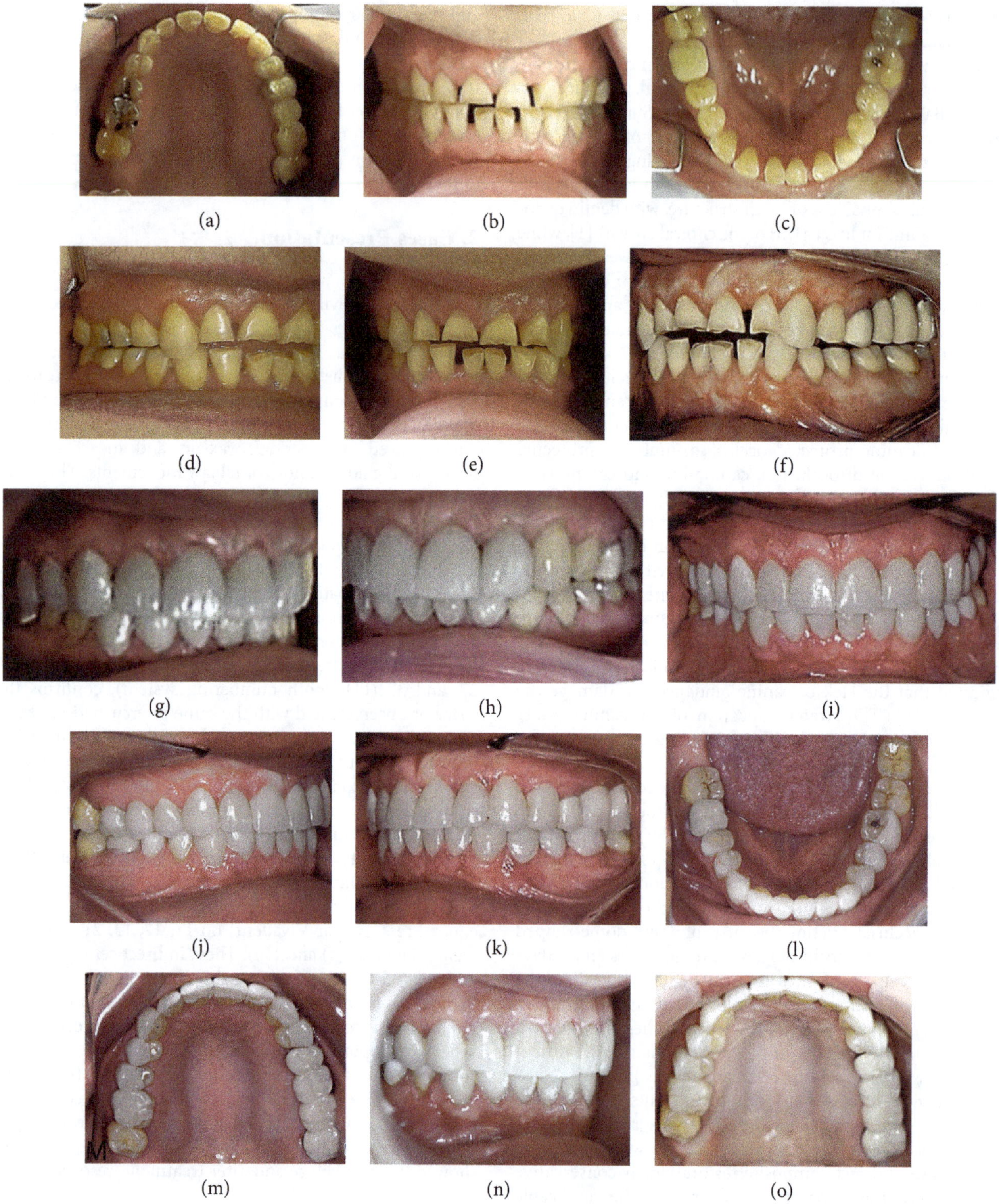

FIGURE 1: Continued.

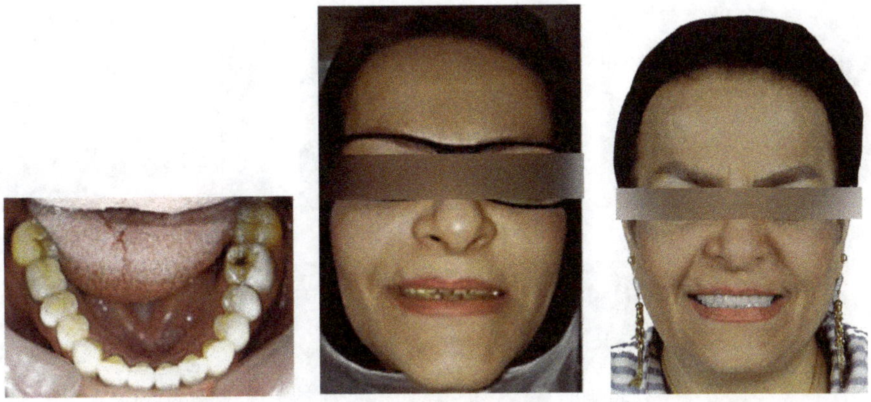

(p) (q) (r)

FIGURE 1: The first case of generalized dental wear. (a)–(c), intraoral view before treatment; (b), frontal view; (d), (e), and (f) show canine rise approach to treat this case using composite resin on upper and lower canines. Definitive restorations (first step) for upper and lower teeth after canine rise approach shown in (g) and (h). Definitive restorations (second step) for veneering upper and lower teeth except some posterior teeth shown in (i), (j), and (k) frontal and lateral views; (l) and (m), occlusal views. Follow-up after three years of initial treatment shown in (n), (o), and (p) occlusal and frontal views. (q) and (r) show facial views before and after treatment.

carried out for 13, 23, 33, and 43 to restrict and guide the horizontal and vertical jaw movements and create an adequate space for direct restorations. Isolation was achieved by inserting a rubber dam. Selective etching with 40% phosphoric acid was used for 20 seconds, and an adhesive agent (G-Premio BOND, GC) was placed; then, composite resin (Essentia, GC) build-up was carried out using the incremental technique. During three appointments, the composite was added only to the attrition sites of all the teeth, and the diastema between 11 and 21 was completely closed with micro- or nanohybrid composite resin material (Essentia Medium Dentin (MD) and dark enamel (DE), GC) without any preparation as seen in Figures 2(f)–2(j). The patient was re-evaluated after six months. In clinical examination, chipping in composite restorations of 11 and 21 was observed, as shown in Figures 2(k) and 2(l). Therefore, composite defects were repaired. The next step was to construct upper and lower removable partial dentures, as seen in Figures 2(m)–2(p). In clinical follow-up after one year, caries (class II disto-occlusal) on 34 was treated by a composite restoration, as seen in Figure 2(q). This case is an example of generalized tooth wear with full-mouth rehabilitation by direct composite restorations based on the canine rise method.

2.3. Cases 3–6. The other four cases with localized dental wear were treated by the same procedure (canine rise method). Permanent restorations were placed on the canines using composite resin, and the other anterior teeth were restored with either direct composite veneers or indirect ceramic veneers (feldspathic porcelain, Noritake, Kuraray Dental Inc.). These cases were followed up from 2 to 5 years, as shown in Figures 3, 4, 5, and 6. Figures 3(a)–3(c) show severe localized dental wear on the anterior segment of the first case with localized dental wear. The treatment of this patient's worn teeth was started by direct build-up composite resin restorations on 13, 12, 11, 21, 22, and 23, without considering the canine rise method as seen in Figure 3(d). After about two years, the crown on 21 was fractured, as shown in Figures 3(e) and 3(f). Based on canine rise method, a proper space was created to restore 13, 12, 11, 21, 22, and 23 by direct composite restorations without increasing vertical dimension of occlusion as seen in Figures 3(g)–3(i). The occlusion in laterotrusive and protrusive movements showed the canine and anterior teeth guidance, respectively, as seen in Figures 3(i)–3(k). Follow-up of the case after five years is shown in Figures 3(l)–3(n). The second case with localized dental wear on anterior teeth was also treated based on the canine rise method with a direct composite restoration, as seen in Figures 4(a)–4(k). The definitive treatment after 2 years of follow-up is shown in Figures 4(i)–4(m), while the lateral extortion movement is seen in Figures 4(n) and 4(o). Also, after 2 years, composite restoration of left central incisor was completely debonded and restored by new composite restoration as shown in Figures 4(p)–4(r). The third case of localized dental wear was also treated based on the canine rise method with direct composite resin restorations for 13 and 23 and porcelain laminate veneers for 11 and 21, as seen in Figures 5(a)–5(e). The follow-up of the patient after four years is shown in Figures 5(f)–5(h). The fourth case of localized dental wear is shown in Figures 6(a)–6(e). The treatment of the patient's dental wear was started by direct composite resin restoration on the 13 and 23 based on the canine rise method. After one month, porcelain laminate veneers were placed on the remaining 12 and 22 without restoration of posterior teeth, as seen in Figures 6(b) and 6(d). The follow-up of the patient after four years shows that the extracted tooth number 35 has been replaced by a dental implant and PFM crown restoration as seen in Figure 6(e).

3. Discussion

Frequently, the occlusal disease remains undiagnosed until severe damage becomes esthetically and functionally discomforting for the patient. It is one of the contributing factors in tooth loss. Treatment planning can be preventive (i.e., controlling the erosive factor), restorative, or a combination.

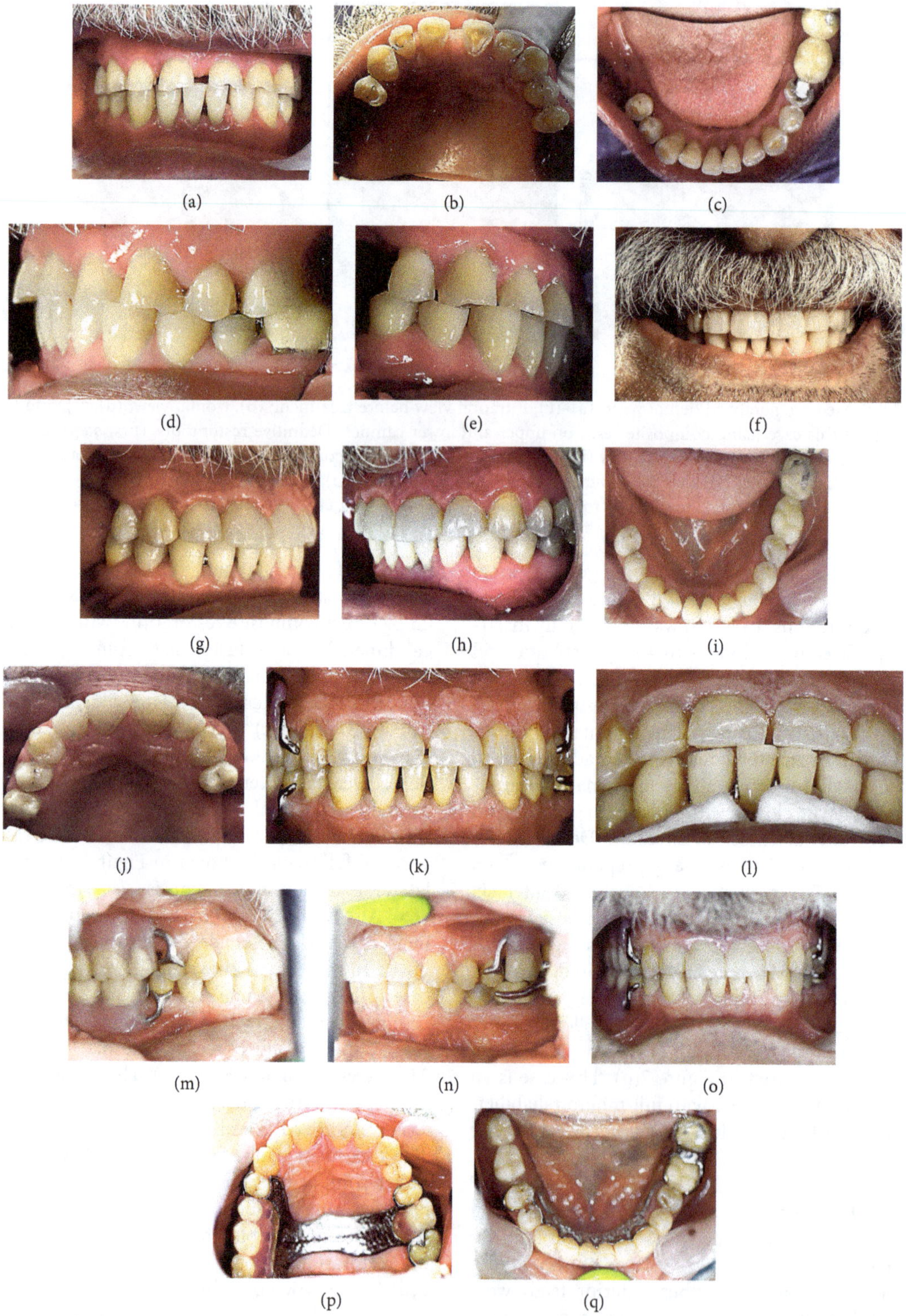

FIGURE 2: The second case of generalized dental wear; before treatment: (a), Frontal view; (b) and (c), occlusal views; (d) and (e), lateral views. After treatment: (f), facial view; (g) and (h), lateral views; (i) and (j), occlusal views of upper and lower dental arches. (k) and (l) show this case six months after treatment; there was a fracture of restorations on maxillary central incisors before constructing upper and lower removable partial dentures. Follow-up one year after treatment; (m) and (n), lateral views; (o), frontal view; (p) and (q), occlusal view of upper and lower jaws. Note: there was a class II disto-occlusal caries in mandibular left first premolar one year after treatment in the last image (q).

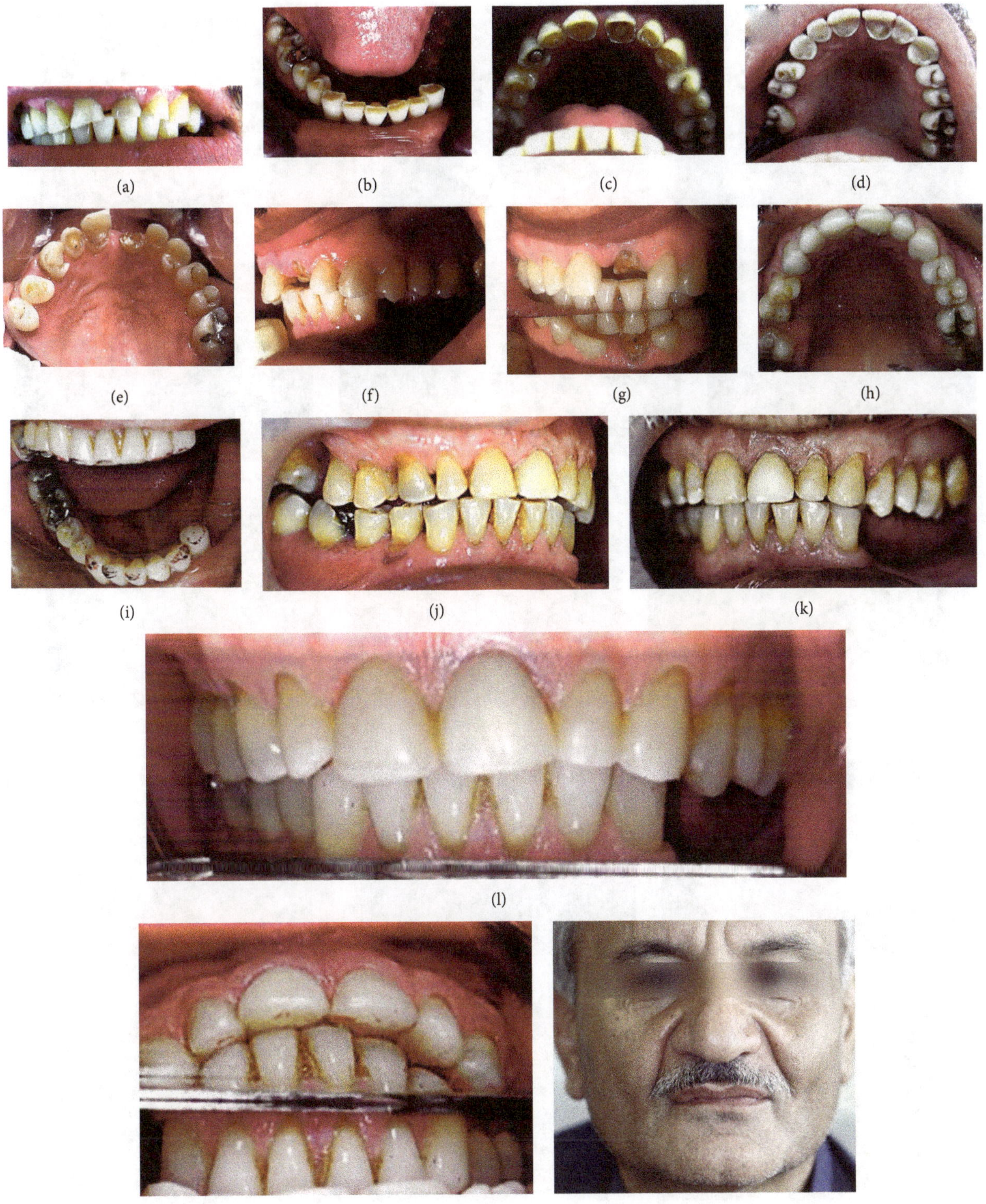

FIGURE 3: First case of localized dental wear. (a)–(c), intraoral and frontal views before treatment; (d), dental wear treatment without considering canine rise method by direct composite restoration seven years ago; (e)–(g), fracture of maxillary left central incisor two years after initial treatment. Therefore, this case was retreated by composite resin with the canine rise method as shown in (h) and (i). The backward position of the mandible is confirmed by comparing (f) and (g). The follow-up five years after initial dental wear treatment by direct composite resin with canine rise method is shown in (j)–(l), intraoral lateral and frontal views; (m) shows the relationship between upper and lower anterior teeth; (n), extraoral facial view.

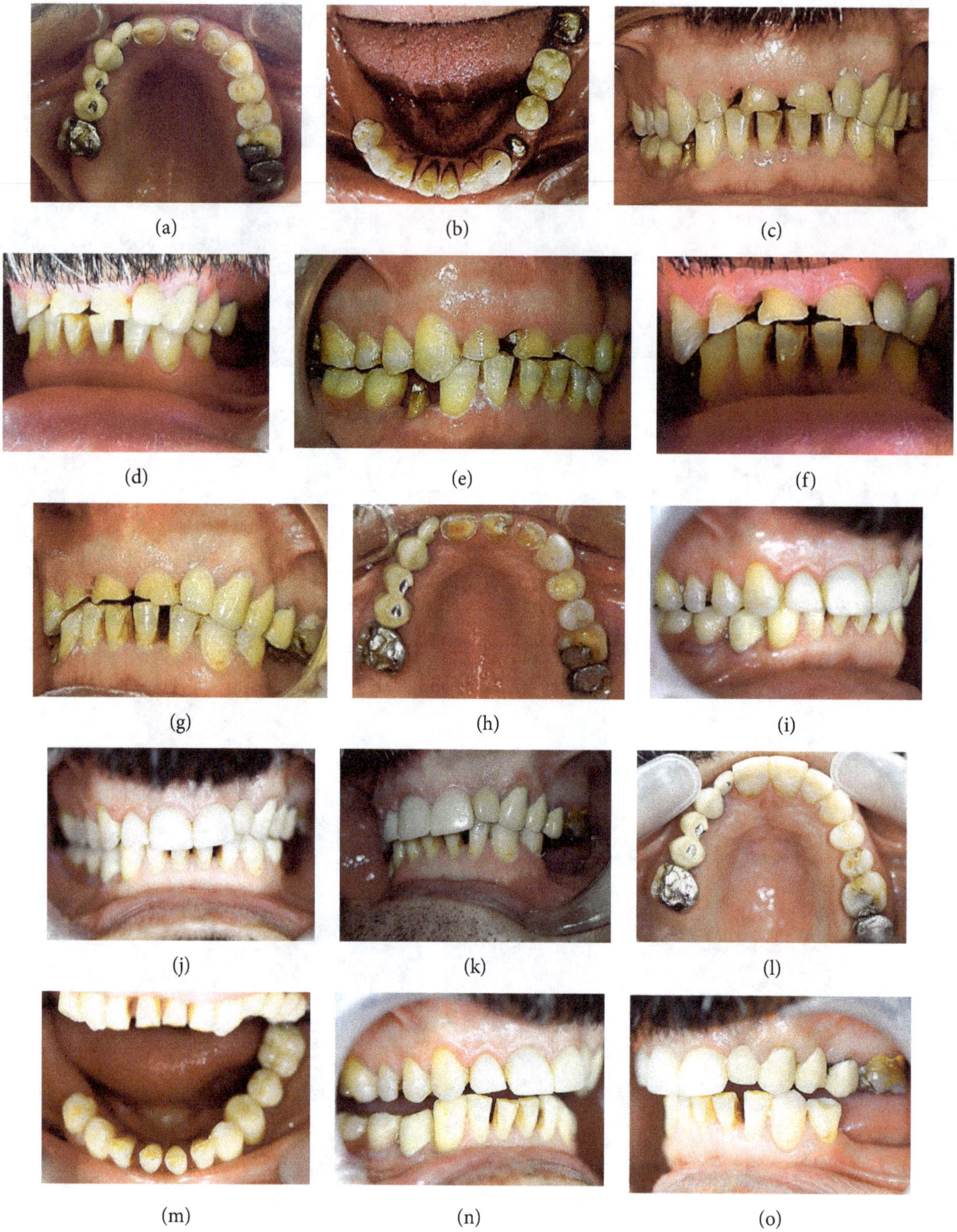

FIGURE 4: Continued.

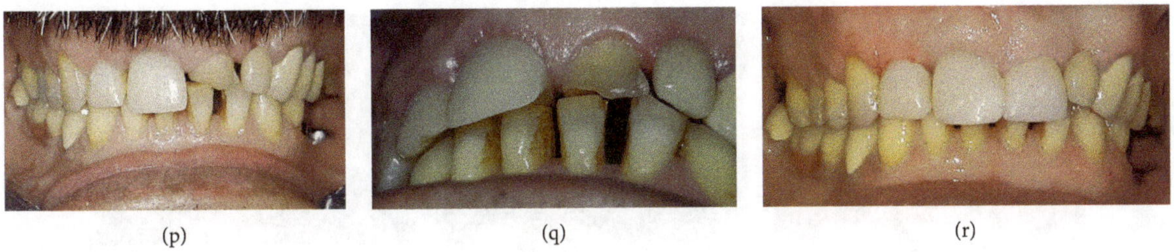

FIGURE 4: The second case of localized dental wear: (a)–(d), occlusal and frontal views before treatment; (e)–(h), frontal, lateral, and occlusal views after the canine rise method and creation of space for the restorative material. After 1.5 years of definitive treatment, (i)–(k), frontal and lateral views; (l) and (m), occlusal views. The lateral excursion is showed with canine rising (n and o). After 2 years, composite restoration of left central incisor was completely debonded, and the created space by the procedure is obvious in (p) and (q). New composite restoration (r).

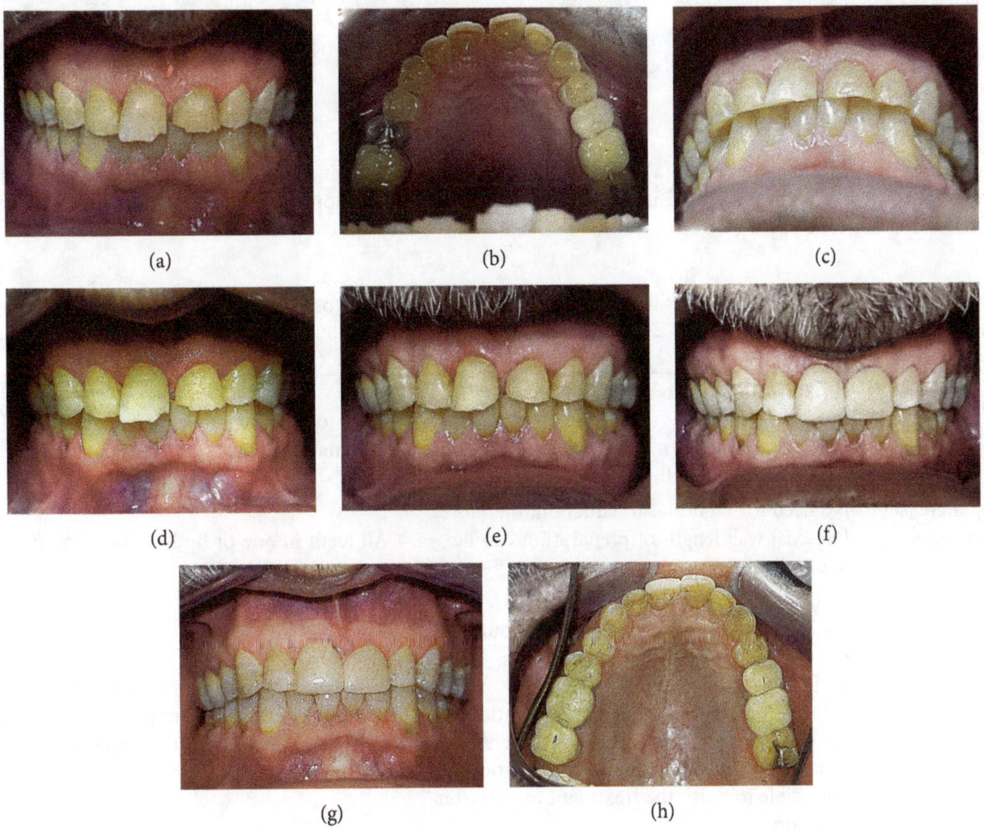

FIGURE 5: The third case of localized dental wear: (a)–(c), before treatment; (d), after the canine rise method; (e), teeth preparation for two ceramic veneers; (f), after cementation of two veneers; (g) and (h), frontal and occlusal views after three years.

To describe an occlusal treatment as a successful one, it should provide a comfortable and stable TMJ position and centric relation; the anterior teeth must be in harmony with the envelope of function without premature contacts in posterior teeth. The position that allows for interference-free contact is the centric relation; this position is an important factor in treatment planning for dental wear, and similarly, anterior guidance is an important factor to be considered [2].

Loss and fracture of posterior restorations has a multifactorial etiology, including loss of anterior guidance and canine protection. The latter increases horizontal stresses on the posterior occlusal surfaces [17]. These problems are usual with dental wear patients since the loss of the guidance and protection mechanism is usually associated with this type of occlusal disease. The treatment for dental wear and associated side effects basically depends on the type of restoration, the guidance, and the protection mechanism. The use of direct composite restorations to restore the worn-away dental surfaces is a conservative and easy-to-maintain method [20].

The most important question during clinical decision making is how to create space for the restorative material. In the literature, five methods are described to create the spaces needed for restorative materials: (1) preparation of worn teeth (with the same intercuspation position of the

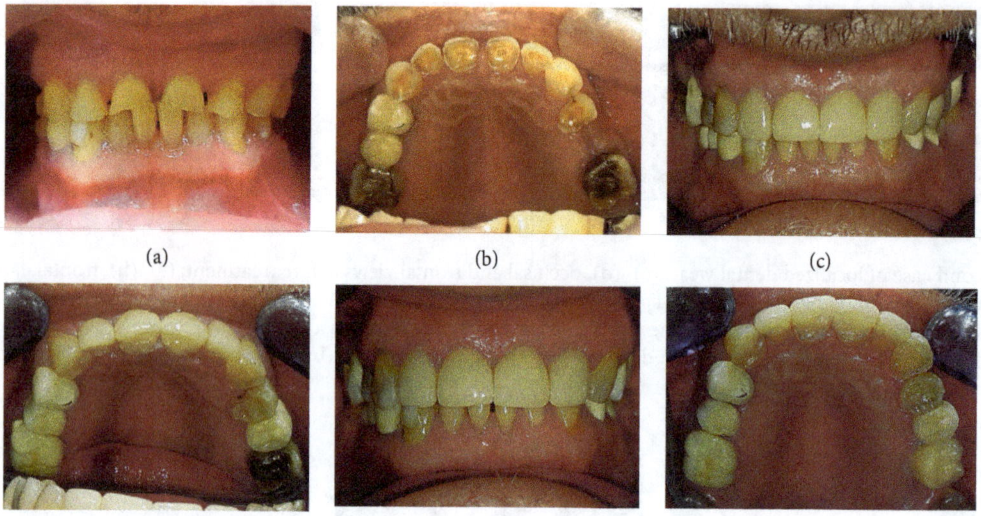

(a) (b) (c)

(d) (e) (f)

FIGURE 6: The fourth case of localized dental wear: (a) and (b), before treatment; (c) and (d), the one-year follow-up shows that the extracted upper left premolar area was restored by a dental implant and PFM crown restoration by another practitioner. (e) and (f); frontal and occlusal views of the case after four years.

TABLE 1: Techniques for creating space to allow the restoration of worn teeth.

Technique	Advantages	Disadvantages
Space creation by distalization of the mandible technique [24].	(i) No (or little) anterior tooth reduction required (ii) Can enable worn teeth to be restored without increasing the vertical dimension	Limited to cases where large horizontal RCP-ICP (retruded contact position-inter cuspal position) slide exists
Space creation by increase the vertical dimension technique [24].	No need for an occlusal reduction; therefore, full axial wall length of preparation can be maintained	All teeth in one or both arches may need restorations
Canine rise method	(i) Conservative and not destructive to teeth (ii) Worn teeth can be restored without an increase in the vertical dimension of occlusion (iii) It is possible to finish the restoration of the worn teeth without articulator devices (iv) Because of neuromuscular regulation, it is possible to finish the treatment in a shorter duration	Monitoring the restored canine teeth is essential because losing the restoration may result in damaging of other anterior restored teeth.

posterior teeth; usually, crown lengthening is needed); (2) increasing the vertical dimension of occlusion (VDO) can be used in localized dental wear (Dahl technique) or generalized dental wear. The tooth will be restored by either an additive method or a destructive method; (3) tooth movement by orthodontic forces or orthognathic surgeries (in limited cases); (4) distalization by occlusal adjustment of defective contact on posterior teeth (in limited cases); and (5) canine rise method (see Table 1) [21]. The canine rise method is a conservative approach for restoring the worn teeth in occlusal disease. It is applicable in many cases of worn teeth; also, it is an opportunity for the operator to restore generalized worn teeth (without an articulator and a technician) in a conservative, accurate, inexpensive, and fast way, as seen in Figure 2. Regardless to vertical dimension, the canine rise method is not suggested in class lll, because canine tooth does not have the guidance. However, in cases such as case no. 2 (full-mouth rehabilitation), to reduce chair time, taking the impression to prepare a silicone matrix or clear stand for the build-up of the affected teeth can be another way. Obviously, canine rise must be implemented before taking the impression (case no. 1 in the temporary stage). This method is indicated for patients with occlusion types Cl I and Cl II Angle's classification (except Cl III due to canine tooth does not have the guidance), where restoring worn teeth can be carried out without increasing the vertical dimension, as shown in Figures 1–6. A healthy periodontium of canine teeth with sufficient tooth structure is critical for this method. It is well-established that canine rise occlusion is superior to group function occlusion

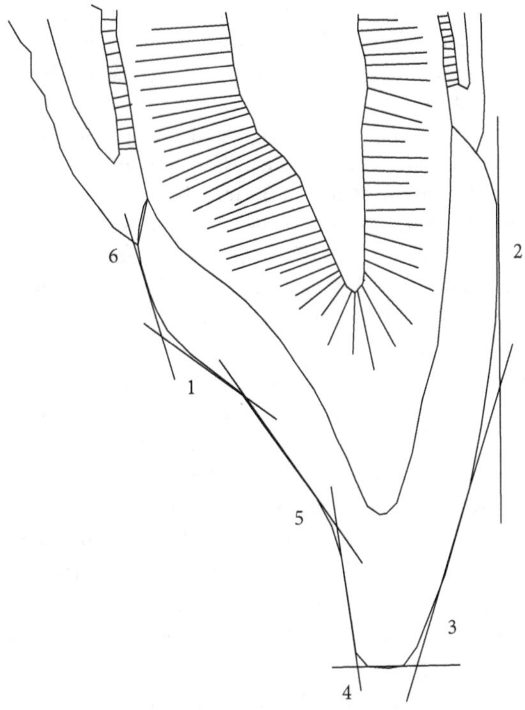

FIGURE 7: The six factors that determine labial and lingual contour and relate them to the correct incisal edge position: 1, mandible-to-maxilla relationship; 2, lip support; 3, lip closure path; 4, tooth-to-lip relationship; 5, the envelope of function; 6, tooth-to-tooth relationship.

in providing better protection against nonphysiologic muscle tension [9]. The canine rise method is based on the biofeedback mechanism through periodontal proprioceptive fibers surrounding the root of the canine teeth [22]. These fibers provide muscle function regulatory impulses during lateral excursion movements; more specifically, when canine teeth come in contact, the ratio of shear forces exerted on the canine teeth is regulated by that mechanism through translating the shear forces to the regulatory impulse that, in turn, is fed to the mesencephalic root of the trigeminal nerve, altering the motor impulses to the musculature [23]. Manns et al. observed that the fewer the occlusal contacts, the lower the amount of elevator muscle activity; on the contrary, more occlusal contact points resulted in higher activity [9]. Based on the previous description, the canine rise method decreased muscle tension in patients with this condition. Moreover, it reduced the tonicity of elevator muscles to provide more freedom for the mandible to slide backward. This mandibular movement provides enough space in the anterior dental region and some of the posterior parts, for example, case no. 3 and 4 shown in Figures 3(a)–3(l) and 4(o) and 4(p). In this way, the worn teeth can be restored without any change in the length of upper and lower posterior teeth, creating an ideal condition for the rehabilitation of worn teeth [2]. This method has the following advantages: (1) it is based on the neuromuscular system; (2) anterior worn teeth can be restored without any change in the cuspal contact of posterior teeth; and (3) finishing the restoration of worn teeth is possible without an articulator.

Based on EMG studies, composite restorations in worn canine teeth serve as a canine ramp in an occlusal splint and decrease muscle activity during excursions [24–26]. Furthermore, composite restorations are more comfortable for the patients. To restore worn anterior teeth accurately, as shown in Figures 1 to 6, the operator can use clinical judgment instead of using an articulator. As Figure 7 shows, all the anterior teeth, including canines, might be involved in one or a combination of six tooth segments in the wear process: mandible-to-maxilla relationship in centric relation depends on restoring segment 1; restoring segment 2 is important for lip support, and restoring segments 3, 4, 5, and 6 are essential for lip closure path, tooth-to-lip relationship during pronouncing F and V sounds, envelope of function, and tooth-to-tooth relationship while pronouncing the S sound, respectively [2].

The articulator is important only for the reconstruction of segment 1, while dynamic, esthetic, and phonetic factors are critical determinants for restoring the labial/lingual contour in other segments. Since it is unlikely for canine teeth to undergo wear in the segment 1, considering the unique role of these teeth in occlusion and reconstruction of worn teeth, in the first step of the canine rise method, canines should be restored with a direct composite resin procedure. However, if segment 1 of canine teeth is affected by wear, it will be necessary to use an articulator to restore them.

4. Conclusion

This report made an effort to present generalized and localized tooth wear rehabilitation with a new method. The images of the patients before and after treatment confirm clinical success. This method is not time-consuming; instead, it is economical and extremely conservative compared to conventional prosthodontic methods. The most important factor in achieving satisfactory clinical results is the ability and experience of the operator. Furthermore, in this method, the presence of a canine tooth with sufficient structure and periodontal support is a key factor. Canine is more resistant to wear than other anterior teeth because of its dome shape of the incisal edge. In our opinion, canine teeth must be considered as a determinant factor for the limitation and guidance of eccentric jaw movements. Increasing the length of canines in this method restricts the occlusal contacts to the canine teeth in eccentric jaw movements and produces adequate space for restorative materials to be added to the other worn teeth with the same intercuspation position of the posterior teeth. In this way, friction and wear of teeth will be reduced.

Consent

The authors declare that they obtained proper patient consent forms. In the form, the patient(s) gave their consent for their images and any other clinical information to be reported in a journal. The patients were reassured that their names and initials would not be published, and due efforts would be made to conceal their identity, but anonymity could not be guaranteed at all.

Acknowledgments

The authors would like to thank Dr. Fateme Amiri, Dr. Bahare Aghamohammadi, and Dr. Marieh Rashidi for their invaluable help and support.

References

[1] B. Loomans, N. Opdam, T. Attin et al., "Severe tooth wear: European consensus statement on management guidelines," *The Journal of Adhesive Dentistry*, vol. 19, no. 2, pp. 111–119, 2017.

[2] P. E. Dawson, *Functional occlusion-e-book: from TMJ to smile design*, Elsevier Health Sciences, 2006.

[3] D. W. Bartlett, "Erosion and tooth surface loss," *The International Journal of Prosthodontics*, vol. 16 Suppl, pp. 87–90, 2003.

[4] B. Smith and J. Knight, "A comparison of patterns of tooth wear with aetiological factors," *British Dental Journal*, vol. 157, no. 1, pp. 16–19, 1984.

[5] E.-J. Muts, H. van Pelt, D. Edelhoff, I. Krejci, and M. Cune, "Tooth wear: a systematic review of treatment options," *The Journal of Prosthetic Dentistry*, vol. 112, no. 4, pp. 752–759, 2014.

[6] A. Milosevic and G. Burnside, "The survival of direct composite restorations in the management of severe tooth wear including attrition and erosion: a prospective 8-year study," *Journal of Dentistry*, vol. 44, pp. 13–19, 2016.

[7] L. J. Thornton, "Anterior guidance: group function/canine guidance. A literature review," *The Journal of Prosthetic Dentistry*, vol. 64, no. 4, pp. 479–482, 1990.

[8] W. E. Shankland II, "Ernest syndrome as a consequence of stylomandibular ligament injury: a report of 68 patients," *The Journal of Prosthetic Dentistry*, vol. 57, no. 4, pp. 501–506, 1987.

[9] A. Manns, C. Chan, and R. Miralles, "Influence of group function and canine guidance on electromyographic activity of elevator muscles," *The Journal of Prosthetic Dentistry*, vol. 57, no. 4, pp. 494–501, 1987.

[10] N. Okano, K. Baba, and T. Ohyama, "The influence of altered occlusal guidance on condylar displacement during submaximal clenching," *Journal of Oral Rehabilitation*, vol. 32, no. 10, pp. 714–719, 2005.

[11] N. O. Domingos, *Análise da atividade elétrica do músculo masseter em diferentes guias laterais*, 2017.

[12] G. Grubwieser, A. Flatz, I. Grunert et al., "Quantitative analysis of masseter and temporalis EMGs: a comparison of anterior guided versus balanced occlusal concepts in patients wearing complete dentures," *Journal of Oral Rehabilitation*, vol. 26, no. 9, pp. 731–736, 1999.

[13] E. Ximinis and D. Tortopidis, "Electromyographic activity changes of jaw-closing muscles in patients with different occlusion schemes after fixed prosthetic restoration," *Balkan Journal of Dental Medicine*, vol. 22, no. 3, pp. 157–162, 2018.

[14] M. Seifi, D. Nodehi, A. Ghahramanloo et al., "Comparing the electromyographic features of the masseter and temporal muscles in patients with full mouth implant-supported FDPs and natural dentition," *Acta Informatica Medica*, vol. 25, no. 1, pp. 49–53, 2017.

[15] S. Valenzuela, R. Miralles, M. I. Muñoz et al., "Awake teeth grinding in participants with canine guidance or group function: effect on diaphragm EMG activity, heart rate, and oxygen saturation," *CRANIO®*., vol. 38, no. 6, pp. 412–418, 2020.

[16] Planning C, *Cuspid Disclusion: Is It Not Academic?*, Inside dentistry, 2006.

[17] K. W. Hemmings, U. R. Darbar, and S. Vaughan, "Tooth wear treated with direct composite restorations at an increased vertical dimension: results at 30 months," *The Journal of prosthetic dentistry*., vol. 83, no. 3, pp. 287–293, 2000.

[18] M. E. Mesko, R. Sarkis-Onofre, M. S. Cenci, N. J. Opdam, B. Loomans, and T. Pereira-Cenci, "Rehabilitation of severely worn teeth: a systematic review," *Journal of Dentistry*, vol. 48, pp. 9–15, 2016.

[19] A. Gulamali, K. Hemmings, C. Tredwin, and A. Petrie, "Survival analysis of composite Dahl restorations provided to manage localised anterior tooth wear (ten year follow-up)," *British Dental Journal*, vol. 211, no. 4, p. E9, 2011.

[20] C. Redman, K. Hemmings, and J. Good, "The survival and clinical performance of resin–based composite restorations used to treat localised anterior tooth wear," *British Dental Journal.*, vol. 194, no. 10, pp. 566–572, 2003.

[21] P. Yule, J. Steele, and R. Wassell, *Occlusal Control*, Springer, 2019.

[22] E. E. Vitria, I. Tofani, E. W. Bachtiar, and L. Kusdhany, "Association of maxillary transverse discrepancies and impacted maxillary canines in patients 10-25 years old," *Journal of International Dental and Medical Research*, vol. 9, p. 322, 2016.

[23] A. D'Amico, "Functional occlusion of the natural teeth of man," *The Journal of Prosthetic Dentistry*, vol. 11, no. 5, pp. 899–915, 1961.

[24] V. A. Kumar and T. Padmanabhan, "Influence of group function and canine guidance on electromyographic activity of elevator muscles in treating subjects for occlusal rehabilitation," in *Proceedings of the conference, the Japan Prosthodontic Society*, Japan, 2007.

[25] E. Williamson and D. Lundquist, "Anterior guidance: its effect on electromyographic activity of the temporal and masseter muscles," *The Journal of Prosthetic Dentistry*, vol. 49, no. 6, pp. 816–823, 1983.

[26] R. Miralles, R. Bull, A. Manns, and E. Roman, "Influence of balanced occlusion and canine guidance on electromyographic activity of elevator muscles in complete denture wearers," *The Journal of Prosthetic Dentistry*, vol. 61, no. 4, pp. 494–498, 1989.

Cosmetic "Gold Thread Therapy": A Nuisance that Decreases the Diagnostic Quality of a Dental Panoramic Image

Mah Eng Ching,[1] Lim Zhi Yin Joan,[2] and Phrabhakaran Nambiar[3,4]

[1]Department of Orthodontics, Faculty of Dentistry, MAHSA University, Bandar Saujana Putra, 42610 Selangor, Malaysia
[2]Department of Restorative Dentistry, Faculty of Dentistry, MAHSA University, Bandar Saujana Putra, 42610 Selangor, Malaysia
[3]Department of Oral Biology and Biomedical Sciences, Faculty of Dentistry, MAHSA University, Bandar Saujana Putra, 42610 Selangor, Malaysia
[4]Department of Oral & Maxillofacial Clinical Sciences, Faculty of Dentistry, University of Malaya, 50603 Kuala Lumpur, Malaysia

Correspondence should be addressed to Phrabhakaran Nambiar; phrabha@um.edu.my

Academic Editor: Maria Beatriz Duarte Gavião

During routine imaging of the craniofacial region, it is recognised that some "cosmetic" procedures with metallic insertions can be revealed radiographically. These objects however make it difficult to obtain a good interpretation of anatomical structures for management of diseases. A 58-year-old female patient visited a private dental facility in Kuala Lumpur for prosthodontic replacement of missing teeth. The dental panoramic image revealed generalized bone loss and numerous unusual multiple thread-like radioopacities. These gold threads made radiographic evaluation difficult and complicated the process of treatment planning for dental implant placement advocated for this patient.

1. Introduction

Digital intraoral images along with other radiographic projection methods such as dental panoramic images, extraoral imaging views, and cone-beam computed tomography (CBCT) scans are employed to diagnose diseases or abnormalities in the craniofacial region. Therefore, any fault or artifact observed on these images affects our interpretations and ultimately the diagnosis. Different types of radiopaque images and artifacts caused by accessory piercings, tongue studs, necklaces, reading glasses, removable prostheses, and earrings have been described. To avoid having these faults on the images, it is essential to remove all metallic objects in the maxillofacial region. However, there are metallic dental materials that cannot be removed. These include amalgam fillings, implants, and metallic braces that cause acquired artifacts on the images [1].

During routine imaging of the craniofacial region, it is recognised that some "cosmetic" procedures can also be demonstrated radiographically. Unexpected foreign metallic talismans inserted into the body, often referred to as "susuk" (charm needles) or acupuncture needles hidden in the body, might become revealed [2–4]. These objects make it difficult to obtain a good interpretation of images for management of the cases. They will also cause scattering on CBCT images and affect the treatment planning for implant placements [5]. In many occasions, the nonexperienced dental practitioner can mistake these faults for electrostatic discharges (on X-ray films), ghost images, or even radiopaque images of orthodontic ligature wires [6].

Another less reported hyperdense, short, thread-like fragments noted on oral and maxillofacial images/radiographs are caused by gold thread therapy or lift. This is also one of the methods of facial rejuvenation to firm up sagging skin in the cheek and jaw line by threading a web of gold fragments in the subdermal soft tissues [7]. As this procedure of face liftings is getting popular, the dental practitioners should be aware of the radiographic appearance of these foreign bodies to avoid any misinterpretation for diagnosis. Patient management will be further improved, and embarrassment will be avoided if these patients are approached gently with tact as the practitioner is aware of this therapy.

2. Case Report

A 58-year-old female patient visited a private dental facility in Kuala Lumpur for replacement of missing teeth and other prosthodontic treatment. Medical history of the patient revealed that the patient was unremarkable. Patient had her teeth extracted because of caries. An extraoral examination of the head and neck region showed no obvious abnormalities. Intraoral examination revealed a few missing teeth and retained root in the maxilla, and quite a few prosthodontic procedures were done in the mandible. Patient was interested to have dental implants done to replace the missing teeth. A dental panoramic image was taken for radiographic investigation. The Pax-i Digital Panoramic Unit (Vatech Imaging Systems, Korea) with the following parameters were used: tube voltage: 74 kVp, tube current: 10 mA, and scan time: 13 secs. The image revealed generalized bone loss and innumerable unusual multiple thread-like radioopacities over a wide area. These fragments were observed located bilaterally over the lower border of the orbits and middle and lower facial soft tissues. Radioopacities were very thin and tortuous and have short fragments.

Patient was enquired about whether she had undergone any kind of surgery before on her face. The patient revealed she had undergone "gold thread therapy" for facial "rejuvenation" (on multiple occasions) during the last 10 years. She mentioned that during the face-lift procedure, very thin needle with the gold thread was inserted under her skin, forming a mesh beneath it. The entire procedure was done under local anaesthesia and took 30 minutes to 1 hour. She also mentioned that she was very satisfied with the results of the procedure. These gold threads were inserted by a foreign medical doctor. The doctor carried his own instruments and visited households where patrons needed this service. All treatment is considered private and confidential and was also illegal as the doctor is not registered with the Malaysian Medical Council. The patient ordered for the service through a cosmetic agent, and procedures were performed whenever the doctor was visiting Malaysia.

The patient is a grandma with children and grandchildren; however, she still looks like a youthful middle-aged woman with firm facial muscles. She appeared to be confident and had high self-esteem. She admitted she has got addicted with the procedure and is very satisfied with it. She did not seem mindful if the doctor is not registered with the national medical council nor his procedure is considered an illegal practice.

3. Discussion

Gold is preferred metal of choice for this therapy as it is biocompatible and is not rejected by human skin and underlying tissues. It can be safely left in place for a long-term face lifting and subsequent skin rejuvenation. The "golden thread lift" was first introduced in dermatology by Dr. Caux in France approximately 30 years ago and then developed in Russia by Dr. Pawel Koziczynski in year 2000 [7–9]. Since then, it has also been adopted and broadly advertised in western countries and Asia. The early procedures involved the implantation of short 0.5 mm diameter gold thread. These procedures were very invasive, had a longer, less appealing recovery time, and required local anaesthesia most of the time.

Nowadays, microfine surgical gold threads (0.1 mm diameter, 24 K gold) are implanted into the subdermal tissues. With the finer/smaller diameter of gold thread, no local anaesthesia is needed [7, 8, 10]. A gold web is weaved to hold the facial tissues in place, provide mechanical support to the tissues, and prevent sagging of the skin. The gold will rejuvenate the skin by initial reaction within the skin tissues to coat the threads with collagen and intensify angiogenesis and blood circulation of the surrounding tissue. The usual sites for gold thread implantation in the face are cheeks, forehead, and mouth. The threads can also be inserted in other parts of the body such as hand, arms, and hips [7, 11]. In addition, in this case, the gold thread lift was not only performed in the cheek and perioral area but also at the periorbital area.

Few case reports about gold lift thread on images/radiographs have been reported in the literature, but the threads showed on the dental panoramic radiograph and periapical radiograph were fewer compared to what has noted in this case. In 2014, Mizrahi and Scully reported one of the earliest unusual linear radioopacities that were evident over a wide area on pantomographs [12]. Garg et al. described them as radiodense string-like artifacts in the posterior aspect of the maxilla and the mandible of a patient who confirmed undergoing gold thread facelift [9]. In addition, Cho and Park reported noticing gold thread therapy in posterior-anterior extraoral radiograph. According to them, this therapy was an adjunct for acupuncture for relieving perennial headaches in a 39-year-old Korean lady [13]. Recently, Negayama and Fujikawa provided a 3-dimensional volumetric rendering of a computed tomography (CT) scan of a patient who had undergone insertion of "gold threads" for facial rejuvenation. Their description of the insertions was very apt—numerous short, hyperdense, thread-like fragments, whose actual thickness was intensified, randomly distributed over the face [5]. Evidently bilateral symmetry in the gold lift was maintained so that the patient is aesthetically outstanding as the person in Figure 1.

Similar to gold thread lifting, implanting susuk subcutaneously is commonly done at the maxillofacial region for aesthetic purposes. Insertion of "susuk" or charm needles is a common practice in Malaysia. When a radiograph is taken for diagnostic purposes, these invisible implanted needles are typically observed by chance. These are often misdiagnosed as foreign bodies, acupuncture needles, fractured endodontic files, or even root fillings and restorative pins [2, 3]. Clinicians should be able to differentiate between these two foreign entities on the face. Gold threads can make radiographic evaluation more difficult because they can obstruct essential anatomical structures and complicate the process of treatment planning in dental procedure—in this case, it was for dental implant placement. A CBCT scan on

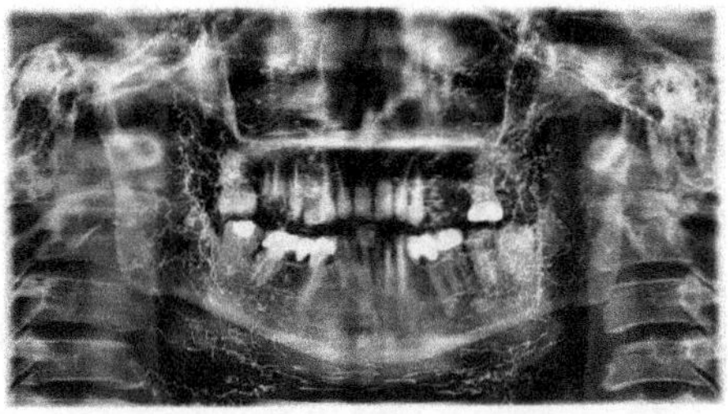

FIGURE 1: Numerous, short, tortuous, hyperdense threads revealed bilaterally in the maxillofacial region.

this person will have limited benefit as there shall be numerous streaking, beam hardening, and cupping artifacts which will render the scan useless [1]. The efficiency of gold thread lifting used for plastic surgery or acupuncture is controversial [14]. The drawback of the gold thread face lift is that the gold threads can migrate and may get fragmented over a period of time.

In addition, a variety of absorbable (collagen, hyaluronic acid, calcium hydroxyapatite, and poly-L-lactic acid) and nonabsorbable (polymethylmethacrylate beads) materials have been developed as dermal fillers for the facial area for cosmetic purposes [15]. These mineralized particles shall be observed to have diverse radiodensities and varying shapes and therefore different from these gold threads.

4. Conclusion

The above case highlights the importance of clinical practitioners working in Southeast Asian countries being aware of such gold thread therapy to reduce adverse and unintended effects during diagnosis and treatment planning. Nowadays, cosmetic procedures in the facial region are getting common as aesthetic awareness increased for the past few decades. The general dental practitioner should be aware of facial rejuvenation procedures and their radiographic appearance. A comprehensive medical history taking of the patient should include questions about utilization of such therapies.

Consent

The authors confirm that they have obtained written consent from the patient to use her clinical history and dental panoramic image for a report in a journal. The patient understands that her name and initials will not be published to conceal her identity.

References

[1] W. C. Scarfe, "Chapter 11. Cone Beam Computed Tomography Volume Preparation," in *White and Pharoah's Oral Radiology-Principles and Interpretation*, S. M. Mallya and L. EWM, Eds., pp. 466–504, St Louis: Elseiver, 2019.

[2] P. Nambiar, N. Ibrahim, Y. R. M. Tandjung, and P. Shanmuhasuntharam, "Susuks (charm needles) in the craniofacial region," *Oral Radiology*, vol. 24, no. 1, pp. 10–15, 2008.

[3] A. Thapasum and F. Mohammed, "Susuk - Black Magic Exposed "White" by Dental Radiographs," *Journal of Clinical and Diagnostic Research*, vol. 8, no. 7, pp. ZD03–ZD04, 2014.

[4] Y. R. M. Tandjung, C. P. Hong, P. Nambiar, and N. Ibrahim, "Uncommon radiological findings: a case report," *International Dental Journal*, vol. 57, no. 3, pp. 173–176, 2007.

[5] R. Negayama and T. Fujikawa, "CT appearance of gold thread facelift," *QJM: An International Journal of Medicine*, vol. 111, no. 1, p. 57, 2018.

[6] A. Sinha, A. Mishra, S. Srivastava, P. M. Sinha, and A. Chaurasia, "Understanding artifacts in cone beam computed tomography," *International Journal of Maxillofacial Imaging*, vol. 2, no. 2, pp. 51–54, 2016.

[7] M. Lichaj and T. Katsnelson, "Gold thread worldwide," May 2021. https://www.goldthread.ru/eng.

[8] G. B. Stark and H. Bannasch, "The "golden thread lift": radiologic findings," *Aesthetic Plastic Surgery*, vol. 31, no. 2, pp. 206–208, 2007.

[9] R. Garg, B. Fernandes, and M. K. Sunil, "Unusual radiopacities spotted in a dental radiograph: case report," *Journal of Indian Academy of Oral Medicine and Radiology*, vol. 29, no. 2, p. 138, 2017.

[10] J. A. Keestra, R. Jacobs, and M. Quirynen, "Gold-wire artifacts on diagnostic radiographs: a case report," *Imaging Science in Dentistry*, vol. 44, no. 1, pp. 81–84, 2014.

[11] K. C. Shin, T. H. Bae, W. S. Kim, and H. K. Kim, "Usefulness of gold thread implantation for crow's feet," *Archives of Plastic Surgery*, vol. 39, no. 1, pp. 42–45, 2012.

[12] B. Mizrahi and C. Scully, "Dental radiography: gold thread therapy," *British Dental Journal*, vol. 216, no. 11, p. 606, 2014.

[13] J. Cho and Y. S. Park, "Gold thread acupuncture for a headache," *The American Journal of the Medical Sciences*, vol. 350, no. 5, p. 420, 2015.

[14] N. M. H. Ainul, "Gold thread implantation," May 2021. file:///-C:/Users/Admin/Downloads/21_gold_thread_implantation%20(3).pdf.

[15] Y. E. Kwon, C. H. An, K. S. Choi, D. H. Lee, and S. Y. An, "Radiographic study of dermal fillers in the facial area: a series of 3 cases," *Imaging Science in Dentistry*, vol. 48, no. 3, pp. 227–231, 2018.

Permissions

All chapters in this book were first published by Hindawi Publishing Corporation; hereby published with permission under the Creative Commons Attribution License or equivalent. Every chapter published in this book has been scrutinized by our experts. Their significance has been extensively debated. The topics covered herein carry significant findings which will fuel the growth of the discipline. They may even be implemented as practical applications or may be referred to as a beginning point for another development.

The contributors of this book come from diverse backgrounds, making this book a truly international effort. This book will bring forth new frontiers with its revolutionizing research information and detailed analysis of the nascent developments around the world.

We would like to thank all the contributing authors for lending their expertise to make the book truly unique. They have played a crucial role in the development of this book. Without their invaluable contributions this book wouldn't have been possible. They have made vital efforts to compile up to date information on the varied aspects of this subject to make this book a valuable addition to the collection of many professionals and students.

This book was conceptualized with the vision of imparting up-to-date information and advanced data in this field. To ensure the same, a matchless editorial board was set up. Every individual on the board went through rigorous rounds of assessment to prove their worth. After which they invested a large part of their time researching and compiling the most relevant data for our readers.

The editorial board has been involved in producing this book since its inception. They have spent rigorous hours researching and exploring the diverse topics which have resulted in the successful publishing of this book. They have passed on their knowledge of decades through this book. To expedite this challenging task, the publisher supported the team at every step. A small team of assistant editors was also appointed to further simplify the editing procedure and attain best results for the readers.

Apart from the editorial board, the designing team has also invested a significant amount of their time in understanding the subject and creating the most relevant covers. They scrutinized every image to scout for the most suitable representation of the subject and create an appropriate cover for the book.

The publishing team has been an ardent support to the editorial, designing and production team. Their endless efforts to recruit the best for this project, has resulted in the accomplishment of this book. They are a veteran in the field of academics and their pool of knowledge is as vast as their experience in printing. Their expertise and guidance has proved useful at every step. Their uncompromising quality standards have made this book an exceptional effort. Their encouragement from time to time has been an inspiration for everyone.

The publisher and the editorial board hope that this book will prove to be a valuable piece of knowledge for researchers, students, practitioners and scholars across the globe.

List of Contributors

Daishi Arai
Department of Orthodontics and Dentofacial Orthopedics, Tokushima University Graduate School of Oral Sciences, Tokushima, Japan

Akihiro Yasue and Eiji Tanaka
Department of Orthodontics and Dentofacial Orthopedics, Tokushima University Graduate School of Biomedical Sciences,Tokushima, Japan

Shinya Horiuchi
Department of Orthodontics and Dentofacial Orthopedics, Tokushima University Hospital, Tokushima, Japan

Adith Venugopal and Anand Marya
Department of Orthodontics, University of Puthisastra, Phnom Penh, Cambodia

Paolo Manzano
10:10 Dental Clinic, Mandaluyong, Manila, Philippines

Sri Rengalakshmi
Department of Orthodontics, Saveetha Dental College, Tamil Nadu, India

Hiroyuki Kimura and Tsuyoshi Kumano
Private Practice, Kumamoto, Kyushu, Japan

Yusuke Hamada
Department of Periodontology, Indiana University School of Dentistry, Indianapolis, IN, USA

Taro Eida and Kazutoshi Okamura
Faculty of Dental Science, Kyushu University, Japan

Makoto Yokota
YDA Yokota Juku, Japan

Luca Casula
Vita Salute University, Milan, Italy

Fahad F. Alsulaimani
Consultant and Professor, Department of Orthodontics, Faculty of Dentistry, King Abdulaziz University Jeddah 21589, Saudi Arabia

Basem Jamal
Consultant and Associate Professor, Oral & Maxillofacial Surgery Department, King Abdulaziz University, Jeddah, Saudi Arabia

Rania Mitwally
North Dental Specialty Center, Orthodontic Department, Orthodontist, Ministry of Health, Jeddah, Saudi Arabia

Abdulkarim A. Hatrom
Ministry of Health, Makkah, Saudi Arabia. Makkah 24359, Saudi Arabia

Ahmed R. Afify
Orthodontic Department, Faculty of Dentistry, King Abdulaziz University, Jeddah 21589, Saudi Arabia
Orthodontic Department, Faculty of Dentistry, Mansoura University, Mansoura, Egypt

Ali H. Hassan
Orthodontic Department, Faculty of Dentistry, King Abdulaziz University, Jeddah 21589, Saudi Arabia
Alfarabi Private College for Dentistry and Nursing, Jeddah 21589, Saudi Arabia

Farnoosh Mohammadi and Hamid Mojtahedi
Craniomaxillofacial Research Center, Oral and Maxillofacial Surgery Department, Shariati Hospital, Tehran University of Medical Sciences, Tehran, Iran

Afrooz Javanmard
Department of Prosthodontics and Dental Research Center, Faculty of Dentistry, Tehran University of Medical Sciences,Tehran, Iran

Joanna Jasnoch, Maria Zielke and Izabela Maciejewska
Department of Dental Prosthodontics, Medical University of Gdansk, Poland

Mohammed K. Badri
Department of Pedodontics & Orthodontics, College of Dentistry, Taibah University, Madinah, Saudi Arabia

A. A. A. K. Wimalarathna
Department of Prosthetic Dentistry, Faculty of Dental Sciences, University of Peradeniya, Sri Lanka

W. B. M. C. R. D. Weerasekara and E. M. U. C. K. Herath
Department of Community Dental Health, Faculty of Dental Sciences, University of Peradeniya, Sri Lanka

Federico Rosti
Private Practice, Cesano Boscone, Italy

Maria Francesca Sfondrini, Marina Consuelo Vitale, Paola Gandini and Andrea Scribante
Unit of Orthodontics and Paediatric Dentistry-Section of Dentistry-Department of Clinical, Surgical, Diagnostic and Paediatric Sciences, University of Pavia, Pavia, Italy

Davide Bressani
Dental Technician, Pavia, Italy

José Antonio Vera-Guerra
Department of Orthodontics, School of Dentistry, Universidad Autónoma de Nuevo León, Nuevo León, Mexico

José Rubén Herrera-Atoche and Gabriel Eduardo Colomé-Ruiz
Department of Orthodontics, School of Dentistry, Universidad Autónoma de Yucatán, Yucatán, Mexico

Mandla Dominic Nyakale
Department of Orthodontics, Faculty of Dentistry, University of the Western Cape, Cape Town, South Africa

M. Srirengalakshmi
Department of Orthodontics, Saveetha Dental College, Tamil Nadu, India

Nikhilesh R. Vaid
European University College, DHCC, Dubai, UAE

S. Jay Bowman
Department of Orthodontics, University of Michigan, USA

Abdulkarim Hatrom
Department of Orthodontic, Ministry of Health, Makkah, Saudi Arabia

Manuel Gustavo Chávez Sevillano and Gina Judith Flores Diaz
Department of Orthodontics, National University of San Marcos, Lima, Perú. Av. GermánAmézaga 375, Cercado de Lima-Lima, Peru

Luciane Macedo de Menezes
Orthodontics Professor of the School of Health and Life Science-Pontifícia Universidade Católica do Rio Grande do Sul (PUCRS), Brazil. Ipiranga Avenue, 6681 Partenon-Porto Alegre RS, Brazil

Livia Kelly Ferraz Nunes, José Augusto Mendes Miguel and Cátia Cardoso Abdo Quintão
Department of Orthodontics, Rio de Janeiro State University, Rio de Janeiro, RJ, Brazil. Boulevard 28 de Setembro, 157; Vila Isabel -Rio de Janeiro, RJ, Brazil

A. Giancotti, P. Mozzicato and G. Mampieri
Department of Orthodontics, University of Rome "Tor Vergata", Rome, Italy

Yahya A. Alogaibi
Bisha Dental Center, Ministry of Health, Bisha 61922, Saudi Arabia
Department of Orthodontic, King Fahad Hospital, Specialized Dental Center, Madina, Saudi Arabia

Ahmad A. Al-Fraidi and Saleh S. Alkhathami
Department of Orthodontic, King Fahad Hospital, Specialized Dental Center, Madina, Saudi Arabia

Manar K. Alhajrasi
Department of Orthodontic, North Jeddah Specialty Dental Center, MOH, Jeddah, Saudi Arabia

Ali A. Hassan
Alfarabi Private College, Jeddah, Western Region, Saudi Arabia
Department of Orthodontics, Faculty of Dentistry, King Abdulaziz University, Jeddah 21589, Saudi Arabia

Lorenzo Rustico, Vincenzo Ronsivalle, Gaetano Isola and Antonino Lo Giudice
Department of Medical-Surgical Specialties, School of Dentistry, University of Catania, Policlinico Universitario "G. Rodolico", Via Santa Sofia 78, 95123 Catania, Italy

Flavia Iaculli and Gianrico Spagnuolo
Department of Neurosciences, Reproductive and Odontostomatological Sciences, University of Naples "Federico II", Via Pansini 5,80131 Naples, Italy

Echeverry Juan Carlos
Faculty of Dentistry, University of Antioquia, Calle 70 #52-21 Medellín, Colombia

Barbosa-Liz Diana
Orthopedic Maxillary and Orthodontic Postgraduate Program, Faculty of Dentistry, Universidad de Antioquia, Calle 70 #52-21 Medellín, Colombia

Stefano Martina
Department of Medicine, Surgery and Dentistry, "Scuola Medica Salernitana", University of Salerno, Via Allende, 84081 Baronissi, Italy

Roberto Martina, Vincenzo D'Antò and Rosa Valletta
School of Orthodontics, Department of Neurosciences, Reproductive Sciences and Oral Sciences, University of Naples Federico II, Via Pansini 5, 80131 Naples, Italy

Lorenzo Franchi
Department of Experimental and Clinical Medicine, University of Florence, Largo Brambilla 3, 50134 Florence, Italy

Hamid Kermanshah
Dental Research Center, Dentistry Research Institute, Department of Restorative Dentistry, School of Dentistry, Tehran University of Medical Sciences, Tehran, Iran

Aws Alzwghaibi
Department of Orthodontics, School of Dentistry, Shahid Beheshti University of Medical Sciences, Tehran, Iran

Maitham Al-Tufaili
Department of Restorative Dentistry, School of Dentistry, Tehran University of Medical Sciences, Tehran, Iran

Sholeh Ghabraei
Department of Endodontics, School of Dentistry, Tehran University of Medical Sciences, Tehran, Iran

Mah Eng Ching
Department of Orthodontics, Faculty of Dentistry, MAHSA University, Bandar Saujana Putra, 42610 Selangor, Malaysia

Lim Zhi Yin Joan
Department of Restorative Dentistry, Faculty of Dentistry, MAHSA University, Bandar Saujana Putra, 42610 Selangor, Malaysia

Phrabhakaran Nambiar
Department of Oral Biology and Biomedical Sciences, Faculty of Dentistry, MAHSA University, Bandar Saujana Putra, 42610 Selangor, Malaysia
Department of Oral & Maxillofacial Clinical Sciences, Faculty of Dentistry, University of Malaya, 50603 Kuala Lumpur, Malaysia

Index

www.ingramcontent.com/pod-product-compliance
Lightning Source LLC
LaVergne TN
LVHW082232200926
848484LV00008B/2342